CW00431499

BIOPHARMACEUTICS OF ORALLY ADMINISTERED DRUGS

ELLIS HORWOOD SERIES IN PHARMACEUTICAL TECHNOLOGY
incorporating Pharmacological Sciences

Series Editor: Michael H. Rubinstein, Professor of Pharmaceutical Technology, School of Pharmacy, Liverpool John Moores University

Series Consultant: Professor C.G. Wilson, J.P. Todd Professor of Pharmaceutics, Strathclyde University

Titles published (still in print) and in press

Armstrong & James	**UNDERSTANDING EXPERIMENTAL DESIGN AND INTERPRETATION IN PHARMACEUTICS**
Cartwright & Matthews	**PHARMACEUTICAL PRODUCT LICENSING: Requirements for Europe**
Cartwright & Matthews	**INTERNATIONAL PHARMACEUTICAL PRODUCT REGISTRATION: Quality, Safety, Efficacy**
Clark & Moos	**DRUG DISCOVERY TECHNOLOGIES**
Cole	**PHARMACEUTICAL PRODUCTION FACILITIES: Design and Application**
Cole, Hogan & Aulton	**PHARMACEUTICAL COATING TECHNOLOGY**
Cook	**POTASSIUM CHANNELS: Structure, Classification, Function and Therapeutic Potential**
Damaini	**SULPHUR-CONTAINING DRUGS AND RELATED ORGANIC COMPOUNDS: Volumes 1-3, Parts A and B**
D'Arcy & McElnay	**PHARMACY AND PHARMACOTHERAPY OF ASTHMA**
Denyer & Baird	**GUIDE TO MICROBIOLOGICAL CONTROL IN PHARMACEUTICS**
Doods & Van Meel	**RECEPTOR DATA FOR BIOLOGICAL EXPERIMENTS: A Guide to Drug Selectivity**
Ford & Timmins	**PHARMACEUTICAL THERMAL ANALYSIS: Techniques and Applications**
Glasby	**DICTIONARY OF ANTIBIOTIC-PRODUCING ORGANISMS**
Hardy et al.	**DRUG DELIVERY TO THE GASTROINTESTINAL TRACT**
Harvey	**DRUGS FROM NATURAL PRODUCTS: Pharmaceuticals and Agrochemicals**
Hider & Barlow	**POLYPEPTIDE AND PROTEIN DRUGS: Production, Characterization, Formulation**
Ioannides & Lewis	**DRUGS, DIET AND DISEASE, Volume 1: Mechanistic Approaches to Cancer**
Izquierdo & Medina	**NATURALLY OCCURRING BENZODIAZEPINES: Structure, Distribution and Function**
Junginger	**DRUG TARGETING AND DELIVERY: Concepts in Dosage Form Design**
Krogsgaard-Larsen & Hansen	**EXCITATORY AMINO ACID RECEPTORS: Design of Agonists and Antagonists**
Kourounakis & Rekka	**ADVANCED DRUG DESIGN AND DEVELOPMENT**
Labaune	**HANDBOOK OF PHARMACOKINETICS: The Toxicity Asssessment of Chemicals**
Macheras, Reppas & Dressman	**BIOPHARMACEUTICS OF ORALLY ADMINISTERED DRUGS**
Martinez	**PEPTIDE HORMONES AS PROHORMONES**
Rainsford	**ANTI-RHEUMATIC DRUGS: Actions and Side Effects**
Ramabhadran	**PHARMACEUTICAL DESIGN AND DEVELOPMENT: A Molecular Biological Approach**
Ridgway Watt	**TABLET MACHINE INSTRUMENTATION IN PHARMACEUTICS: Principles and Practice**
Roth et al.	**PHARMACEUTICAL CHEMISTRY, Volume 1: Drug Synthesis**
Roth et al.	**PHARMACEUTICAL CHEMISTRY, Volume 2: Drug Analysis**
Rubinstein	**PHARMACEUTICAL TECHNOLOGY, Volume 1: Controlled Drug Release**
Russell & Chopra	**UNDERSTANDING ANTIBACTERIAL ACTION AND RESISTANCE**
Taylor & Kennewell	**MODERN MEDICINAL CHEMISTRY**
Theobald	**RADIOPHARMACEUTICALS: Using Radioactive Compounds in Pharmaceutics and Medicine**
Vergnaud	**CONTROLLED DRUG RELEASE OF ORAL DOSAGE FORMS**
Washington	**PARTICLE SIZE ANALYSIS IN PHARMACEUTICS AND OTHER INDUSTRIES**
Washington et al.	**PHARMACOKINETIC MODELLING USING STELLA ON THE APPLE MACINTOSH (TM)**
Wells	**PHARMACEUTICAL PREFORMULATION**
Wells & Rubinstein	**PHARMACEUTICAL TECHNOLOGY Controlled Drug Release, Volume 2**
Wells & Rubinstein	**PHARMACEUTICAL TECHNOLOGY Tableting Technology, Volume 2**
Wilson & Washington	**PHYSIOLOGICAL PHARMACEUTICS**
Woolfson & McCafferty	**PERCUTANEOUS ANAESTHESIA**

BIOPHARMACEUTICS OF ORALLY ADMINISTERED DRUGS

P. Macheras, C. Reppas and J.B. Dressman

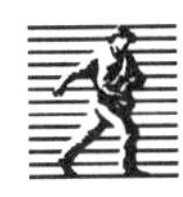

Ellis Horwood

London New York Toronto Sydney Tokyo Singapore

Madrid Mexico City Munich

First published 1995 by
Ellis Horwood Limited
Campus 400, Maylands Avenue
Hemel Hempstead
Hertfordshire, HP2 7EZ
A division of
Simon & Schuster International Group

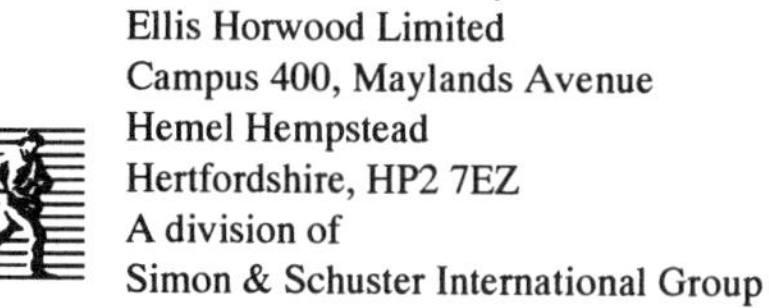

Printed and bound in Great Britain by
Bookcraft (Bath) Ltd.

Library of Congress Cataloging-in-Publication Data

Available from the publisher

British Library Cataloguing in Publication Data

A catalogue record for this book is available
from the British Library

ISBN 0-13-108093-8

1 2 3 4 5 99 98 97 96 95

Table of contents

Preface

Most drugs on the market today are taken orally. Provided a drug is well absorbed, this route of administration results in effective therapy with a minimum of inconvenience to the patient. Therefore, much effort in pharmaceutical research has been devoted to developing oral dosage forms which can deliver the drug to the systemic circulation in a timely and efficient manner. In this book, we describe the series of events that occur after oral administration of a drug, including its release from the dosage form, uptake across the gastrointestinal mucosa, delivery to the systemic circulation and site of action, and metabolism and removal from the body.

Unlike many other routes of administration, a dosage form designed for oral use must deliver the drug to an absorptive region that is remote from its point of application. This means that the formulator must pay special attention to how the physiological conditions between the oral cavity and the absorptive region will affect the ability of the dosage form to release the drug. This requires a knowledge of which regions in the gastrointestinal tract are capable of absorbing the drug. And since the time during which the dosage form is passing through the absorptive region is limited, one must design a dosage form which releases the drug in a timely and efficient manner. The fundamental aspects of physical properties and kinetics needed as a basis for assessing absorption and disposition characteristics are provided in chapter 2, while the concept of bioavailability is introduced in chapter 3. Chapters 4 and 5 address the release kinetics specific to oral dosage forms, and the interaction between the physiological conditions and the ability of the dosage form to release the drug. A second important physiological consideration is the mechanism by which the drug is taken up across the gastrointestinal mucosa. The pathway by which a drug is taken up will determine in which regions the drug is best absorbed, the kinetics of uptake and the capacity of uptake. These pathways are presented in chapter 6.

For completeness, chapters 7–9 describe post-uptake factors that affect the concentration–time profile of the drug in the body. These include protein binding, distribution to the tissues and elimination from the body.

Throughout the book, we have provided working examples and problems to illustrate the various concepts. These should help the reader to better understand and apply the concepts presented. Wherever possible, we have also described the research methodologies that are usually applied, and given appropriate references to more detailed literature on these topics. Finally, statistical background essential to the concepts presented and proper treatment of experimental data are provided in chapter 10.

We hope that this book will provide a useful resource for those involved in formulation research of oral dosage forms, and for those interested in drug delivery and bioavailability.

We are greatly indebted to many individuals who helped with the preparation of this book. Those to whom we extend special thanks for their help include Drs A. Angelakou, E. Sideris and G. Valsami. We finally give our deepest appreciation to the authors and publishers who generously granted permission to reproduce illustrations from other books and journals and to Ellis Horwood for the publication of this book.

PANOS MACHERAS,
CHRISTOS REPPAS,
JENNIFER B. DRESSMAN

January, 1995

1

Introduction

Up until the middle of the century, the design, development and production of oral pharmaceutical dosage forms was based mostly on experience and art. The scientific era for pharmacy in the field of oral formulation began in the 1950s, when the principles of physical chemistry were first applied to each step in design, development and production. At this time, attention was also directed to the quality testing of the dosage forms. The main focus, however, was on optimizing the formulation with respect to the physicochemical characteristics of the drug. Later it was realized that not all formulations designed from the physicochemical standpoint resulted in delivery of the drug to the systemic circulation at the desired rate and extent. This divergence of design and result was addressed by the birth of two new disciplines within pharmacy, *biopharmaceutics* and *pharmacokinetics*, in the 1960s. The main object of these two new disciplines was to close the gap between the *in vitro* data collected in the laboratory and the *in vivo* performance of the pharmaceutical formulation. Biopharmaceutics refers to the study of the effect of formulation characteristics, the physicochemical properties of the drug, and the physiology on both drug absorption and drug disposition. In pharmacokinetics, the mathematical analysis of the overall kinetics of drug in the body is carried out, usually using data for plasma concentration versus time. This book is intended to introduce the reader to the basic concepts of biopharmaceutics, focusing on the most frequent route of administration, i.e. oral drug delivery.

For a pharmacologically active compound to be able to exert its action in a safe and timely manner, it must first be delivered efficiently to its specific site of action, which is usually intracellular. A second important consideration is the ability of the body to eliminate the compound after its action is no longer desired. Direct administration of drugs at the specific site(s) where they exert their pharmacological effect is rarely possible on a practical basis. Although drugs are sometimes administered purely for local action, for example topical antibiotics or artificial tears, most drugs are intended to act at a location remote from the site of administration, where the interaction with their target receptor molecules takes place.

The efficiency of transfer from the site of administration to the site of action may be limited by several factors. These include:

(a) **Release of the drug from the administered formulation**. Drugs are usually administered in formulations which are designed to protect their stability and facilitate contact with their absorptive sites while retaining patient convenience in terms of administration. The dosage form itself rarely accompanies the drug to its final destination, but rather releases the drug in a way that is conducive to optimal delivery of drug to the target receptor.

(b) **The changing conditions that the drug has to pass on its way to the target receptor**. For example, an orally administered drug must pass through gastrointestinal fluids of varying composition, the epithelial layer which constitutes the gut wall, the blood and/or lymph, and in most cases be distributed into a tissue remote from the gastrointestinal tract, in order to reach its target site. As these environments vary widely in terms of lipophilicity and ability to bind the drug, it is possible that part or all of the drug may become trapped in a region far from its target receptor and therefore not to be able to exert the desired effect.

Elimination of the compound from the site(s) of action usually involves a combination of transport away from the site (a function of lipophilicity and binding characteristics, as for delivery to the site of action) and conversion to less active, easier to eliminate metabolites.

Thus, the intensity and duration of the therapeutic effect of a given drug are determined not only by its pharmacology, but also by its delivery to and removal from the site of action. The properties of both the drug and, up to a point, the dosage form can affect these processes. Fig. 1.1 illustrates the relationships between delivery, disposition and pharmacological action of a drug after oral administration. Absorption is often more variable than disposition. This is because absorption, apart from physiological and drug physicochemical characteristics, can also be highly dependent on formulation characteristics. In some cases, large changes in absorption can indirectly affect the disposition kinetics, since disposition may be ongoing during the absorption phase.

The contents of this book are divided into four parts. The first part describes the physical processes relevant to drug absorption from the mathematical standpoint. Part II covers all processes which are involved in the oral absorption of drugs, with special emphasis on the concept of bioavailability. Phenomena which occur after the drug arrives in the general circulation are discussed in Part III. These include disposition processes, such as protein binding and distribution, and elimination processes. Finally, since the study of all processes described in Parts II and III is limited by both the inherent variability in biological parameters and the variations in the experimental techniques, an additional chapter, which constitutes Part IV, has been included at the end of the book to provide an introduction on the basic statistical procedures used in biopharmaceutics to analyse experimental data.

FURTHER READING

Higuchi T. The Undergraduate Curriculum from the Viewpoint of Graduate Instruction in Pharmacy. *Am. J. Pharm. Educ.* **16**: 239–240 (1952).

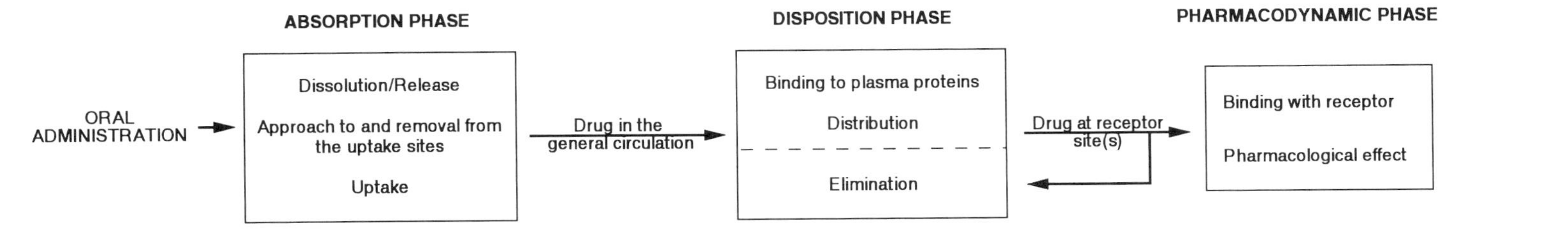

Fig. 1.1. The main processes that an orally administered drug must undergo before it reaches its intracellular receptor site(s) and exerts its pharmacological action.

Stella VJ. Evolution of Formulation Practices. *Drug Dev. Ind. Pharm.* **16**: 2627–2633 (1990).

Wagner JG. Biopharmaceutics: Absorption Aspects. *J. Pharm. Sci.* **50**: 359–387 (1961).

Wagner JG. History of Pharmacokinetics. *Pharmacol. Ther.* **12**: 537–562 (1981).

PART I

2

Rate parameters and physical processes relevant to drug absorption

Objectives
At the end of this chapter the reader should be familiar with:

— *Procedures for the assessment of transport rates*
— *The concept of half-life and mean time*
— *The kinetics of drug transport*

2.1 BASIC KINETICS RELEVANT TO DRUG TRANSPORT

2.1.1 Order of a process

The rate of drug transport in the various processes described in this book can be expressed in the same way as the kinetics of chemical reactions. Consider for example the general reaction

$$A \rightarrow B$$

where A is a drug chemically transformed to compound B. The rate of this reaction can be followed either as a decrease in the amount of drug A, X_A, as a function of time, i.e.

$$\text{Rate of reaction} = -\,\mathrm{d}X_A/\mathrm{d}t$$

or, as an increase in the amount of compound B, X_B, as a function of time, i.e.

$$\text{Rate of reaction} = \mathrm{d}X_B/\mathrm{d}t$$

Similarly, the rate of change of the amount of drug at a particular site in the body can be expressed with these simple general relationships. In biopharmaceutics, a change in the amount of a drug at a particular site may be a result of drug transport from one region to another (e.g. from the gastrointestinal tract to the blood capillaries), or chemical (e.g. hydrolysis), biochemical (e.g. oxidation and/or glucuronidation) or physical (e.g. dissolution) transformation of drug.

An important objective in establishing the kinetics of the various processes is to quantitatively evaluate the rate of each process. This assessment is usually based on the calculation of the *rate constant* of the process. Using the principles of chemical kinetics, the rate of change of the amount of drug during a non-reversible process can be expressed with the equations

$$-\mathrm{d}X_A/\mathrm{d}t = kX_A^n \qquad \mathrm{d}X_B/\mathrm{d}t = kX_A^n \tag{2.1}$$

with A and B indicating the initial and the final states of the drug molecule; k is the rate constant and n is a positive number which corresponds to the *order* of the reaction. When reversible processes are encountered equations (2.1) are written as

$$-\mathrm{d}X_A/\mathrm{d}t = k(X_A - X_{A(E)})^n \qquad \mathrm{d}X_B/\mathrm{d}t = k(X_A - X_{A(E)})^n \tag{2.2}$$

with E indicating the equilibrium state at the end of the process; k in this case corresponds to the apparent rate constant, which is equal to the algebraic sum of the two real rate constants of the forward and reverse reactions.

Depending on the value of n in equations (2.1) or (2.2) the process is characterized as zero order ($n = 0$), first order ($n = 1$), second order ($n = 2$) etc. Biopharmaceutical processes are most often first or zero order. According to equations (2.1) or (2.2), for a zero-order process the rate is constant throughout the process and independent of the amount of drug present, i.e.

$$-\mathrm{d}X_A/\mathrm{d}t = k \qquad \text{or} \qquad \mathrm{d}X_B/\mathrm{d}t = k$$

By contrast, the rate of a first order process decreases exponentially with time. Plots of rate versus time and amount versus time for zero- and first-order processes are shown in Fig. 2.1.

From equations (2.1) and (2.2) and Fig. 2.1 it is clear that, if the same initial quantity of drug is considered, a zero-order process will be completed sooner than a first-order process. This difference arises from the fact that the rate of the zero-order process remains constant while the rate of the first-order process diminishes with time.

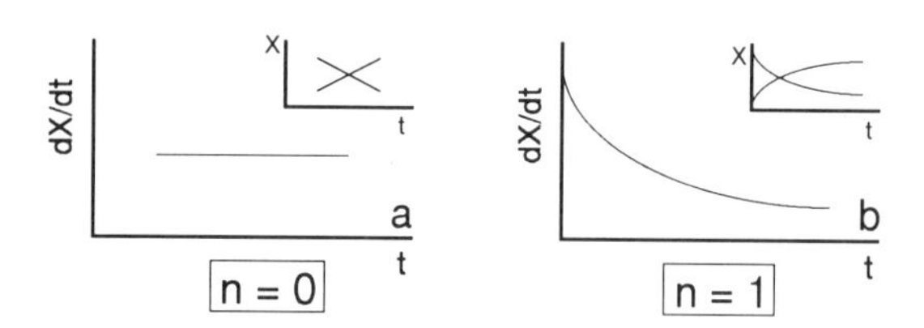

Fig. 2.1. Rate of change of the amount of drug as a function of time for a zero-order (a) process and a first-order (b) process. The inserts show the change (increase or decrease) of the amount versus time.

2.1.2 Calculation of rate constants

2.1.2.1 Calculation of zero-order rate constant

For $n = 0$, equations (2.1) and (2.2) yield

$$-dX_A/dt = k_0 \qquad dX_B/dt = k_0 \tag{2.3}$$

where k_0 is the zero-order rate constant. Equations (2.3) reveal that the rate of reaching state B is constant and not dependent on the quantities of compounds A and B throughout the process. Integrating the first of the two equations (2.3) from time $t = 0$ (i.e. $X_A = X_{A(0)}$) and $t = t$ (i.e. $X_A = X_A$) the following equation results:

$$X_A = X_{A(0)} - k_0 t \tag{2.4}$$

Similarly, integrating the second of the two equations (2.3) from $t = 0$, ($X_B = X_{B(0)} = 0$) and $t = t$, ($X_B = X_B$) one obtains

$$X_B = k_0 t \tag{2.5}$$

Fig. 2.2 gives a graphical depiction of equations (2.4) and (2.5). The magnitude of the slope of the two linear graphs corresponds to the value of the zero-order rate constant, k_0.

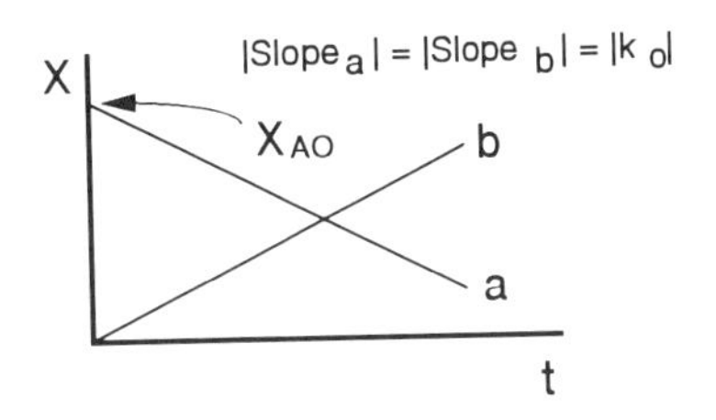

Fig. 2.2. Graphical representation of equations (2.4) (a) and (2.5) (b).

When zero-order kinetics prevail, the study of the rate can be readily based on either the amount or the concentration of drug. In the former case the units of k_0 are [mass] [time]$^{-1}$ while in the latter case the units for k_0 are [concentration] [time]$^{-1}$.

A simple example of the usefulness of the knowledge of the zero-order rate constant in biopharmaceutical problems can be now considered. Let us suppose that the release of a drug from an oral extended-release formulation obeys zero-order kinetics. We assume that the formulation contains 80 mg of a drug and the value of the zero-order rate constant is 8 mg h^{-1}. According to equation (2.4) the release of drug from the formulation is completed in 10 h. If the transit time through the small intestine is 5 h and the drug is readily absorbed in this region, then an amount of (5 h) × (8 mg h^{-1}) = 40 mg will be absorbed. Unless the drug is well absorbed at more distal sites in the gastrointestinal tract, incorporating more than 40 mg of drug in such a formulation would result in inefficient absorption.

2.1.2.2 Calculation of first-order rate constant

For a first order process the value of n in equations (2.1) and (2.2) is 1. The rate of a first-order process is dependent on the amount present in the system and therefore reversible and non-reversible processes require different analyses.

Non-reversible process

Based on equations (2.1) for state A we obtain

$$-dX_A/dt = k_1 X_A$$

Integrating this equation results in

$$\ln X_A = \ln X_{A(0)} - k_1 t \tag{2.6}$$

Equation (2.6) can also be written in exponential form:

$$X_A = X_{A(0)} e^{-k_1 t} \tag{2.7}$$

Plots of equations (2.6) and (2.7) are shown in Fig. 2.3.

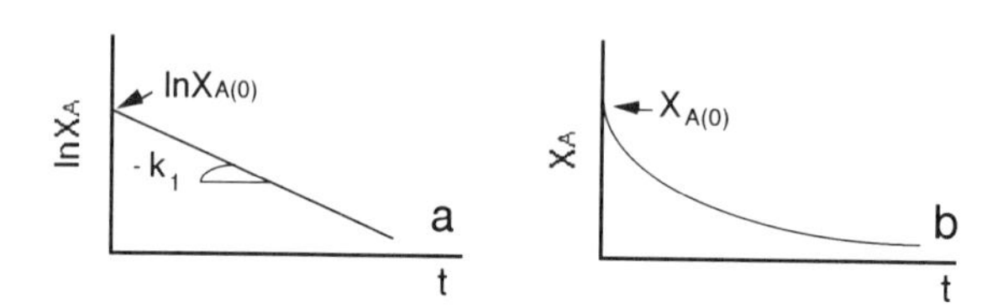

Fig. 2.3. Graphical representation of equations (2.6) (a) and (2.7) (b).

Similarly for state B we have: $dX_B/dt = k_1 X_A$. Combination of this equation with equation (2.7) gives

$$dX_B/dt = k_1 X_{A(0)} e^{-k_1 t}\, dt \tag{2.8}$$

Integrating equation (2.8) we have

$$X_B = X_{A(0)}\left(1 - e^{-k_1 t}\right) \tag{2.9}$$

which can also be written in logarithmic form:

$$\ln\left(X_{A(0)} - X_B\right) = \ln X_{A(0)} - k_1 t \tag{2.10}$$

Plots of equations (2.9) and (2.10) are shown in Fig. 2.4.

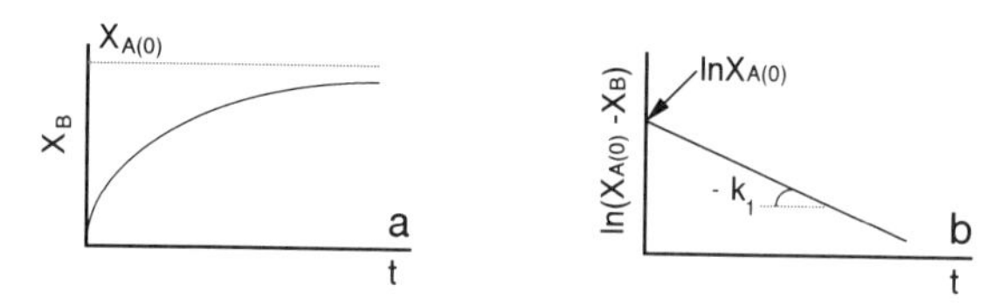

Fig. 2.4. Graphical representation of equations (2.9) (a) and (2.10) (b).

The calculation of the first order rate constant, k_1, can be accomplished from the slopes of the lines in Figs 2.3a and 2.4b.

Let us consider again the problem used to illustrate zero-order kinetics, now assuming that the rate of release from the formulation follows first-order kinetics with a first order rate constant 0.20 h^{-1}. Supposing that the formulation takes 5 h to pass through the absorptive region in the small intestine, the amount of drug released during this time is calculated from equation (2.9) to be $X_B = 80(1 - e^{-0.20\times5}) = 51$ mg. An important distinction from zero-order kinetics is that here the amount of drug released depends on the initial amount of drug incorporated into the formulation. Thus, if the drug content of the formulation was 100 mg, then in 5 h the amount of drug released would increase to $X_B = 100(1 - e^{-0.20\times5}) = 63$ mg whereas from the zero-order formulation the amount released would still be 40 mg.

Reversible process

An example of a reversible first order process is the dialysis experiment in which the drug is transported across a membrane from a donor compartment, without removal from either compartment. In such cases, according to Fick's first law of diffusion (see section 2.3.1), the driving force for drug transport is the concentration gradient between the two compartments and not the amount difference.

Let us consider the case of reversible transport of a drug between the two sides of a dialysis membrane, in which the volumes of the two compartments are equal as depicted in Fig. 2.5. The rate of the decrease in the concentration C_A in compartment A follows the equation

$$-\mathrm{d}C_A/\mathrm{d}t = k_1(C_A - C_{A(E)}) \tag{2.11}$$

where k_1 is the first-order rate constant and $C_{A(E)}$ is the concentration of drug in compartment A at equilibrium. Similarly, the rate of the increase of the concentration of drug in compartment B is given by equation (2.12):

$$\mathrm{d}C_B = k_1(C_A - C_{A(E)}) = k_1(C_{A(0)} - C_B - C_{A(E)}) = k_1(C_{A(E)} - C_B) \tag{2.12}$$

since the volumes of the two compartments A and B in Fig. 2.5 are equal. Integrating equation (2.11) for $t = 0$ and $C_A = C_{A(0)}$ and $t = t$, $C_A = C_A$ we have

$$\ln(C_A - C_{A(E)}) = \ln(C_{A(0)} - C_{A(E)}) - k_1t = \ln C_{A(E)} - k_1t \tag{2.13}$$

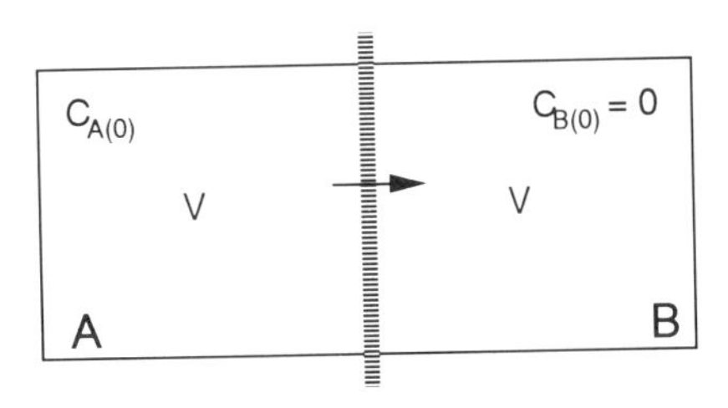

Fig. 2.5. Transport of a drug from compartment A to compartment B across a dialysis membrane. The volumes of the two compartments are equal; the initial drug concentrations in compartments A and B are $C_{A(0)}$ and $C_{B(0)}$, respectively.

According to equation (2.13) a plot of $\ln(C_A - C_{A(E)})$ versus time will yield a straight line with slope equal to k_1 as illustrated in Fig. 2.6a. Equation (2.13) can be also written as follows:

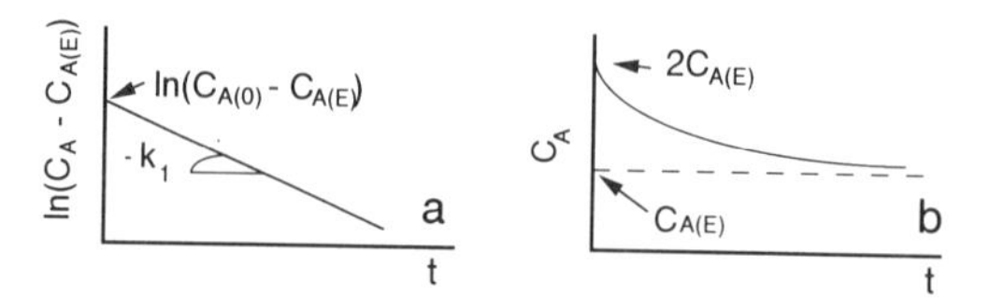

Fig. 2.6. Graphical representation of equations (2.13) (a) and (2.14) (b).

$$C_{\mathrm{A}} = C_{\mathrm{A(E)}}\left(1+e^{-k_1 t}\right) \tag{2.14}$$

which is depicted in Fig. 2.6b.

Similarly, integration of equation (2.12) shows that the amount of drug in compartment B can be calculated from

$$\ln\left(C_{\mathrm{A(E)}} - C_{\mathrm{B}}\right) = \ln C_{\mathrm{A(E)}} - k_1 t \tag{2.15}$$

Equation (2.15) can also be written in exponential form:

$$C_{\mathrm{B}} = C_{\mathrm{A(E)}}\left(1-e^{-k_1 t}\right) \tag{2.16}$$

Graphical representations of equations (2.15) and (2.16) are shown in Fig. 2.7. A basic conclusion which can be drawn from equations (2.15) and (2.16) is that the rate of increase of drug concentration in the receiving compartment in a closed system such as a dialysis experiment depends on the equilibrium concentration.

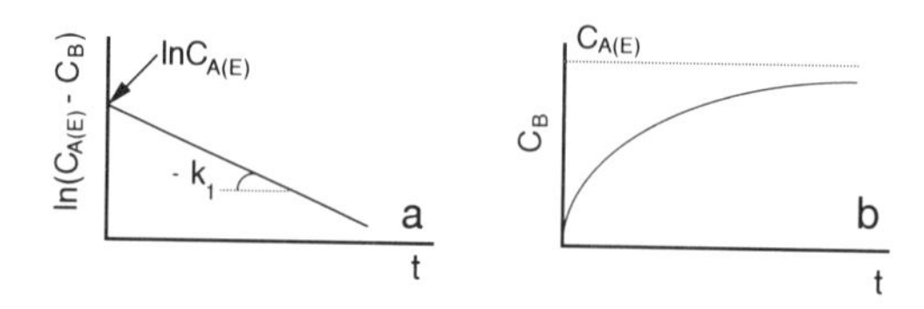

Fig. 2.7. Graphical representation of equations (2.15) (a) and (2.16) (b).

Regardless of the reversibility of the process, the rate constant of a first order process, k_1, is always expressed in $[\text{time}]^{-1}$ units. The value of the first-order rate constant can be related roughly with the percentage of completion of the process at a given time point. For example, a value of $0.300\ \mathrm{h}^{-1}$ for a non-reversible first-order process means that roughly 30% of the process is completed in 1 h. More precisely, from equation (2.9) for $k_1 = 0.300\ \mathrm{h}^{-1}$ and $t = 1$ h one can conclude that $X_{\mathrm{B}}/X_{\mathrm{A(0)}} = 1 - e^{-0.300} = 0.259$, i.e. the process is 26% complete after 1 h. The same result can be easily obtained assuming a reversible process and using equation (2.16).

2.2 CHARACTERISTIC TIMES: APPLICATION TO FIRST- AND ZERO-ORDER PROCESSES

2.2.1 Half-life

A time commonly used to characterize a process is its half-life, $t_{1/2}$, which corresponds to the time needed for 50% completion of the process. The relationship between the half-life and the rate constant of a process is dependent on the order of the process.

For *zero-order processes* the use of equation (2.4) for $X_A = X_{A(0)}/2$ and $t = t_{1/2}$ yields

$$t_{1/2} = X_{A(0)}/2k_0 \tag{2.17}$$

It is interesting to note that the half-life for zero-order processes is dependent on the initial amount (or concentration) of drug.

For *non-reversible first-order processes* the calculation of half-life can be derived from equation (2.7):

$$X_{A(0)}/2 = X_{A(0)}e^{-k_1 t_{1/2}}$$

which leads to

$$t_{1/2} = \ln 2/k_1 \tag{2.18}$$

Equation (2.18) reveals that the half-life for non-reversible first-order processes is not dependent on the initial quantity or concentration of drug. An important use of the half-life concept is in the characterization of elimination of drugs from the body. The value of the biological half-life (time for 50% elimination of drug from the body) is a very useful indicator for the kinetic profile of drug in the body. Two relevant examples are listed in Table 2.1 for drugs administered in two separate occasions with an intravenous bolus dose. The two drugs have biological half-lives $t_{1/2,A} = 4.0$ h and $t_{1/2,B} = 11.0$ h. The fractions of the initial dose remaining in the body for each drug are calculated from equation (2.7) expressing time in multiples of half-life. Although identical *fractions* of the two drugs remain in the body for a given number of multiples of half-life, this time differs enormously (contrast columns 2 and 3) for the two drugs examined when expressed chronologically.

Table 2.1. First-order elimination of drugs A and B from the body with $t_{1/2,A} = 4.0$ h and $t_{1/2,B} = 11.0$ h

Time after administration in multiples of half-life	Time (h) after administration of drug A	Time (h) after administration of drug B	% of drug (A or B) remaining to be eliminated
0	0	0	100
1	4.0	11	50.0
2	8.0	22	25.0
3	12	33	12.5
4	16	44	6.25
5	20	55	3.12
6	24	66	1.56
7	28	77	0.781

For *reversible first-order processes*, the calculation of half-life depends on the conditions of the process and a general equation cannot be derived. For example, the following equation applies at equilibrium for the transport process of Fig. 2.5 (i.e. if the volumes of two compartments are equal):

$$X_{A(0)}/2 = X_{A(E)} \qquad \text{and therefore} \qquad C_{A(0)}/2 = C_{A(E)} \tag{2.19}$$

It can be concluded from equation (2.19) that in this particular case the time for drug to reach half its initial concentration in the donor compartment is identical to the time needed for the completion of the process. However, the process is 50% complete when the concentration in the donor compartment becomes $(C_{A(0)} + C_{A(E)})/2$, i.e. $3C_{A(0)}/4$ (from equation (2.19)). If we consider a case in which unequal volumes are, say $V_B = 2V_A/3$, then at equilibrium we have in the two compartments $C_{AE} = C_{B(E)}$ or $X_{A(E)}/V_A = X_{B(E)}/V_B$. Since $X_{A(0)} = X_{A(E)} + X_{B(E)}$, at equilibrium $X_{A(E)} = 3X_{A(0)}/5$ or $C_{A(E)} = 3C_{A(0)}/5$. In this example the amount of drug in compartment A never decreases to 50% of its initial value and the process will be 50% complete when concentration in the donor compartment becomes $(C_{A(0)} + C_{A(E)})/2 = (C_{A(0)} + 3C_{A(0)}/5)/2 = 4C_{A(0)}/5$.

It is apparent from these sample calculations that, regardless of the volumes of the donor and receiving compartments, in reversible first-order processes the time needed for 50% completion of the process cannot be identical to the time at which the amount of drug becomes one half of its initial value.

2.2.2 Mean time

The concept of mean time of a process is linked with the stochastic consideration of a process. The stochastic approach can be applied to the analysis of a process whose mechanism is random. Consider for example the emptying of a multiparticulate (pelletized) dosage form from the stomach. Individual pellets will empty randomly, according to their orientation in the stomach relative to other contents of the stomach and the motility pattern. Since the probability of emptying is different for each particle at a given time, the mean time of the overall emptying process is the mean of the times required for each individual pellet to empty. Hence, the overall pattern may be first or zero order in terms of the percentage of pellets emptied per unit time.

The calculation of the mean time of a process depends on the order of the process. For zero-order kinetics, the mean time of the process is equal to the half-life, $t_{1/2}$. In this case the mean time and the half-life are identical. For first-order kinetics, the mean time corresponds to the reciprocal of the rate constant of the process. When the order of the process is not known, a numerical method can be applied to the calculation of the mean time from the experimental data.

2.3 MECHANISMS OF DRUG TRANSPORT

In the great majority of cases in biopharmaceutics, the driving force for the transport of drug from one area to another, e.g. from the gastrointestinal tract to the blood capillaries, is the concentration gradient between these areas. Under these conditions the process is characterized as *passive transport* and follows the principles of first order kinetics. However, in several cases the drug may be transported by *a carrier-mediated transport* process. This means that the mechanism of the drug transport is founded on the interaction of drug with a carrier.

2.3.1 Passive transport

Passive transport is described mathematically by Fick's first law of diffusion, which refers to the diffusion of molecules due to the change in concentration as a function of distance. This kind of transport is the result of the kinetic energy of the molecules and is termed 'passive diffusion' since a supply of energy is not required for the transport. Diffusion is better understood with the following classical example.

Let us assume that a drop of a solution of the indicator methyl red is placed in a flask full of water so carefully that no convection (mixing) is induced. The intensity of the red colour of the aqueous solution will be inversely proportional to the distance from the initial placement of the drop. With time, the colour of the solution will become homogeneous, i.e. the system will reach equilibrium. According to Fick's law, the flux, J, of the diffusing molecules is defined by the following equation:

$$J = -D(\mathrm{d}C/\mathrm{d}x) \tag{2.20}$$

where D is the diffusion coefficient with units [area] [time]$^{-1}$ and $\mathrm{d}C$ is the change of concentration as a function of distance, $\mathrm{d}x$. The flux, J, is expressed in units of [quantity] [time]$^{-1}$[area]$^{-1}$. The negative sign in equation (2.20) indicates the decrease of colour density as a function of distance from the original placement of the drop of dye. The law of diffusion finds extensive application for the description of passive transport of a drug between two compartments separated by a dialysis membrane (Fig. 2.5). Thus, the rate of drug transport across a membrane with a specific surface area, A, obeys the following equation:

$$\mathrm{d}m/\mathrm{d}t = AJ = AD(\mathrm{d}C/\mathrm{d}x) \tag{2.21}$$

where m is the mass of the transferred drug, D is the diffusion coefficient in the membrane, $\mathrm{d}x$ is the membrane thickness and $\mathrm{d}C$ is the concentration gradient.

2.3.1.1 Non-reversible passive transport

Parallel transport pathways

At any given time during the residence of the drug in the body it may be subject to several reactions and transport processes. The diagram shows a simple example, in which two processes proceed simultaneously in a parallel fashion:

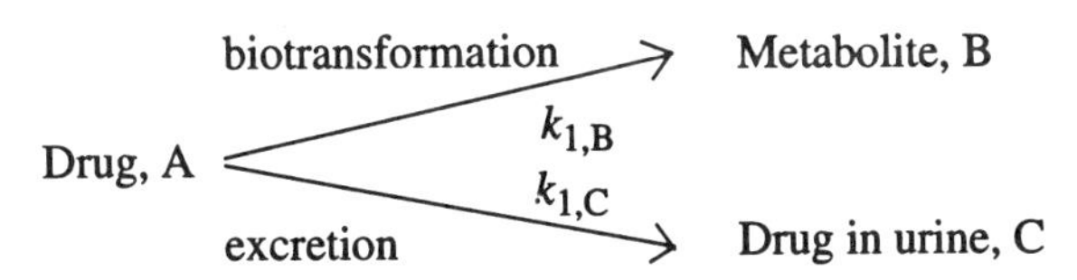

where $k_{1,B}$ and $k_{1,C}$ are the first-order rate constants for the two processes. A typical example of parallel processes occurs when a drug can be either metabolized or excreted unchanged in the urine. The mathematical treatment of a system with parallel first-order processes relies on the equations describing the rate of change of drug at the different states or compartments. The rate of decrease in the amount of drug A is given by the equation

$$-\mathrm{d}X_A/\mathrm{d}t = (k_{1,B}X_A + k_{1,C}X_A) = (k_{1,B} + k_{1,C})X_A \tag{2.22}$$

After integration of equation (2.22) and in full analogy with equation (2.6) we have

$$\ln X_A = \ln X_{A(0)} - (k_{1,B} + k_{1,C})t \tag{2.23}$$

The rate of appearance of the metabolite, B, can be written on the basis of equation (2.8):

$$\mathrm{d}X_B/\mathrm{d}t = k_{1,B}X_A = k_{1,B}X_{A(0)}e^{-(k_{1,B}+k_{1,C})t} \tag{2.24}$$

Integration of equation (2.24) results in an expression for the quantity of metabolite B, as a function of time:

$$X_B = \frac{k_{1,B}X_{A(0)}}{k_{1,B} + k_{1,C}}\left[1 - e^{-(k_{1,B}+k_{1,C})t}\right] \tag{2.25}$$

As $t \to \infty$

$$X_{B(E)} = X_{A(0)}\left[k_{1,B}/(k_{1,B} + k_{1,C})\right] \tag{2.26}$$

where $X_{B(E)}$ is the total amount of drug metabolized to B. Combining equations (2.25) and (2.26) we obtain

$$X_B = X_{B(E)}\left[1 - e^{-(k_{1,B}+k_{1,C})t}\right] \tag{2.27}$$

which can also be written in logarithmic form:

$$\ln(X_{B(E)} - X_B) = \ln X_{B(E)} - (k_{1,B} + k_{1,C})t \tag{2.28}$$

Applying the same approach, an analogous equation for the amount of drug excreted unchanged in the urine, *C*, can be derived:

$$\ln(X_{C(E)} - X_C) = \ln X_{C(E)} - (k_{1,B} + k_{1,C})t \tag{2.29}$$

Plots of the left-hand sides of equations (2.23), (2.28) and (2.29) versus time give straight lines with a common slope corresponding to the sum of the two rate constants. This means that a treatment of data using equations (2.23), (2.28) and (2.29) will provide an apparent first order rate constant k_1:

$$k_1 = k_{1,B} + k_{1,C}$$

Processes in series

Processes in series are frequently encountered *in vivo*. A typical example of processes in series is drug dissolution prior to uptake from the small intestine. The following diagram describes this situation:

$$\mathrm{A} \xrightarrow{k_1} \mathrm{B} \xrightarrow{k_1'} \mathrm{C}$$

where k_1 and k_1' are first order rate constants of the transfer of drug from compartment A to B and from compartment B to C, respectively. The fundamental processes of absorption and elimination during the time course of drug in the body can be also considered as processes operating in series, with compartments A, B and C representing in this case the gastrointestinal tract, the blood and the urine, respectively.

The loss of drug from compartment A can be described by equation (2.6) or (2.7). However, the rate of change of the quantity of drug in compartment B is described by the differential equation (2.30) which expresses the simultaneous arrival of drug from compartment A and loss to compartment C:

$$\mathrm{d}X_B/\mathrm{d}t = k_1 X_A - k_1' X_B \tag{2.30}$$

Combining equations (2.7) and (2.30) we obtain

$$\mathrm{d}X_B/\mathrm{d}t = k_1 X_{A(0)} e^{-k_1 t} - k_1' X_B \tag{2.31}$$

Integration of equation (2.31) yields

$$X_B = \frac{X_{A(0)} k_1}{k_1 - k_1'}\left(e^{-k_1' t} - e^{-k_1 t}\right) \tag{2.32}$$

Equation (2.32) is a biexponential equation where X_B rises to a maximum and then declines as a function of time. The relative magnitude of the rate constants k_1 and k_1' determines the shape of the curve of the quantity of drug in compartment B, X_B, as a function of time. In general, the higher the ratio k_1/k_1' the steeper the ascending limb of the curve. Finally, the quantity of drug in compartment C is given by the mass balance equation

$$X_C = X_{A(0)} - (X_A + X_B) \tag{2.33}$$

Combining equations (2.7), (2.32) and (2.33) we obtain

$$X_C = X_{A(0)}\left[1 - \frac{1}{k_1' - k_1}\left(k_1' e^{-k_1 t} - k_1 e^{-k_1' t}\right)\right] \tag{2.34}$$

The last equation reveals that as $t \to \infty$ all of the initial quantity of drug in compartment A, $X_{A(0)}$, will have been transported in compartment C. In other words, the plot of X_C as a function of time will be monotonically increasing towards a plateau value, $X_{A(0)}$.

The concept of the rate-limiting step

Consider the case of drug absorption from the gastrointestinal tract after administration of a tablet. The drug must dissolve from the tablet before it becomes available for uptake across the intestinal mucosa. Dissolution corresponds to the first step, and uptake to the second step, in the series of processes shown in Fig. 4.3. If dissolution is very slow compared to uptake the overall rate of absorption will be dependent on the dissolution rate. Conversely, if the mucosa is not very permeable to the drug, it will be slowly absorbed irrespective of how quickly the drug dissolves from the tablet. Thus, the slower of the two steps in a series process will control the overall rate at which the process occurs and, as such, it may be referred to as the *rate-limiting step*.

2.3.1.2 Reversible passive transport

In Fig. 2.5 the two compartments of equal volume contain the same quantity of drug at equilibrium. Under *in vivo* conditions, however, reversible processes often take place between two compartments which are quite different in size. In this case, almost the entire quantity of drug can be found in the larger of the two compartments. Furthermore, in some instances only a portion of drug is able to permeate the membrane(s) between the two compartments. Under these conditions equilibrium is established when the concentrations of the permeable form of the drug become equal in the two compartments. Two examples of such behaviour follow.

Passive transport and ionization

Many drugs are weak acids or bases. Consequently, the degree to which they are ionized depends on the pK_a value and the pH of the surrounding environment. The ratio of the ionized and non-ionized concentrations of drugs can be calculated using the Henderson–Hasselbach equations:

For acids

$$pH = pK_a + \log[\text{ionized form/unionized form}] \qquad (2.35)$$

For bases

$$pH = pK_a + \log[\text{non-ionized form/ionized form}] \qquad (2.36)$$

Penetration of physiological membranes is usually favoured for the non-ionized fraction of the drug. The following diagram shows an equilibrium of this type:

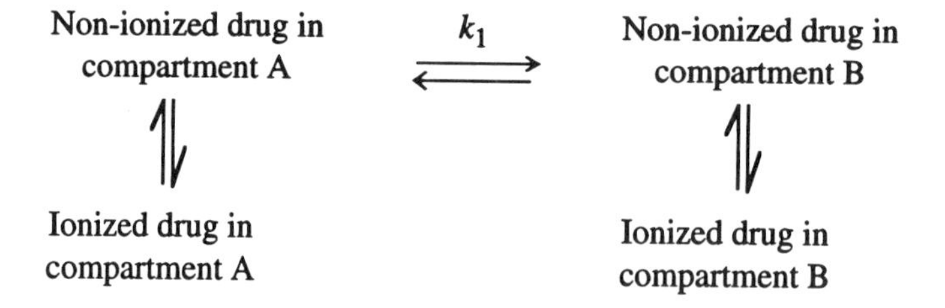

The equilibrium between non-ionized and ionized forms of the drug will be influenced by the pH of the fluids on each side of the membrane. For example distribution of drugs between plasma and breast milk depends on the value of the drug's pK_a and the pH values in plasma (pH = 7.4) and in milk (pH = 6.6) (see section 8.3.1).

Passive diffusion and complexation of drug with a macromolecule

In some cases the drug is bound to a macromolecule which, owing to the size limitations, cannot permeate the membranes. This happens very frequently in plasma. The drug bound to plasma proteins cannot cross the blood capillaries, thereby limiting the distribution of drug to the body tissues. The effect is very significant when strong and extensive binding is observed.

2.3.2 Carrier-mediated transport

Carrier-mediated transport processes rely on the reversible interaction of the drug with a component of the membrane, most likely a protein, acting as a carrier. Although the mechanisms of carrier-mediated transport processes have not been fully elucidated several potential explanations have been advanced. At one time it was thought that this type of transport involved three successive steps, the first of which was the formation of a complex between the drug and the carrier on the external part of the membrane. The second step involved the transport of the complex to the internal part of the membrane by the carrier, while the third step was the release of drug from the carrier complex. This mechanism, however, is not compatible with the current view of the arrangement of carrier proteins in the membrane. These proteins appear to span the membrane from one side to the other with little evidence for their movement relative to other membrane components. To accommodate these observations, a translocation model has been recently proposed to interpret carrier-mediated transport. The so-called *alternating access model* of transfer assumes that there are 'uptake' and 'discharge' conformational states for the carrier protein at the outer and inner surfaces of the membrane, respectively. A complex is initially formed between the solute and a carrier protein in the uptake conformation. The change from the uptake to discharge conformation of the carrier protein permits the passage of the solute through the membrane. This operation is energetically coupled with the hydrolysis of ATP.

Carrier-mediated transport processes have the following unique characteristics.

(a) *Specificity*: In passive processes the membrane acts as a simple physical barrier for the diffusion of drug molecules with general drug properties such as lipophilicity determining the efficiency of the process. However, in the case of carrier-mediated transport the carrier must be able to specifically recognize the structure in order to interact with and transport the drug across the membrane. Even slight changes in the chemical structure may critically affect this recognition.

(b) *Competition*: When two compounds share the same carrier their individual rates of transfer may be diminished owing to competition for sites of recognition on the carrier. In this case the decrease in the rate of transport will be more significant for the substance with the lower affinity for the carrier. A typical example of a reduced rate of transport due to competition is the decrease in uptake of L-dopa when it is coadministered with food. This drug is an amino acid and must compete for uptake with structurally similar amino acids produced by digestion of proteins.

(c) *Saturation kinetics*: For passive processes a linear relationship exists between the initial rate of transport and the concentration of drug. A non-linear relationship between the rate of transport and the concentration of drug may indicate that uptake requires a carrier. Fig. 2.8 provides a general schematic representation of the relationships between the rate of transport and the drug concentration for carrier-mediated kinetics.

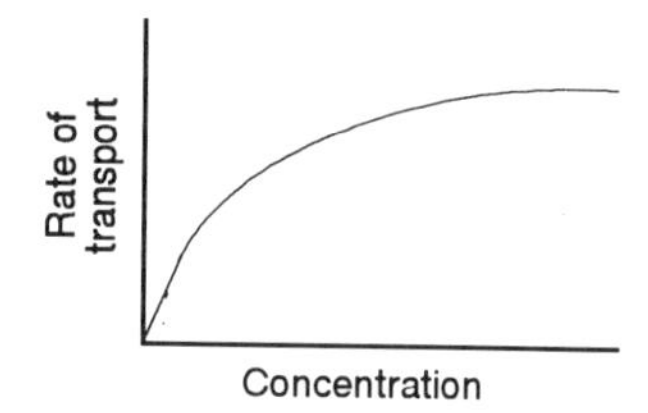

Fig. 2.8. Transport rate versus drug concentration for carrier-mediated transport processes. The rate of transport is non-linearly related to the drug's concentration; at low drug concentrations the carrier is not saturated and the rate is proportional to the concentration, while at high drug concentrations the rate of transport reaches a maximum due to saturation of the carrier.

At sufficiently low drug concentrations there is an excess of carrier molecules available for the active transfer of drug. Under these conditions the rate of transfer increases with the increase of the concentration of drug and the kinetics are linear (initial linear portion in Fig. 2.8). However, the number of carrier molecules is finite. Therefore, at high enough concentration of drug, the ability of the carrier to transport the drug becomes saturated and the rate of transport reaches a maximum value which remains unaltered with further increases in the concentration of drug (plateau in Fig. 2.8). Saturation kinetics are frequently encountered in the biotransformation reactions of drugs in the liver and sometimes during drug uptake through membranes. In all these cases the relation between rate and concentration can be described by Michaelis–Menten kinetics as described in section 2.3.2.1.

(d) *Energy requirement*: The ability to transfer a substance against a concentration gradient is used as a criterion to distinguish between the two types of carrier-mediated transport, i.e. *facilitated diffusion* and *active transport*. The term 'facilitated diffusion' is used for all carrier-mediated processes which cannot proceed against a concentration gradient. The term 'active transport' is used for the carrier-mediated processes which can operate against a concentration gradient and therefore are net energy-consuming processes. Both types of carrier-mediated transport require an initial supply of energy to overcome the energy threshold. In the case of facilitated diffusion, the downhill transfer requires only the initial supply of energy to overcome the energy barrier and there is no net energy requirement. In active transport, by contrast, net consumption of energy from a metabolic system coupled with the transfer process is observed. Thus, inhibition of the transport can be observed when the energy supply is blocked by metabolic inhibitors. Examples of metabolic inhibitors include the glycosides phlorizin and ouabain. Phlorizin inhibits absorption of glucose while ouabain inhibits sodium transport from the small intestine.

The supply of energy appears to be based on the transformation of ATP to ADP. The enzyme responsible for this transformation may also act as the carrier. The energy threshold per mole of the transferred compound, ΔE, for a non-ionized compound is dependent on its concentration gradient:

$$\Delta E = RT \ln (C_2/C_1) \tag{2.37}$$

where R is the universal gas constant (8.31 J mol deg^{-1}), T is the absolute temperature (K) and C_1, C_2 are the concentrations of the transferred molecule from compartment 1 to compartment 2, e.g. from the gastrointestinal fluids into the enterocyte. For ionized compounds the energy threshold corresponds to the electrochemical potential which can be expressed per mole of the transferred compound with equation 2.38:

$$\Delta E = RT \ln (C_2/C_1) + ZF(E_2 - E_1) \tag{2.38}$$

where Z is the valence of the ion, F is the Faraday constant (96 487 coulombs/gram equivalent) and $(E_2 - E_1)$ is the potential difference at the two sides of the membrane.

2.3.2.1 Carrier-mediated transport kinetics

The kinetics of carrier-mediated transport processes follow the principles of the kinetics of enzyme action. This theory assumes that the enzyme E (in our case, the carrier protein) combines with the substrate S (drug) to form the complex ES, which then is cleaved to products and the enzyme (carrier) E:

$$\mathrm{E} + \mathrm{S} \rightleftharpoons \mathrm{ES} \longrightarrow \text{Products} + \mathrm{E}$$

In 1913, Michaelis and Menten derived the following equation for an enzyme-catalysed reaction:

$$u = (V_{max} C_{sub})/(K_M + C_{sub}) \tag{2.39}$$

where u is the rate of the reaction, V_{max} is the maximum rate of the reaction, C_{sub} is the substrate concentration, and K_M is the Michaelis–Menten constant. The units for u and V_{max} are either [concentration/time] or [mass/time] according to the experimental system used. K_M is always expressed in the same units as those for the substrate (drug), C_{sub}, which is usually expressed in concentration or, more rarely, in mass units. Equation (2.39) finds extensive application in biotransformation reactions as discussed in chapter 9. By analogy, a Michaelis–Menten type equation can be used to describe the rate of transport dC/dt of a carrier-mediated transport process:

$$dC/dt = (T_{max} C_{sub})/(K_M + C_{sub}) \tag{2.40}$$

where T_{max} is the maximum rate of transfer.

FURTHER READING

Bull HB. *An Introduction to Physical Biochemistry*, 2nd edn, FA Davis, Philadelphia (1971).

Cox DR and Miller HD. *The Theory of Stochastic Processes*, Wiley, New York (1965).

Lippold BH. Simulierung der Gastro-Intestinale Resorption von Dissozierenden Arzneistoffen mit einem Membranmodell. *Pharm. Ind.* **38**: 208–215 (1976).

Notari RE. *Biopharmaceutics and Pharmacokinetics. An Introduction*, Marcel Dekker, New York (1971).

Pratt WB and Taylor P (eds). *Principles of Drug Action: The Basis of Pharmacology*, 3rd edn, Churchill Livingstone, New York (1990).

Stricker H. Drug Absorption in the Gastrointestinal Tract II, In vitro Investigations on Lipophilic Substances. *Drugs Made Germ.* **14**: 93 (1971).
Wagner JG. Biopharmaceutics: Absorption Aspects. *J. Pharm. Sci.* **50**: 359–387 (1961).

PART II

3

Bioavailability

Objectives

After completing this chapter the reader will be familiar with:

- *The concepts of bioavailability and bioequivalence*
- *The processes controlling the arrival of drug at the systemic circulation after oral administration*
- *The key bioavailability parameters*

3.1 INTRODUCTION TO BIOAVAILABILITY

The mode of drug administration is of great importance for the onset, intensity and duration of pharmacological action. The barriers to systemic delivery encountered in most frequently used routes of administration are compared in Fig. 3.1. Intravenous administration ensures rapid arrival of the entire dose in the systemic circulation. Other routes of administration require that the drug crosses a number of physical barriers (membranes, tissues) prior to arrival in the systemic circulation. As a consequence,

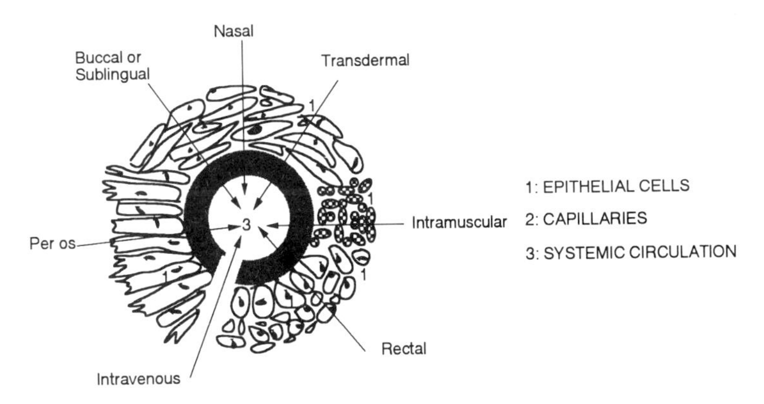

Fig. 3.1. Comparison of barriers to drug arrival in the general circulation after administration at various sites.

complete delivery of the administered dose to the systemic circulation is guaranteed only when the drug is administered intravenously. When the drug is administered by another route of administration, the rate and extent of absorption compared to that observed after intravenous dosing is called the *bioavailability*.

Although the concept of bioavailability refers to all extravascularly administered dosage forms it is of particular importance for the oral route. Until the end of the 1950s there was no scientific speculation concerning the absorption of drug after oral administration. There was a general impression that the entire quantity of the dose administered was absorbed from the gastrointestinal (GI) tract. This belief wavered and then collapsed in the early 1960s when a plethora of scientific reports demonstrated that in many cases the amount of drug reaching the general circulation was less than the administered dose. At that time the term *bioavailability* was introduced to describe the fraction of dose reaching the general circulation. During the same period comparative studies revealed that formulations of the same drug from different pharmaceutical companies do not necessarily exhibit similar bioavailabilities. These observations prompted the beginning of *bioequivalence studies* which specifically compare the bioavailability of a drug from different formulations.

The scientific knowledge accumulated over the years from bioavailability studies unmasked the mechanisms which may cause a reduction of the fraction of the dose that reaches the systemic circulation. Such mechanisms were found to occur prior to, during and/or after the permeation of drug through the GI epithelium. The luminal processes that affect bioavailability after oral dosing can be discussed on the basis of Fig. 3.2 and include:

— the inability of the drug to dissolve in a timely and efficient manner in the GI fluids;
— the inability of drug to cross the GI epithelium efficiently; and/or
— the biotransformation of drug in the GI lumen or the GI mucosa.

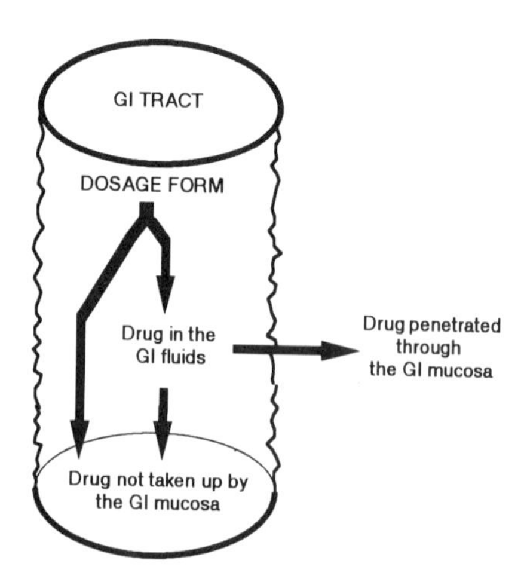

Fig. 3.2. Luminal processes that affect oral bioavailability.

These three factors can be grouped in terms of general processes which control the GI absorption of drugs, namely, the *supply* of the GI fluids with drug, the *delivery* to the uptake sites and the *uptake* of the drug by the GI mucosa.

Apart from these three processes, GI absorption and, consequently, the arrival of the drug at the systemic circulation may also be controlled by post-uptake processes, the two most important of which are:

(a) Biotransformation of the drug during passage through the GI epithelium and/or liver, en route to the systemic circulation via the liver. This type of biotransformation is referred to as the *first-pass effect*.
(b) *Enterohepatic circulation of the drug*. During the first pass through the liver, the drug may be excreted to the bile, re-enter the GI tract via the gallbladder, and be reabsorbed.

It is evident that both of these post-absorptive processes can contribute to alterations in bioavailability.

An overall view of the processes controlling the arrival of drug to the general circulation is presented in Fig. 3.3. In this figure, F denotes the *bioavailability coefficient*, which expresses the fraction of dose reaching the general circulation ($0 < F \leqslant 1$). At this point the distinction between the terms 'fraction absorbed' and 'bioavailability coefficient' should be clarified. For example, if 80 mg from the 100 mg of the orally administered dose are absorbed then the fraction absorbed is 0.80 and the bioavailability coefficient is 0.80. However, if 20% of the absorbed drug is biotransformed during its first passage through the liver, then the 'fraction absorbed' is 0.80 and the 'bioavailability coefficient' is 0.64. The two terms become equivalent when both the first-pass effect and enterohepatic circulation are negligible.

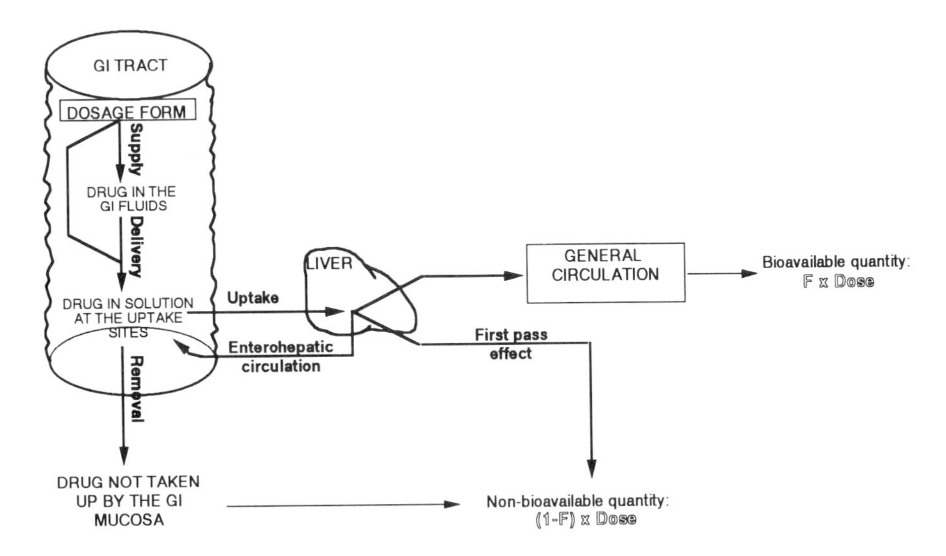

Fig. 3.3. Luminal and post-absorptive processes involved in the arrival of drug to the systemic circulation after oral administration.

3.2 PROCESSES THAT AFFECT THE BIOAVAILABILITY OF DRUGS AFTER ORAL ADMINISTRATION

3.2.1 Luminal processes that affect oral bioavailability

3.2.1.1 Supply of the gastrointestinal fluids with drug

The supply of the GI fluids with drug depends not only on the dosage form characteristics but also on the GI physiological conditions.

In the case of conventional dosage forms the rate of drug dissolution depends on the physicochemical properties of both the drug and the excipients. Modified-release systems are designed so that the rate of release is controlled entirely from the formulation. The ability of the dosage form to release drug within its residence time is key to the bioavailability of drug from modified-release dosage forms.

The physiological GI conditions which are directly related to dissolution or release of drug usually include the volume of the GI contents, type and quantity of other substances (physiological or not) which are present in the GI lumen, and the GI motility pattern when the dosage form is administered.

3.2.1.2 Delivery of the drug to and removal of drug from uptake sites

A key process in the delivery of drug to the uptake sites is gastric emptying. The small intestine usually constitutes the most favourable absorption site and, therefore, delivery of drug to this region is a prerequisite for absorption.

There are also processes which tend to remove drug from the absorptive sites. These include the chemical or enzymatic transformation of drug, the complexation of drug in the GI lumen, the precipitation of drug in the GI fluids and/or physical elimination due to the transit of GI contents, all of which reduce the availability of drug for uptake from the GI mucosa.

Biotransformation in the GI lumen can be catalysed by compounds of exogenous or physiological origin. For example, penicillins and erythromycin are decomposed in the stomach by hydrochloric acid. Enzymes secreted from the stomach, from the pancreas (into the small intestine) and from bacteria in the large intestine can also catalyse the biotransformation of drugs. Peptides are especially sensitive to luminal transformation in the stomach and small intestine. Obviously, in all these cases biotransformation reduces the bioavailability of the compound administered.

On the other hand, chemical or biochemical modification in the GI lumen may be desirable if this is a prerequisite for pharmacological action. A typical example is the prodrug sulfasalazine, which is used in the treatment of ulcerative colitis. The larger portion of the administered dose is not absorbed in the small intestine owing to insufficient solubility; in the large intestine the drug undergoes enzymatic hydrolysis to sulfapyridine and 5-aminosalicylic acid, a reaction which is catalysed by bacterial enzymes. The selective release of 5-aminosalicylic acid enhances local action in the large intestine while minimizing upper GI side-effects.

Colonic flora

Sulfasalazine → Sulfapyridine + 5-amino-salicylic acid

Complexation reactions are rather difficult to predict because of the heterogeneity of the GI contents. Nevertheless, such interactions are not uncommon. A classic example is the complexation of tetracyclines with Ca^{2+}, in cases where tetracyclines are coadministered with dairy products. Precipitation of the drug in the GI fluids may also occur owing to the large differential in the pH between the stomach and small intestine. The category of drugs most likely to be affected is that of the poorly soluble weak bases.

Finally, the rate of GI transit affects the absorption of drugs as in most cases it is the major factor which determines the residence time to the uptake sites. This physiological process is mostly controlled by the motility state of the GI tract, the type of dosage form and the composition of the accompanying fluids.

3.2.1.3 Uptake of the drug by the gastrointestinal mucosa

In the majority of cases, drug uptake from the GI epithelium follows the principles of passive diffusion. In some cases, however, carrier-mediated transport or both passive and carrier-mediated mechanisms may be operating.

The lipophilicity of the drug is the determining factor for passive permeation of the GI mucosa by the transcellular route. Thus, the assessment or the prediction of the degree of the drug's uptake depends on the non-ionized (more lipophilic) fraction of drug, with the ionization in turn depending on the drug pK_a value and the pH of the environment (Henderson–Hasselbach equations, section 2.3.1.3). In essence, these two factors, i.e. the fraction of drug in the non-ionized form and the lipophilicity of the drug, determine its ability to partition into the lipoidal membrane of the enterocytes. Since the pH, and hence fraction of drug in the non-ionized form, may vary with location in the gut, even drugs that are absorbed by transcellular diffusion may exhibit differences in absorption rate with location in the gut.

Whenever carrier-mediated transport is encountered, the affinity of drug for the carrier and the capacity of the carrier determine the efficiency of transport.

Irrespective of the uptake mechanism(s), another important factor may be the ability of the drug to diffuse through the GI contents to the surface of the epithelial cells. This process may become the rate-limiting step for absorption when the drug has very poor aqueous solubility, the drug is associated with a slow-diffusing moiety (e.g. complexed with a macromolecule or solubilized into micelles) or the GI contents have high viscosity.

3.2.2 Post-absorptive processes that affect oral bioavailability

3.2.2.1 First-pass effect and enterohepatic circulation

After the uptake of drug from the GI epithelium and prior to its arrival in the general circulation, the drug can be biotransformed during its passage through the epithelial cell, and/or during its first passage through the liver. Occasionally, during its (first and subsequent) pass through the liver, the drug is excreted in the bile. When the gallbladder contracts in response to consumption of a meal, the drug is secreted with the bile back into the duodenum.

3.3 METHODS OF ASSESSING AND PARAMETERS USED TO CHARACTERIZE BIOAVAILABILITY

3.3.1 Bioavailability parameters

From the aforementioned discussion it can be concluded that the fraction of dose reaching the general circulation depends on a number of processes occurring in the GI tract. Since absorption phenomena in the GI tract are difficult to measure experimentally indirect methods of calculating bioavailability were developed. The concentration versus time profile of drug in plasma is partially a reflection of absorption phenomena and can be used to estimate bioavailability. For a given drug, the higher the fraction of the dose reaching the general circulation the larger will be the area under the concentration versus time curve (AUC, Fig. 3.4). Consequently, the magnitude of this area (expressed in units of [concentration] × [time]) is a measure of the quantity of drug reaching the general circulation, i.e. the extent of absorption. The experimentally determined maximum concentration, C_{max}, and the time which this occurs, t_{max}, are measures of the kinetic characteristics of bioavailability, since both are related to the rate of drug absorption. A low value for t_{max} indicates a fast rate of absorption. The parameters AUC, C_{max}, and t_{max} can be calculated either by pharmacokinetic modelling of the experimental data or by visual inspection of C_{max} and t_{max}, and application of the trapezoidal rule for the AUC.

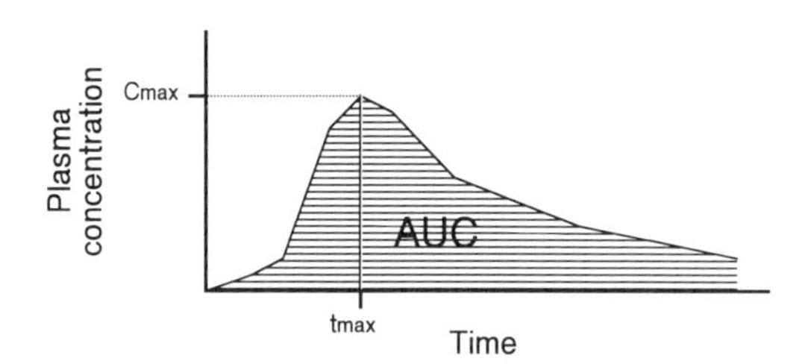

Fig. 3.4. Typical plasma concentration–time plot after oral administration. The fundamental bioavailability parameters AUC, C_{max}, and t_{max} are also shown.

It should be noted that the magnitude of the parameters C_{max} and t_{max} are often related to therapeutic effect. For analgesics, antihistaminics and many other drugs used for symptomatic relief, therapeutically effective plasma levels should be achieved with a single dose. In these cases fast and complete absorption (short t_{max}, effective C_{max}) is the main target. At the other end of the scale, in the case of antiepileptics or antihypertensives, the maintenance of therapeutic blood concentrations over a long period of time is the clinically desirable goal. Under these circumstances the extended release of drug, implying a slow rate of absorption with a correspondingly large value for t_{max}, is the main characteristic sought in the formulation.

3.3.2 Absolute and relative bioavailability

Bioavailability can be broadly divided to relative and absolute. In the former case the bioavailability study involves comparison of extravascularly administered formulations while in the latter an extravascularly administered formulation is compared with a dose of drug given intravenously. Relative bioavailability studies provide only a relative measure of the bioavailability of the formulations and not an estimate for the fraction of dose absorbed. By contrast, in absolute bioavailability studies one is able to calculate the amount of drug reaching the general circulation. This can be accomplished because the reference formulation is administered intravenously thereby ensuring the complete delivery of the entire dose to blood.

The evaluation of either relative or absolute bioavailability is based on the calculation of the bioavailability coefficient, F, which corresponds to the ratio of AUCs of the two formulations:

$$F = (\mathrm{AUC})_{\mathrm{test}}/(\mathrm{AUC})_{\mathrm{ref}} \tag{3.1}$$

where $(\mathrm{AUC})_{\mathrm{test}}$ and $(\mathrm{AUC})_{\mathrm{ref}}$ are the areas under the plasma concentration versus time curve for the test formulation and the reference formulation, respectively. Equation (3.1) is valid only when the two formulations contain the same doses. For the more general case of unequal doses, equation (3.1) is written as

$$F = (\mathrm{AUC})_{\mathrm{test}}(\mathrm{dose})_{\mathrm{ref}}/(\mathrm{AUC})_{\mathrm{ref}}\,(\mathrm{dose})_{\mathrm{test}} \tag{3.2}$$

It should be clarified that in the great majority of cases the AUC is proportional to dose and this proportionality justifies the use of equation (3.2) for calculation of the extent of bioavailability. However, in some cases, dose and AUC are non-linearly related. This can be observed with drugs having either a saturable first pass effect or when the uptake of drug is carrier mediated, with saturation of the carrier at doses studied. Vitamins B_2 and B_{12} are two examples of compounds with saturable uptake kinetics and which exhibit lower bioavailability coefficient at higher doses.

For the calculation of absolute bioavailability, relationships analogous to equations (3.1) and (3.2) are used:

$$F = (\mathrm{AUC})_{\mathrm{test}}/(\mathrm{AUC})_{\mathrm{iv}} \tag{3.3}$$

$$F = (\mathrm{AUC})_{\mathrm{test}}(\mathrm{dose})_{\mathrm{iv}}/(\mathrm{AUC})_{\mathrm{iv}}\,(\mathrm{dose})_{\mathrm{test}} \tag{3.4}$$

The only difference lies in the reference formulation; here, an intravenous dose is administered as a reference formulation. Equations (3.3) and (3.4) are applied to bioavailability studies with equal and unequal doses, respectively. A typical concentration–time profile after an intravenous bolus administration is shown in Fig. 3.5.

Finally, it should be noted that the use of equations (3.1)–(3.4) assumes that the body clearance (chapter 9) is the same when the two formulations are administered. Under this assumption the differences in AUCs can be reliably attributed to bioavailability

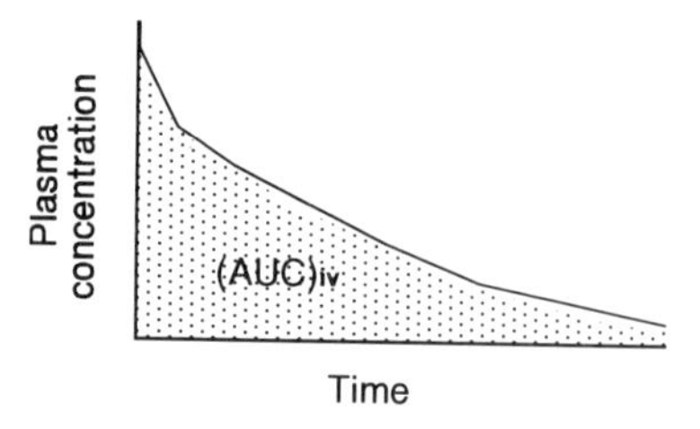

Fig. 3.5. Typical plasma concentration–time plot after intravenous bolus administration.

differences and not to changes associated with the rate of drug elimination. In order to reduce the effect of clearance on the evaluation of bioavailability, both formulations can be administered to the same group of volunteers on separate occasions, in a crossover study design.

Example 3.1: Two formulations of griseofulvin G_1 and G_2, were given to the same group of volunteers on two separate occasions; the mean values of AUCs found, based on plasma concentration versus time plots for 24 h, were $(AUC)_1 = 12.0\ \mu g \times h \times ml^{-1}$ and $(AUC)_2 = 9.0\ \mu g \times h \times ml^{-1}$. Assuming that the formulations G_1 and G_2 contain 500 and 250 mg of griseofulvin, respectively, calculate the relative bioavailability of G_1 versus G_2.

Answer: According to equation (3.2)

$$F = (12.0 \times 250)/(9.0 \times 500) = 0.67$$

Thus, the relative bioavailability of formulation G_1 versus G_2 is 0.67 or 67%.

Example 3.2: To study the absolute bioavailability of an extended-release formulation of 300 mg of theophylline, this formulation and an intravenous bolus dose of 250 mg of theophylline were administered to the same group of volunteers on two separate occasions. The mean AUC_{0-12h} values calculated were 70 and $100\ \mu g \times h \times ml^{-1}$ after the per os and i.v. administration, respectively. Calculate the absolute bioavailability of the per os formulation.

Answer: According to equation (3.4)

$$F = (70 \times 250)/(110 \times 300) = 0.53$$

This figure corresponds to 53% absolute bioavailability, which is equivalent to an absorbed quantity of 159 mg of theophylline from the dose of 300 mg contained in the dosage form.

3.3.3 Bioequivalence

Two formulations can be characterized as *bioequivalent* when the values of the parameters AUC, C_{max}, and t_{max} are statistically equivalent. As a general rule of thumb, bioequivalence of two formulations is justified when the difference in the mean values of the bioavailability parameters of the two formulations is less than 20%. This is defined mathematically with one of the three relationships:

$$0.8\mu_{\text{ref}} < \mu_{\text{test}} < 1.2\mu_{\text{ref}} \tag{3.5}$$

or
$$|\mu_{\text{ref}} - \mu_{\text{test}}| < 0.2\mu_{\text{ref}} \tag{3.6}$$

or
$$0.8 < \mu_{\text{test}}/\mu_{\text{ref}} < 1.2 \tag{3.7}$$

where μ_{ref} and μ_{test} are the mean values of the bioavailability parameters (AUC, C_{max}, t_{max}) for the reference and test formulation, respectively. The mean values are calculated from the values of the parameters estimated in the individuals participating in the study. When the criterion of equivalence is not satisfied the statistical inference is that the formulations are *bio-inequivalent*.

Due to the many sources of variability in bioequivalence studies (e.g. intra- and inter-subject variability and experimental error) the decision rules for bioequivalence rely on strict statistical analysis of data. Currently the most common decision rules are the classical *t*-based and the Westlake's symmetric confidence intervals. Both approaches are based on the computation of a certain percentage of confidence level (most frequently 90%) around the sample mean of the bioavailability parameter. These intervals are computed and compared with the acceptable range for bioequivalence in accordance with one of the equations (3.5)–(3.7). The reader is referred to the bibliography below for further reading on the various statistical aspects of the bioequivalence issue.

FURTHER READING

Skelly JP, Amidon GL, Barr WH, Benet LZ, Carter JE, Robinson JR, Shah VP and Yacobi A. Workshop Report. *Pharm. Res.* **7**: 975–982 (1990).

Stenijans VW (guest ed.). *Int. J. Clin. Pharmacol. Ther. Toxicol.* **30**: S1–S68 (1992).

Welling PG, Tse FLS and Dighe SV (eds). *Pharmaceutical Bioequivalence*, Marcel Dekker, New York (1991).

4

Supply of the gastrointestinal fluids with drug

Objectives

After completing this chapter the reader will have an understanding of:

- *The processes involved in the transfer of drug from the dosage form to the gastro-intestinal fluids*
- *The mathematics of mass transfer of drug from the dosage form to the gastointestinal fluids*
- *The methods used for studying release of drug from the dosage form and drug dissolution, in media simulating gastrointestinal fluids*

Drug molecules can penetrate the epithelial barrier of the gastrointestinal (GI) tract by diffusion and carrier-mediated mechanisms only if they are in solution. Therefore, effective oral administration of solid, suspension or semi-solid dosage forms requires the dissolution of drug in the GI fluids. Ideally, the active ingredient of the dosage form should be released before it reaches the region of the GI tract in which its uptake is optimum. The term *release* encompasses several processes which contribute to the transfer of drug from the administered dosage form to the GI fluids. Figs 4.1 and 4.2 illustrate these processes, according to formulation type.

The most common type of formulation administered orally is the solid dosage form. Using US Pharmacopoeia (USP; Edition XXII, 1990) terminology, solid dosage forms can be classified into two categories: *immediate* and *modified* release. Immediate-release dosage forms are designed to release the drug rapidly after administration, and the rate of drug transfer to the GI fluids depends mainly on the properties of the drug and the conditions prevailing in the region where release occurs. Modified-release dosage forms are designed to deliver the drug to the GI fluids at a rate that is governed more by the dosage form and less by drug properties and conditions prevailing in the GI tract. Modified-release dosage forms may be designed to *extend* and/or *delay* release. One way to define extended release is in terms of ability to reduce the frequency of administration by a factor of two compared to the frequency at which the immediate-release dosage form

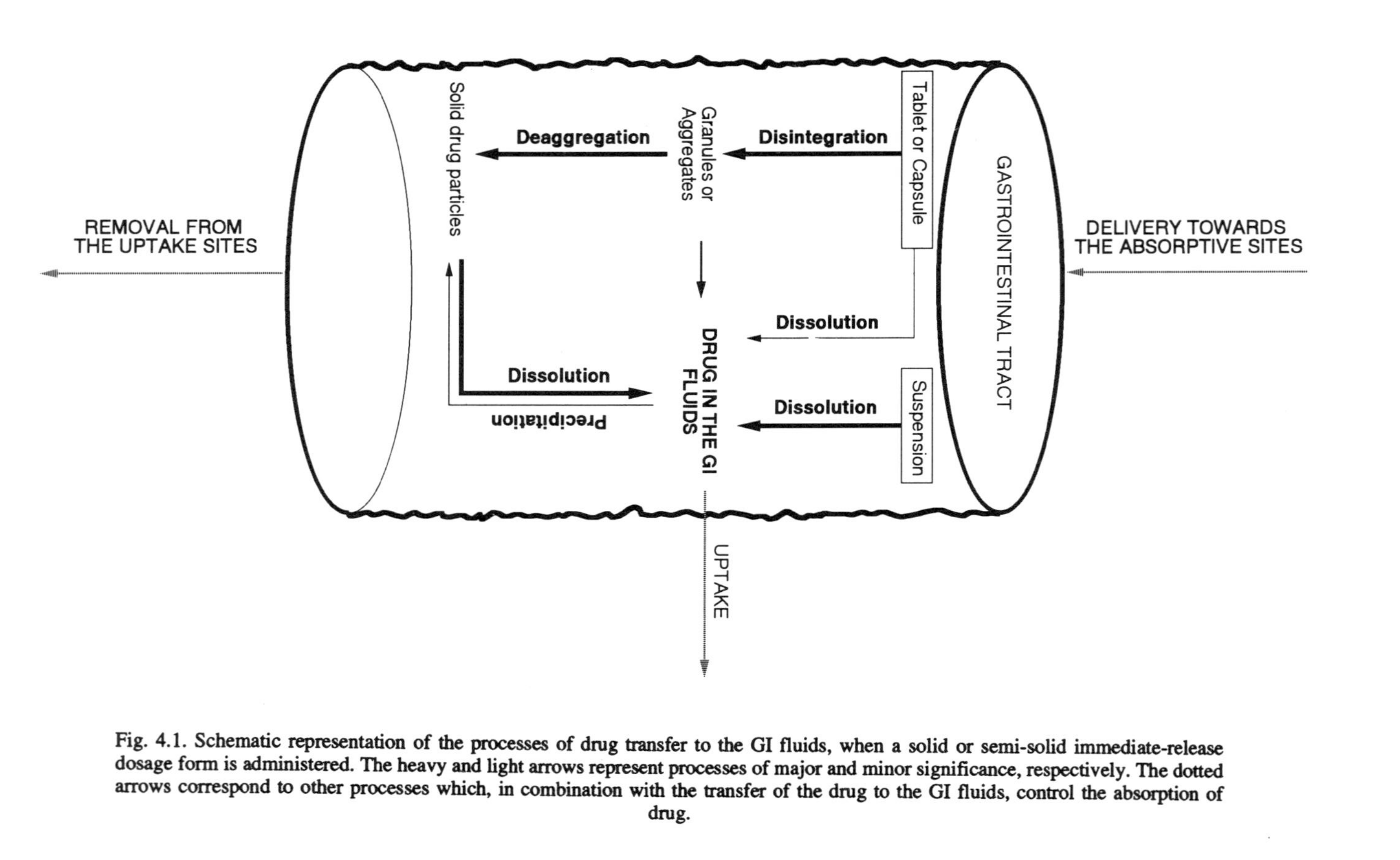

Fig. 4.1. Schematic representation of the processes of drug transfer to the GI fluids, when a solid or semi-solid immediate-release dosage form is administered. The heavy and light arrows represent processes of major and minor significance, respectively. The dotted arrows correspond to other processes which, in combination with the transfer of the drug to the GI fluids, control the absorption of drug.

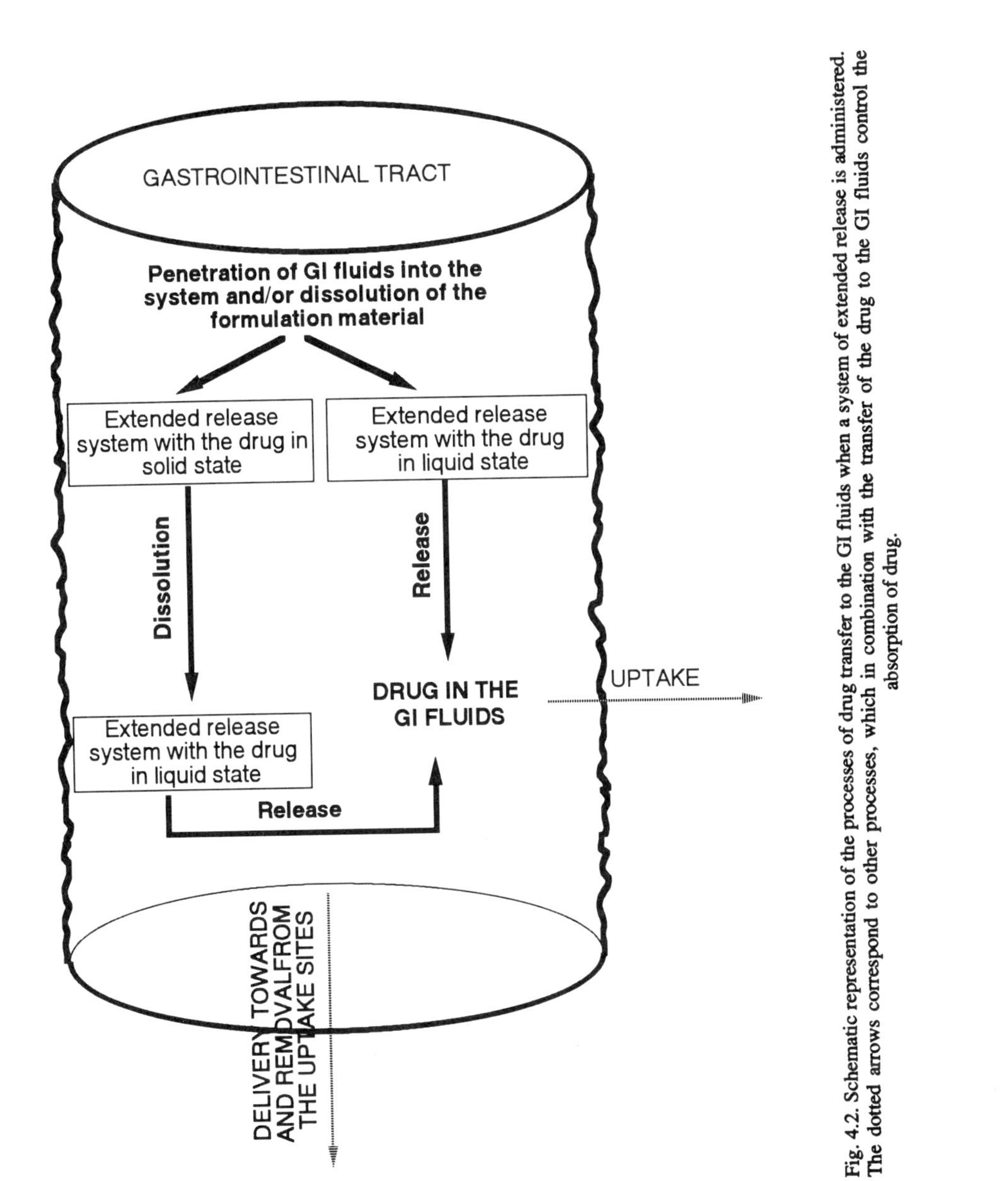

Fig. 4.2. Schematic representation of the processes of drug transfer to the GI fluids when a system of extended release is administered. The dotted arrows correspond to other processes, which in combination with the transfer of the drug to the GI fluids control the absorption of drug.

of the drug is usually administered. As the name suggests, delayed-release dosage forms are designed to wait to release the drug until either a certain time has elapsed, or until a specific location in the GI tract is reached. A typical way to delay release is to enteric coat the dosage form, which then releases the active ingredient soon after it enters the small intestine.

4.1 PROCESSES WHICH TRANSFER DRUG TO THE GASTROINTESTINAL FLUIDS AND THEIR IMPACT ON ABSORPTION

Drug transfer from immediate-release tablets to the gastrointestinal (GI) fluids requires (1) disintegration, the initial rupture of the tablet, (2) deaggregation, a separation of the tablet fragments into finer particles, and (3) dissolution of the drug in the GI fluids. Analogous processes occur in the mass transfer of drug from capsules, suspensions, and semi-solids (Fig. 4.1). These processes mainly occur in series but may also occur in parallel, e.g. direct dissolution from the tablet surface may occur while the tablet is still in the process of disintegrating and deaggregating.

The processes involved in transfer of drug from an extended-release dosage form to the GI fluids are shown in Fig. 4.2. In general, the GI fluids penetrate the dosage form and release of drug is accomplished by solvation, diffusion, osmosis and/or ion-exchange mechanisms.

Although Figs 4.1 and 4.2 illustrate that drug transfer from the dosage form to the GI fluids can be quite complex, one can usually identify one or two steps which govern the overall rate of release.

In the case of immediate-release dosage forms, disintegration and dissolution control the rate at which drug is transferred to the GI fluids. Disintegration depends almost exclusively on formulation factors, while dissolution of drug from deaggregated particles depends on the physicochemical properties of the drug, the composition of the GI fluids, and on properties related to manufacture of the drug product, such as excipient choice and processing variables.

The dependency of disintegration characteristics on the excipients and the manufacturing process permits a large degree of control of this process by the formulator, with the result that disintegration times are usually short. Although rapid disintegration facilitates dissolution, it does not ensure the dissolution of the drug. For suspensions, dissolution is the only barrier to transfer of the drug to the GI fluids. This is also true for capsules which contain powdered drug as the dissolution of standard gelatin housing is not a time-consuming process, and is relatively easy to control. Dissolution is usually the crucial step for the transfer of drug to the GI fluids.

For extended-release dosage forms the mechanism and driving force for release govern the rate at which drug is released from the dosage form. These factors are influenced by the type of system used, the physicochemical properties of drug and the conditions prevailing in the GI tract during release. Drugs which are candidates for extended-release products are usually soluble in aqueous media, and the aim is to formulate them so that the rate of drug release is slower than the dissolution rate from the immediate-release dosage form. Approaches include trapping the drug in a slowly dissolving matrix; coating the tablet/granules with an insoluble polymer coating which retards release; and binding the drug to an ion-exchange resin.

Fig. 4.3, shows the key steps in supply of the GI fluids from solid, suspension and semi-solid dosage forms, for both immediate and extended-release products. If the rate of supply of the drug to the GI fluids is much lower than the uptake rate, then supply will be rate limiting to absorption. Under these circumstances, if the processes involved obey first-order kinetics, the following relationship holds:

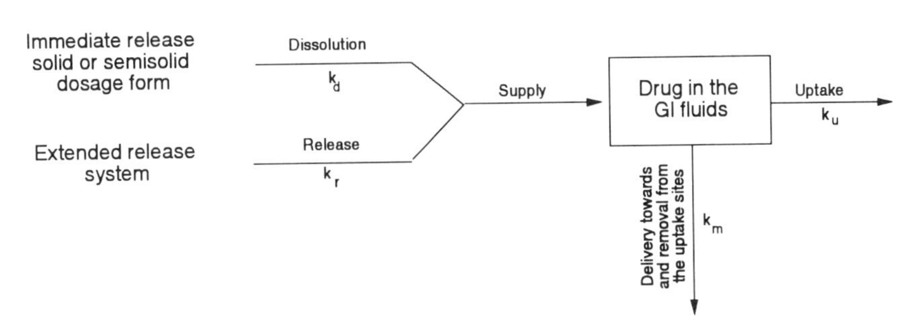

Fig. 4.3. Simplified model for the supply of the GI fluids with drug, from an immediate-release solid dosage form, and from a system of extended release; k_d, k_r, k_t and k_u, are the dissolution, release, transit and uptake rate constants, respectively.

$$R_{0,s} \ll R_{0,u}$$

where $R_{o,s}$ and $R_{o,u}$ are the initial supply rate of the drug to the GI fluids and its initial uptake rate by the GI epithelium, respectively. The initial supply rate can be expressed as follows:

$$R_{0,s} = k_{1,s} C_s V$$

where $k_{1,s}$ is the first-order constant of the supply rate of the drug (dissolution or release) to the GI fluids, C_s is the solubility of drug in the GI fluids, and V is the volume of the GI fluids. If supply is the rate-limiting step, it follows that

$$R_{0,a} = k_{1,s} C_s V$$

where $R_{0,a}$ is the initial absorption rate observed.

It is important to note that the parameters $k_{1,s}$, C_s and V, which control the supply rate, are governed by the physicochemical properties of the drug and the physiological characteristics of the GI tract. For this reason, $R_{0,s}$ can be different in the various regions of the GI tract. For example, the saturation solubility (which affects, as shown later in this chapter, the dissolution of the drug, and therefore the concentration of drug in the GI fluids), may depend on the pH, which varies with location in the GI tract from 1.8 to 7.5, and the bile concentration. Similarly, the volume of fluid in the small intestine has been estimated to range between about 200 and 500 ml. It is thus evident that:

(a) uptake of sparingly soluble drugs administered in immediate-release solid forms may be limited by slow dissolution; and
(b) for extended-release dosage forms, differences in the physiological features of the various segments of the GI tract may make it difficult to design systems which can supply the drug to the GI fluids at a desired rate.

4.2 RELEASE OF THE DRUG FROM A SOLID IMMEDIATE-RELEASE FORMULATION

4.2.1 Disintegration and deaggregation

Until the mid-1950s, release of the active ingredient from tablet dosage forms was assessed by the disintegration time. The assumption that absorption depends only on disintegration, while inaccurate, led to an improvement in the quality of immediate-release dosage forms since much research was focused on improving disintegrants and controlling manufacturing processes which affect disintegration. However, at the end of the 1950s it was realized that disintegration only secures the contact of the solid drug particles with the GI fluids, and not the dissolution of the drug. In the early 1960s it was established that dissolution is the most important process for the transfer of drug to the GI fluids and thus the more important factor in drug absorption. Only in cases where the drug has a high aqueous solubility and therefore facile dissolution in the GI tract is the disintegration time a substantial proportion of the total time it takes to transfer the drug from the formulation to the solution.

The disintegration test for immediate-release dosage forms and for enteric coated products is carried out *in vitro* using the equipment shown in Fig. 4.4. At the lower end of each tube there is a 10 mesh (0.025 inch) stainless-steel wire screen. The system is raised and lowered at a constant frequency (29–32 complete motions per minute), covering a distance of 5.5 ± 0.2 cm, in a 1000 ml beaker, which may contain distilled water, simulated gastric fluid or simulated intestinal fluid, depending on the type of dosage form tested (Table 4.1). The median temperature is held at 37 ± 2°C to simulate body temperature. The disintegration of the dosage form is considered to be complete when

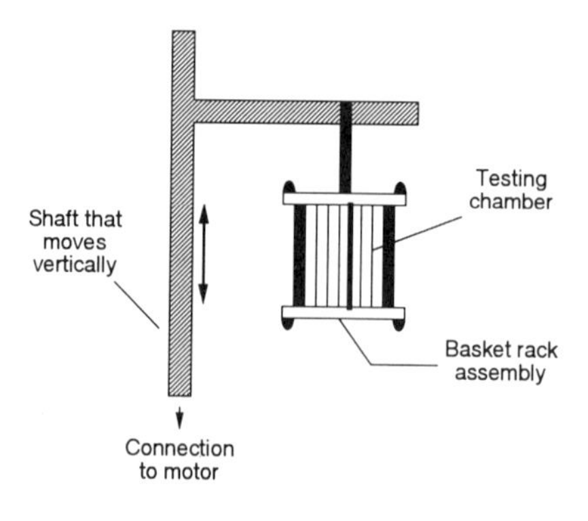

Fig. 4.4. Schematic representation of the *in vitro* system used to assess disintegration time.

any residue, except for fragments of a coating or the capsule housing, remaining on the screen of the test apparatus is a soft mass having no palpably firm core.

Table 4.1. Composition of simulated gastric and intestinal fluids of the USP

Simulated gastric fluid (pH 1.2)	Simulated intestinal fluid (pH 7.5)
Sodium chloride 2.0 g	Pancreatin 10.0 g
Pepsin 3.2 g	0.2 M potassium dihydrogen phosphate 250 ml
Conc. hydrochloric acid 7.0 ml	0.2 M sodium hydroxide 140 ml
Distilled water q.s. 1000 ml	Distilled water q.s. 1000 ml

As well as tablets, many drugs are formulated as powders packed in hard gelatin capsules. Although there is no disintegration step involved in release of drugs formulated this way, poor deaggregation of the powdered contents can adversely affect transfer of the drug to the GI fluids. Processing and formulation variables, such as inclusion of a small amount of surfactant in the formulation, can be used to circumvent any deaggregation problems.

The factors affecting disintegration and deaggregation are summarized in Table 4.2. As they are mainly associated with formulation and processing variables, they can usually be controlled to a large degree. Consequently, as already mentioned, disintegration and deaggregation do not normally limit drug transfer from the dosage form to the GI fluids.

Table 4.2. The most important factors affecting disintegration and deaggregation

Tablets for immediate release	Hard gelatin capsules	Enteric coated tablets
Diluent	Diluent	Coating material
Tableting method	Grinding process	Method of coating
Size of granules	Coating properties	Pre-coating material
Disintegrant	Pressure during filling	Plasticizer
Ageing and storage conditions	Ageing and storage conditions	Ageing and storage conditions
Lubricant	Lubricant	

4.2.2 Dissolution

Dissolution of the active ingredient from an immediate-release solid dosage form or a suspension is a critical step in the transfer of drug to the GI fluids. When the drug is readily taken up by the epithelium of the GI tract, the time to reach the absorptive site (a function of GI motility) and/or the dissolution rate may be rate-limiting to absorption (Fig. 4.3). For drugs which are sparingly soluble in aqueous media, dissolution is often the primary limitation (see Table 4.3). Research has shown that when the saturation

Table 4.3. Some drugs with dissolution rate limited absorption

Chloramphenicol	Phenylbutazone
Danazol	Phenytoin
Digoxin	Prednisolone
Griseofulvin	Prednisone
Hydrochlorthiazide	Quinidine
Hydrocortisone	Sulfadiazine
Mefenamic acid	Spironolactone
Nitrofurantoin	Tetracyclines
p-Aminosalicylic acid (PAS)	Tolbutamide
Penicillin V	Triamterene

solubility of the drug in an aqueous solution with a pH similar to that of the intestinal fluids (i.e. about pH 6–7) is much smaller than 0.1 mg/ml, then poor or at least inconsistent absorption is expected, due to slow dissolution. A classical example is digoxin, which is very poorly soluble in water; it has been shown clinically that the maximum digoxin concentration in plasma of various formulations is proportional to its dissolution rate.

For compounds with low inherent aqueous solubility, dissolution changes due to apparently insignificant modifications of the formulation may affect product performance significantly. For example, in Australia and New Zealand in 1968, phenytoin toxicity occurred in a large number of patients when the manufacturer replaced the excipient calcium sulfate with lactose in the immediate-release phenytoin tablets. The higher hydrophilicity of lactose, compared to calcium sulfate, promoted the dissolution rate of phenytoin resulting in a higher bioavailability and consequently higher concentrations of phenytoin in plasma, exceeding its narrow therapeutic range of 10–20 μg/ml. The results of an independent study, conducted to confirm the excipient effect on the observed levels of phenytoin in plasma, are presented in Fig. 4.5A.

Another example is chloramphenicol. Fig. 4.5B shows the mean plasma concentration of chloramphenicol in 10 volunteers who received four different formulations. The large differences among the concentration–time profiles observed were directly related to the different dissolution rates of drug from each formulation. This study was one of the earliest to demonstrate the effect of dissolution on the bioavailability of drugs. In the 1960s and 1970s many similar studies were reported in the literature for other drugs, such as phenylbutazone, tolbutamide and oxytetracycline. These reports prompted the initiation of bioequivalence studies since more and more generic drug products[†] were becoming available in the market.

The study of dissolution rate is therefore one of the most important tests, not only during the pre-formulation stage, but also in quality-assurance testing of solid dosage forms.

† The increase in generic drug products resulted from the expiration of patents for drugs already on the market.

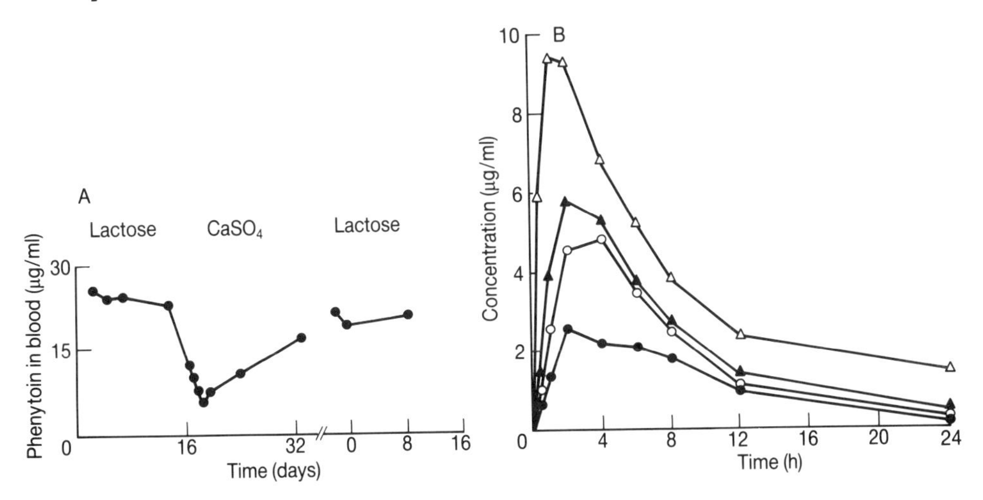

Fig. 4.5. (A) Effect of lactose and calcium sulphate (as excipients in the dosage form) on the phenytoin plasma concentrations of a patient, receiving orally phenytoin at a dose of 400 mg/d (reprinted with permission from *Drug Disposition and Pharmacokinetics with Consideration of Pharmacological and Clinical Relationships* (2nd edn), p. 139, Blackwell Scientific Publications, London, 1977). (B) Mean values of the plasma concentrations of chloramphenicol of 10 volunteers after oral administration of various dosage forms, containing 0.5 g of the drug (reprinted with permission from *Clinical Pharmacology and Therapeutics* **9**: 472–483 (1968)).

4.2.2.1 Theory of dissolution

During the dissolution process the initial transfer of drug molecules from the surface of the solid particle to the surrounding fluid layer is followed by movement of the dissolved molecules to the bulk solution. Based on these two steps, several models have been proposed for the mechanism(s) of the dissolution process as a whole.

The first quantitative study of the dissolution process was published in 1897 by Noyes and Whitney. In their experiments they studied the dissolution of lead chloride and benzoic acid in water using rotating cylinders with a constant surface area. They collected a number of samples and determined the concentration of the solutes in the water at constant time intervals. Their main conclusion was that the dissolution rate is proportional to the difference of the solubility, C_s, and the concentration of the dissolved substance, C, at any time, t:

$$J_d = \alpha(C_s - C) \tag{4.1}$$

where J_d, is the *dissolution rate per unit surface area*, also called *flux* of the dissolving substance, while α is a proportionality constant. The dissolution rate per unit surface area is defined by the following equation:

$$J_d = \frac{dm/dt}{A} = \frac{(dC/dt)V}{A} \tag{4.2}$$

where m is the mass of the solid which has been dissolved by time t; A is the surface area of the solid and V is the volume of the dissolution medium. In conjunction with equation (4.1), Noyes and Whitney proposed the model shown in Fig. 4.6. According to this model

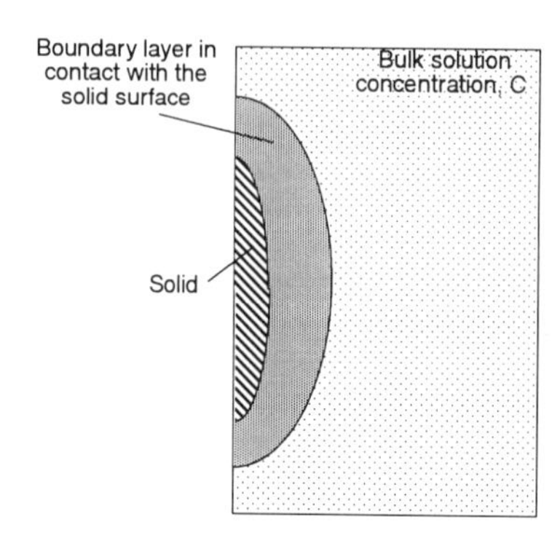

Fig. 4.6. Schematic representation of the dissolution process, according to the Noyes–Whitney model.

a thin layer of saturated solution covers the solid particles and the dissolution rate is controlled by the transfer of the dissolved substance from the saturated layer to the solution. They assumed that the formation of the saturated layer occurs much faster than the transfer of the solute to the bulk solution, and therefore the dissolution rate depends on the diffusion of the substance from the saturated layer to the bulk solution.

A disadvantage of the Noyes–Whitney model is that it does not provide a sound explanation concerning the mechanism of formation of the saturated layer. For this reason, two other models based on the results of Noyes and Whitney's experiments have been proposed. It must be noted that these models, like the Noyes–Whitney model, are directly applicable only if the dissolving solid does not decompose or react with components of the dissolution medium while the dissolution progresses. If not, a modified version of the model must be used.

The most important of these models is in essence an improvement of the Noyes–Whitney model. The dissolution process is considered to be controlled by diffusion of the dissolved substance away from the surface of the solid towards the bulk solution, in accord with Fick's law of diffusion (Fig. 4.7A). This is the model most commonly used today. However, the inability of this model to interpret certain experimental data led to the model depicted in Fig. 4.7B. According to this model, the initial transfer of the molecules of the solid from the solid surface to the liquid medium is assumed to be much slower than the diffusion towards the bulk solution, in which case the initial transfer controls the rate at which the overall process occurs. From the mathematical point of view, both models predict the dissolution rate is proportional to the concentration difference $(C_s - C)$ since in all cases the transfer to the bulk solution is accomplished by diffusion. However, the conceptual differences between the models are significant.

Diffusion boundary layer model

This model was developed by Nernst and Brunner in the 1900s and proceeds directly from the Noyes–Whitney model. According to the diffusion boundary layer model (or, more simply, the diffusion layer model), there is a stagnant liquid layer in contact with the solid. The transfer of drug through this layer occurs by a diffusion process because of

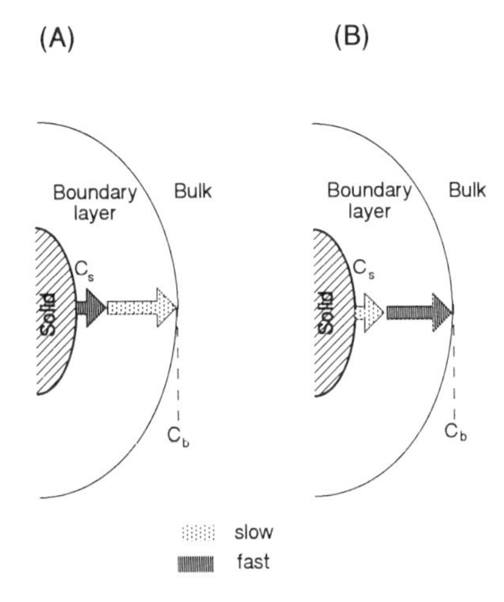

Fig. 4.7. The two main models for the interpretation of the dissolution mechanism: (A) diffusion layer model, and (B) interfacial barrier model.

the concentration gradient between the two sides of the layer. The concentration of the drug decreases gradually over the width of the layer, starting from a maximum close to the solid surface, where the concentration is equal to the solubility, and reaching a minimum at the interface between the stagnant liquid layer and the bulk solution, where the concentration equals the concentration throughout the drug in the bulk solution (Fig. 4.7A). This model assumes that complete mixing takes place immediately after the molecules of the dissolved solid traverse the interface between the layer and the bulk solution. Beyond the interface, the concentration in the dissolution medium is homogeneous. It is also assumed that transfer of the drug molecules from the solid surface to the stagnant liquid layer is fast, and that equilibrium in this region is rapidly established. Consequently, the step which limits the rate at which the dissolution process occurs is the rate of diffusion of the molecules through the stagnant liquid layer rather than the initial release of the molecules from the solid surface. Fig. 4.8 illustrates the Nernst–Brunner model.

The mathematical expression for the dissolution rate according to this model is given by equation (4.3):

$$J_{\mathrm{d}} = \frac{(\mathrm{d}m/\mathrm{d}t)}{A} = \frac{D}{h_{\mathrm{N}}}(C_{\mathrm{s}} - C) = k_{\mathrm{N}}(C_{\mathrm{s}} - C) \tag{4.3}$$

where D is the diffusion coefficient of the drug, h_{N} is the width of the diffusion layer and $k_{\mathrm{N}} = D/h_{\mathrm{N}}$ is the *intrinsic dissolution rate constant* based on the diffusion layer model. The value of h_{N} can be calculated from equation (4.3) if the diffusion coefficient, D, and the surface area, A are known, and if data for the quantity of the dissolved substance as a function of time are available.

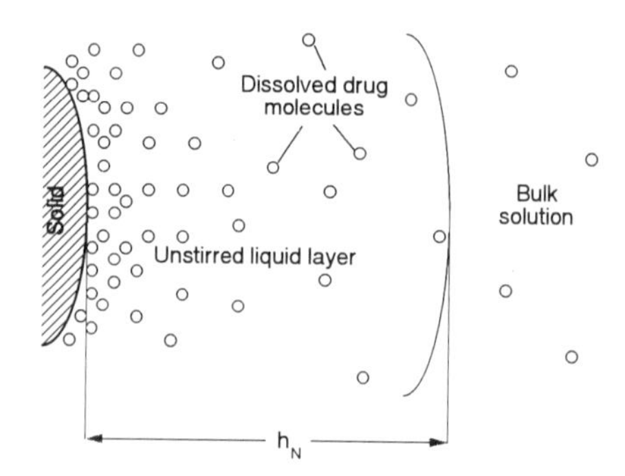

Fig. 4.8. Schematic representation of the distribution of dissolved drug molecules in the diffusion layer.

Current views on the diffusion layer model

Although the diffusion layer model developed by Nernst and Brunner enjoys widespread acceptance, it is a somewhat simplistic interpretation of dissolution. The assumption of a stagnant boundary layer interfacing with a well-mixed bulk solution is used because it results in a mathematically analytical solution to the dissolution equation. Physically, however, there is a gradient region over which mixing becomes less and less complete as the solid surface is approached, and the extent of this region depends on the hydrodynamics (e.g. rate of stirring) in the bulk medium. Thus, the so-called boundary layer thickness has a mathematical rather than a physical meaning. Depending on the experimental conditions, the calculated boundary layer thickness may be as large as several hundred micrometres, which would be physically unreasonable.

An alternative hydrodynamic model to the stagnant layer/well-mixed bulk of Nernst and Brunner is the laminar flow model. When a liquid flows along a solid surface, the velocity close to the surface is low owing to friction. The velocity profile over the solid surface in Fig. 4.9 indicates that the velocity becomes lower as the distance from the surface is reduced and is equal to zero at the solid surface. The layer of the stream which is in contact with the solid surface and in which the velocity of the liquid is lower than the velocity in the main stream, v_b, constitutes the *hydrodynamic boundary layer*. The width of this layer is defined as the distance between the solid surface and the point where the velocity of the liquid approaches 90% of the velocity of the main stream. Under conditions of laminar flow, the width of the hydrodynamic layer increases proportionally to the square root of the distance from the leading edge of the solid (point E in Fig. 4.9). In the hydrodynamic layer the liquid moves in two directions: vertically (at a velocity v_y) and parallel (at a velocity v_x) to the solid surface with the magnitude of v_x constantly increasing as the distance from the solid† increases.

† Levich, one of the major contributors in the revision of the diffusion boundary layer model, proved that the width of the hydrodynamic layer, h_h, can be calculated from the following equation: $h_h = 5.2(x\eta_k/v_b)^{1/2}$, where x is the distance along the surface and η_k is the kinematic viscosity in units of $[\text{length}]^2/[\text{time}]$ (recall that: $\eta_k = \eta/\rho$, where η is the viscosity and ρ is the density of the solution).

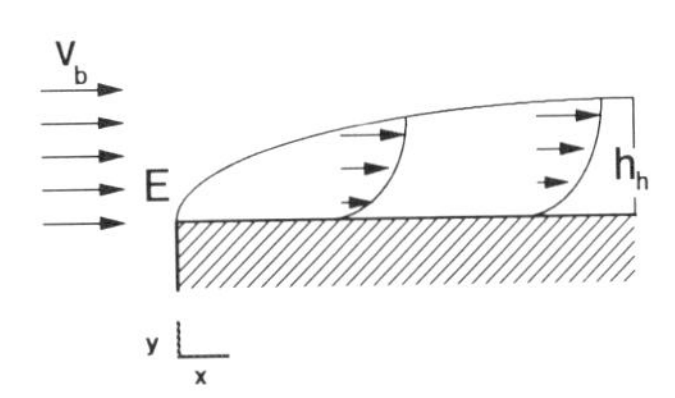

Fig. 4.9. The hydrodynamic boundary layer along an even surface of infinite length under laminar flow conditions; v_b is the velocity of the main stream, h_h is the width of the hydrodynamic layer, while y and x denote the coordinates (vertically and parallel to the surface of the solid).

Based on these hydrodynamic considerations the principle of the *effective diffusion boundary layer* was formulated in the 1960s and 1970s. This principle emphasizes that even under moderate conditions of stirring the transfer of the solid to the solution is controlled by a combination of liquid flow and diffusion. Using the Levich treatment, the width of the effective diffusion boundary layer can be calculated from a knowledge of the hydrodynamic conditions,‡ independent of dissolution data. In this way, a modified version of the diffusion layer model was completed and the relevant theory accompanying Levich's model is called today the *convection–diffusion theory.*

The mathematical expression of the dissolution rate on the basis of the convection–diffusion theory requires, among others, the explicit definition of hydrodynamic conditions prevailing during the experiment. An example of the use of such an equation is given in section 4.4, along with the *in vitro* methods of dissolution testing and in particular for the rotating disk apparatus. This device, although not standard (it is not included in pharmacopoeias), is often used in research because the hydrodynamic conditions can be completely defined, and for this reason it is useful for investigating the kinetics of dissolution of solids under conditions of constant surface area.

In summary, the main differences between the Nernst and Brunner model and the modifications of Levich are:

(1) In the classic diffusion layer model, the layer surrounding the solid, through which the dissolved drug diffuses, is assumed to be static. This assumption leads to a simple mathematical description of the process. However, it is not an accurate representation of the fluid physics near the solid surface.
(2) The effective diffusion boundary layer model assumes that both convection and diffusion contribute to transfer of drug from the solid surface into the bulk solution. The boundary layer thickness can only be calculated accurately if the hydrodynamics are well defined.

Interfacial barrier model

The interfacial barrier model is diagrammatically represented in Fig. 4.7B. It was developed initially by Wilderman at the beginning of the century and was refined by

‡ In 1962, the following equation relating the width of the effective diffusion layer, h, with the width of the hydrodynamic layer, h_h, was proposed by Levich: $h = 0.6h_h(D/\eta_k)^{1/3}$. To obtain this equation Levich assumed that the liquid flows on a surface of 'infinite length'.

Sdanovski and Higuchi after the Second World War. In this case, transfer of the molecules from the solid to the adjoining liquid phase is considered to take place slowly, because of a high activation energy for the transfer. As with the Nernst–Brunner model, there is a stagnant layer through which the drug subsequently diffuses, but in this case the diffusion is relatively rapid. Thus, the rate-limiting step of the total process of transport of the dissolving solid is the initial transfer of drug from the solid phase to the solution. For this model no satisfactory equation has been proposed. The equation proposed by Higuchi simply denotes (as the classic Noyes–Whitney equation does) that dissolution is a first-order process:

$$J_{\mathrm{d}} = \frac{\mathrm{d}m/\mathrm{d}t}{A} = k_{\mathrm{I}}(C_{\mathrm{s}} - C) \tag{4.4}$$

where k_{I} is the *intrinsic dissolution rate constant* based on the interfacial barrier model. A generalized constant, k_{I} is used because of the lack of ability to express the energy of activation in kinetic terms.

Combinations of the basic dissolution models

In certain cases, the inability of any one of the models discussed above to describe the dissolution process of a solid adequately has led to the use of combinations of these models. For example, the dissolution rate of prednisolone has been proved to be better modelled with the following equation:

$$J_{\mathrm{d}} = \frac{D(C_{\mathrm{s}} - C)}{h_{\mathrm{N}}\left[1 + \dfrac{D}{h_{\mathrm{N}} k_{\mathrm{I}}}\right]} \tag{4.5}$$

Equation (4.5) is the mathematical expression of the *double barrier model*, which is a combination of the interfacial barrier and diffusion layer models. It is interesting to note that equation (4.5) collapses to equation (4.3) when $k_{\mathrm{I}} \gg D/h_{\mathrm{N}}$, and to equation (4.4) when $k_{\mathrm{I}} \ll D/h_{\mathrm{N}}$.

4.2.2.2 Equations used in the study of dissolution

From the equations expressing the basic dissolution models it can be concluded that for a nondisintegrating solid, which does not react with the dissolution medium (e.g. by ionization, micellar uptake or enzyme reaction), the dissolution rate per unit surface area is proportional to the concentration difference $(C_{\mathrm{s}} - C)$, with the dissolution rate constant dependent on the model considered. Based on equations (4.2), (4.3) and (4.4), the following equations can be written for the two models:

Diffusion layer model

$$\frac{\mathrm{d}C}{\mathrm{d}t} = \frac{k_{\mathrm{N}} A}{V}(C_{\mathrm{s}} - C) \tag{4.6}$$

Interfacial barrier model

$$\frac{dC}{dt} = \frac{k_I A}{V}(C_s - C) \tag{4.7}$$

These equations are widely used in *in vitro* dissolution studies, where the dissolution medium has a constant volume. If the parameters A and V can be considered constant, then a generalized constant, k_d, can be used to generalize equations (4.6) and (4.7):

$$\frac{dC}{dt} = k_d(C_s - C) \tag{4.8}$$

where k_d is a generalized first order constant, called the *dissolution rate constant*, which is expressed in units of $[\text{time}]^{-1}$ and is equal to

$$k_d = k_i \frac{A}{V} \tag{4.9}$$

where k_i is the *intrinsic dissolution rate constant*, which is equivalent to k_N or k_I, depending on the model applied, and has units of $[\text{length}][\text{time}]^{-1}$.

Equation (4.8) can be rearranged as follows:

$$\frac{dC}{(C_s - C)} = k_d dt$$

and then integrated between $t = 0$, $C = 0$ and $t = t$, $C = C$ to yield

$$-\int_0^C \frac{(C_s - C)'}{(C_s - C)} dC = k_d \int_0^t dt$$

and

$$[-\ln(C_s - C)]_0^C = k_d[t]_0^t$$

Therefore

$$\ln(C_s - C) = \ln C_s - k_d t \tag{4.10}$$

The semi-logarithmic plot of equation (4.10) gives a straight line with a slope equal to $-k_d$, as shown in Fig. 4.10A. When the solution reaches 50% saturation, i.e. $C = C_s/2$, equation (4.10) yields

$$\ln\left(C_s - \frac{C_s}{2}\right) = \ln C_s - k_d t_{1/2}$$

and therefore

$$k_d = \frac{\ln 2}{t_{1/2}} \tag{4.11}$$

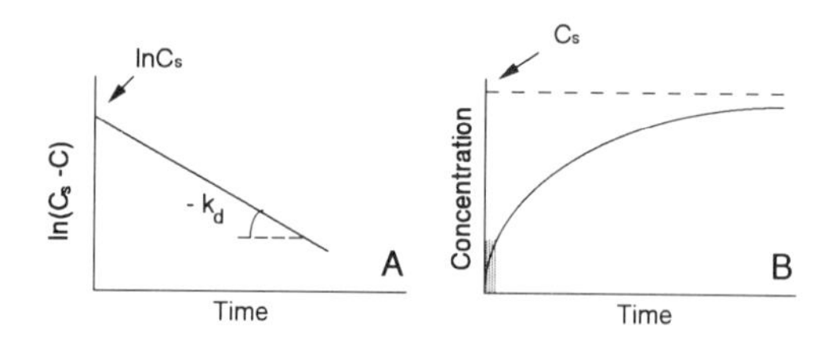

Fig. 4.10. (A) Plot of equation (4.10). (B) Concentration of the dissolved compound versus time, according to equation (4.12). The shaded part of plot B is explained in the text.

where $t_{1/2}$ is the half-life time for the dissolution process. Equation (4.10) can also be written in an exponential form:

$$C = C_s\left(1 - e^{-k_d t}\right) \tag{4.12}$$

As shown in Fig. 4.10B, the concentration of drug in the dissolution medium approaches the solubility in an asymptotic manner.

The reader is reminded that these equations are useful only when the surface area is maintained constant, since k_d is only constant when A is constant (equation (4.9)). In practice, the surface area can be considered constant only when $A_t = A_0$, i.e.

(a) in the initial stages of dissolution;
(b) when a large excess of solid is used; or
(c) when the *in vitro* test conditions meet this requirement (e.g. rotating disk apparatus, section 4.4).

Example 4.1: In a dissolution study using 100 mg of a drug and 1 litre of HCl 0.1 N, the following equation was found to describe the concentration (in μg/ml) of a drug in the dissolution medium as a function of time (in hours):

$$C = 10\left(1 - e^{-0.20t}\right)$$

Assuming that the experiment was carried out under conditions of constant surface area, calculate the amount of the drug which remains undissolved when the study is complete.

Answer: Comparing the equation given with equation (4.12), $C_s = 10\ \mu$g/ml. As the volume of the dissolution medium is 1000 ml, the amount of the drug which will be dissolved at the end of the experiment will be

$$10\ \mu\text{g/ml} \times 1000\ \text{ml} = 10^4\ \mu\text{g} = 10\ \text{mg}$$

Therefore the undissolved quantity will be

$$100 - 10 = 90\ \text{mg}$$

Example 4.2: For a quantity, m, of a drug which consists of spherical particles all having the same radius, r_0:

(a) demonstrate that during dissolution the decrease of the volume of solid drug is not equal to the decrease of its surface area; and
(b) calculate the decrease in the surface area corresponding to 50% dissolution.

Answer: (a) The initial total volume, V_0, of the N particles of the same size is

$$V_0 = N(4/3)\pi r_0^3$$

After time t, the volume of the particles will be

$$V_t = N(4/3)\pi r_t^3$$

The relative change of the volume is therefore

$$1 - V_t/V_0 = 1 - (r/r_0)^3$$

Applying the same methodology for the relative change of the surface area, we have

$$1 - A_t/A_0 = 1 - N(4\pi r_t^2)/N(4\pi r_0^2) = 1 - (r_t/r_0)^2$$

Combining the last two equations

$$1 - V_t/V_0 = 1 - \left[(r_t/r_0)^2 (r_t/r_0)\right] = 1 - \left[(A_t/A_0)(r_t/r_0)\right] = 1 - \left[(A_t/A_0)(V_t/V_0)^{1/3}\right]$$

or

$$(A_t/A_0) = (V_t/V_0)^{2/3}$$

The decrease in volume is accompanied by a smaller decrease in surface area. As dissolution proceeds the remaining surface area available for dissolution is relatively larger than the remaining relative volume.

(b) Since mass is proportional to volume ($m = \rho V$, where ρ is the density of the solid), changes in mass correspond to changes in volume. Consequently

$$(A_t/A_0) = (0.50\, V_0/V_0)^{2/3} = 0.63$$

Therefore, when the mass of drug is decreased by 100–50 = 50%, the decrease in surface area of the solid will be (100–63)% = 37%.

Sink conditions

A convenient simplification of equation (4.8) can be applied in two cases:

(1) in the initial stages of dissolution; and/or
(2) if the drug in solution is continuously removed from the dissolution medium.

In these two cases, the concentration of drug, C, is much smaller than the solubility, i.e. $C \ll C_s$. Under these conditions we say that *sink conditions*† prevail and equation (4.8) can be approximated by the following:

$$\frac{dC}{dt} = k_d C_s$$

which after integration gives

$$C = k_d C_s t \tag{4.13}$$

Equation (4.13) reveals that in this case the concentration of the dissolved drug increases as a linear function of time. The approximately linear character of the dissolution profile at the initial stages of dissolution in Fig. 4.10B (shaded area) demonstrates case (1) above. As a rule of thumb, sink conditions are considered to prevail when the concentration of the drug does not exceed 20% of the solubility, i.e. when $C \leqslant 0.2C_s$.

It is important to emphasize that when the GI epithelium is permeable to the drug, the concentration of drug in the GI fluids is kept negligible in comparison to its solubility. In this case, sink conditions for dissolution are approximated. Some *in vitro* devices have been designed to maintain low drug relative concentrations during the dissolution experiment, to mimic the expected *in vivo* conditions. The reader should note, however, that the use of equation (4.13) requires a constant surface area throughout the dissolution experiment as well low drug relative concentrations in the bulk solution. Although maintenance of a constant surface area can be achieved *in vitro*, it is unlikely under *in vivo* conditions.

Example 4.3‡: A dissolution experiment is carried out in 1 litre of a buffer solution using 30 g of a drug. The solubility of the drug in the buffer is 10 mg/ml, and its surface area of 1 m^2/g is maintained constant during the experiment. It was found experimentally that 10 min after the beginning of the experiment 0.90 g of the drug were dissolved. Calculate:

(a) whether sink conditions prevail at 10 min;
(b) the intrinsic dissolution rate constant;
(c) at what time the assumption of sink conditions is no longer valid; and
(d) the concentration of the drug after 1 h.

Answer: (a) Since $C_s = 10$ mg/ml, sink conditions prevail as long as the drug concentration is less than $0.20 \times 10 = 2.0$ mg/ml = 2.0 g/l. Therefore, sink conditions prevailed at 10 min, when the drug concentration was 0.90 g/l.

(b) The generalized dissolution rate constant is related to the intrinsic dissolution rate constant by equation (4.9), which in combination with equation (4.13) yields

† Although this concept is presented and explained in this book in the context of dissolution, it must be noted that such conditions exist in every first order process. Depending on the process, the appropriate term for the concentration difference varies, e.g. $(C_s - C)$ for dissolution, and $(C_g - C_b)$ for uptake by the GI mucosa, where C_g is the concentration in the GI fluids and C_b is the concentration in blood.

‡ This is a modified version of an example taken from the book by J. Carstensen, *Pharmaceutics of Solids and Solid Dosage Forms*, p. 64, Wiley, New York (1977).

$$k_i = (CV)/(AC_s t)$$

Based on the above equation

$$k_i = \frac{0.9 \times 10^3}{30 \times 10^4 \times 10 \times 10} \frac{(g/l)\ (ml)}{cm^2 (g/l)\ min} = 3 \times 10^{-5}\ cm/min$$

(c) The relationship of concentration and time during sink conditions is linear (equation (4.13):

$$C = \frac{C}{C_s k_d} = \frac{0.2V}{k_i A} = \frac{0.2 \times 1000}{3 \times 10^{-5} \times 30 \times 10^4} \frac{ml}{cm/min \times cm^2} = 22\ min.$$

(d) At time $t = 60$ min sink conditions do not prevail; the general equation (4.12) can be used to describe the process. Therefore

$$C = C_s\left(1 - e^{-k_d t}\right) = C_s\left(1 - e^{-k_i At/V}\right)$$
$$= 10\left[1 - \exp(-3 \times 10^{-5} \times 30 \times 10^4 \times 60/10^3)\right]$$
$$= 4.2\ mg/ml$$

4.2.2.3 Factors affecting the dissolution rate

The equations most commonly used to describe the dissolution rate are equations (4.6) and (4.7). These equations indicate that the change in concentration of the dissolved drug is (1) inversely proportional to the volume of the dissolution medium and (2) proportional to the intrinsic dissolution rate constant, the surface area and the difference $(C_s - C)$. Consequently, any change of one or more of these variables or parameters will affect the rate of dissolution.

Volume of the dissolution medium

Although an increase in the volume of the dissolution medium results in a lower rate of increase of drug concentration in the luminal fluid, the rate of mass transfer is unaffected as long as there is sufficient fluid to maintain sink conditions for dissolution. This will depend on whether the volume of liquid available exceeds the dose administered divided by the drug's solubility, the so-called dose : solubility ratio. The volume of the liquids of the upper GI tract stays within fairly narrow limits. In the fasted state this volume is approximately 250 ml, to which an extra 50–300 ml can be added to account for fluid administered with the dosage form. In the fed state, ingested fluid and GI secretions (gastric, bile and pancreatic fluids) combine to provide a higher volume available for dissolution. Due to extensive water reabsorption in the small intestine, this volume increase is most important in the proximal GI tract.

Intrinsic dissolution rate constant

The potential to influence the intrinsic dissolution rate constant is limited, especially under *in vivo* conditions. In the case of the diffusion layer model, k_N depends on the width of the diffusion layer, which is influenced by the hydrodynamics in the GI tract, the particle size of the drug and the drug's diffusion coefficient. Of these only the particle size can be easily manipulated. For the interfacial barrier model, the overall rate of transfer is determined by the energetics of the interfacial barrier, which may again prove difficult to alter.

In *in vitro* experiments, the rate of dissolution can be affected by the stirring rate, since the width of the diffusion layer of a given particle is a function of the hydrodynamic conditions. The following empirical equation, which relates the intrinsic dissolution rate constant, k_i, to the stirring rate, N, is frequently used:

$$k_i = a(N)^b$$

where a and b are constants. The values of b depend on the model considered. For the interfacial barrier model where dissolution is not diffusion rate limited, $b = 0$ and therefore k_i is not dependent on the stirring conditions, since $k_i = a$. For the diffusion layer model $b = 1$ and therefore $k_i = aN$; thus, in diffusion-controlled processes k_i is proportional to the stirring rate. A lesser dependence of k_i on the agitation rate, N, is observed when the process is described by a combination of the two models (equation (4.5)). If the value of b lies between zero and unity, a combination model should be considered. Under *in vivo* conditions, however, hydrodynamic conditions are controlled by GI motility, and have not been well characterized.

The effect of various factors on the value of the diffusion coefficient can be explored by considering the Stokes–Einstein equation, derived for an approximately spherical molecule:

$$D = (RT)/(6N\pi\eta r)$$

where R is the universal gas constant, T is the absolute temperature, N is Avogadro's constant, η is the viscosity and r is the radius of the molecule in solution. Since the dissolution rate is proportional to the diffusion coefficient, the Stokes–Einstein equation reveals that the rate of dissolution is inversely proportional to the viscosity of the liquid medium but proportional to temperature. It is very likely that the viscosity *in vivo* is higher than in typical *in vitro* test solutions, owing to the presence of the mucus, which covers the interior of the GI tract (section 5.2) and exogenous substances. Under *in vivo* conditions, the effect of temperature on the diffusion coefficient is negligible because body temperature is constant.

Surface area of the solid

For a given quantity of a solid, the surface area is inversely proportional to the particle size. Increasing the surface area by reducing the size of the solid particles is the most common way of increasing the dissolution rate. Data from the literature are particularly impressive for slightly soluble drugs. For example, a two-fold increase in the bioavailability of digoxin was observed when the mean radius of the particles was decreased from 100 μm to approximately 10 μm. The following example quantitatively illustrates the effect of reducing the particle size of a drug on its surface area.

Example 4.4: A sample of 3.000 g of a drug with density $\rho = 1.376$ g/ml consists of elongated crystals, which have approximately cylindrical shape with radius, $r = 2.00\ \mu$m and length, $l = 5.00\ \mu$m.

(a) Calculate the total surface area.
(b) Assuming that each crystal is cut in two pieces in the middle, calculate the new total surface area and the percentage increase in the surface area as a result of size reduction.

Answer: (a) The total volume of the sample is

$$\text{volume} = \text{mass/density} = 3.000/1.376 = 2.180 \text{ ml}$$

The volume of each crystal is

$$\pi r^2 l = 3.14 \times 4.00 \times 5.00 = 62.8\ \mu\text{m}^3 = 62.8(10^{-4}\ \text{cm})^3 = 0.628 \times 10^{-10}\ \text{cm}^3$$

Therefore, the number of crystals in the sample is

$$2.180/(0.628 \times 10^{-10}) = 3.47 \times 10^{10}$$

Each crystal has a surface area of

$$2\pi r^2 + 2\pi rl = 2 \times 3.14 \times 4.00 + 2 \times 3.14 \times 2.00 \times 5.00 = 87.9\ \mu\text{m}^2$$

Therefore, the total surface area will be

$$\begin{aligned}&(\text{number of crystals}) \times (\text{surface area of each crystal})\\ &= 3.47 \times 10^{10} \times 87.9 = 3.05 \times 10^{12}\ \mu\text{m}^2\\ &= 3.05 \times 10^{12}(10^{-4}\ \text{cm})^2 = 3.05 \times 10^4\ \text{cm}^2\end{aligned}$$

(b) The surface area of each of the crystals after size reduction is

$$2\left(\pi r^2/2\right) + (2r)l + \left(2\pi rl/2\right) = 2 \times 6.28 + 4.00 \times 5.00 + 62.8/2 = 64.0\ \mu\text{m}^2$$

As the number of crystals has doubled, the total surface area is

$$2 \times (3.47 \times 10^{10}) \times 64.0 = 444 \times 10^{10}\ \mu\text{m}^2 = 4.44 \times 10^4\ \text{cm}^2$$

Thus, the percentage of increase of the surface area is

$$\left[\left(4.44 \times 10^4 - 3.05 \times 10^4\right)/\left(3.05 \times 10^4\right)\right] \times 100 = 45.6\%$$

Many drugs exhibit increased dissolution rate when the size of the particles is decreased, e.g. griseofulvin, chloramphenicol, certain sulfonamides, spironolactone, tetracycline. However, reduction of particle size is not a guarantee for improvement of the dissolution rate and subsequent bioavailability of drug. Several problems associated with small crystal sizes have been reported in the literature. The two following examples concerning phenacetin and nitrofurantoin are illustrative.

(a) When *in vitro* dissolution experiments were carried out on granules containing the slightly water-soluble analgesic phenacetin and the hydrophilic diluent gelatin, the phenacetin dissolution rate increased as the size of the drug particles was decreased. By contrast, when the dissolution of plain thin crystals of phenacetin was studied in the same medium, the dissolution rate increased as the size of the drug crystals increased. The situation returned to the expected behaviour when the surfactant Tween 80 was added to the dissolution medium. The effects of the particle size and Tween 80 addition on the *in vitro* dissolution rate of phenacetin were confirmed with *in vivo* studies. The anomalous behaviour of the untreated drug crystal was attributed to better wetting of large compared to small crystals. The small crystals were observed to float on aqueous medium and therefore offer less available surface area in contact with the liquid. Hydrophobic powders with small particle sizes have a general tendency to form aggregates which float on the surface of the aqueous solutions. The lack of wetting is caused by the entrapment of air in the pores of the aggregates. Addition of surfactants such as Tween 80 help to expel air from the pores, and replace it with liquid. From the experiments described above, it is clear that the determining factor for the dissolution rate is the *effective* surface area and not the *total* surface area of the solid. The term *effective*† refers to the portion of the total surface which is in actual contact with the dissolution medium.

(b) When nitrofurantoin (an antimicrobial agent used for urinary tract infections, slightly soluble in water) is administered as small particles having a mean radius of about 10 μm, nausea, vomiting and headache symptoms are frequently encountered. The undesired effects are thought to be due to irritation of the GI mucosa by high local concentrations of the drug. Whatever the mechanism(s) involved, the frequency of the undesired effects have been linked to the rapid dissolution rate. Administration of larger-sized particles (macrocrystals with a mean radius 0.4–0.6 mm) results in a decrease in the overall fraction of the dose absorbed, but at the same time eliminates the undesired effects in 80% of subjects.

The concentration difference ($C_s - C$)

The concentration difference ($C_s - C$) can be controlled either by modifying the solubility, C_s, or by maintaining the concentration, C, of the drug in the dissolution medium, at very low levels. Up to this point, the term solubility was used to describe the concentration of drug in a saturated aqueous solution in which the drug is not ionized or otherwise reacted. However, when a component of the liquid medium reacts with the drug, the total solubility, $C_{s,T}$, equals the solubility plus the drug (expressed in terms of concentration) which has reacted.

The solubility is affected by the temperature and drug's crystal structure.‡ The ability of a drug to crystallize in several forms, which are eventually converted with time to the most stable form, is called *polymorphism*. When this conversion is rather slow, the

† Increase of the effective surface area is usually performed by reducing the size of the particles or by dispersing the drug in an inactive hydrophilic carrier (solid dispersion). The latter method, a popular approach in solid dosage form development, is applied to enhance the dissolution of slightly soluble drugs due to rapid wetting of the carrier. An example is the dispersion of sulfathiozole in urea.

‡ It has been shown that the solubility can be increased by drastic reduction of the size of the particles (to sizes much smaller than 0.1 μm). Such small-sized particles can be achieved by certain methods, e.g. solid dispersion. However, sizes of the solid particles encountered in pharmaceutics normally range between 5 and 500 μm. Accordingly, the solubility is considered here as a thermodynamic property, and therefore independent from the size of the particles.

unstable forms are called *metastable*. In some cases, the preparation of new metastable forms is possible using methods like recrystallization from various solvents, melting and appropriate freezing rate, etc. The metastable polymorphs differ, among other ways, in stability and solubility. However, the amorphous powder of a drug (which has little or no crystal arrangement) is always more soluble than any crystal structure. For many drugs, the use of a certain metastable crystalline form or the amorphous powder is used to improve drug absorption. Examples include chloramphenicol, sulfathiazole, novobiocine, methylprednisolone, hydrocortisone and prednisolone.

The total solubility can be affected by the pH of the solution, salt formation, and presence of solubilizing agents.

(a) pH: Many drugs are weak electrolytes and ionize according to the pH of the dissolution medium. Changes in the pH of the bulk solution can affect the total solubility of the drug, as a result of the change in extent of ionization. Changes in total solubility with pH are particularly important given the wide range of pH values in the GI fluids. The ionization constant, K_a, of a drug which is a weak acid, HA, is given by the following equation:

$$K_a = (H^+)(A^-)/(HA) \tag{4.14}$$

The total solubility, $C_{s,T}$, will be the sum of the concentrations of the two forms of the drug: the non-ionized acid, HA, and the ionized form, A^-. Therefore

$$C_{s,T} = (HA) + (A^-) = C_s + (A^-) \tag{4.15}$$

Combination of the last equation with equation (4.14), gives

$$C_{s,T} = C_s\left(1 + \frac{K_a}{[H^+]}\right) \tag{4.16}$$

Based on the definition of pH and pK_a, the previous equation can also be written as

$$C_{s,T} = C_s\left(1 + 10^{pH - pK_a}\right) \tag{4.17}$$

The corresponding equation for a weak base is

$$C_{s,T} = C_s\left(1 + 10^{pK_a - pH}\right) \tag{4.18}$$

Equations (4.17) and (4.18) reveal that the total solubility of a weak acid increases with the pH of the bulk solution, while the total solubility of a weak base increases with decreasing pH. Considering equations (4.6) and (4.7) in accordance with equations (4.17) or (4.18), one sees that changes in the ionization are directly reflected in the dissolution rate. These effects have been affirmed both *in vitro* and in clinical studies. To predict *in vivo* effects from *in vitro* experiments, care must be taken to simulate the conditions in the GI tract. The fluid in the stomach consists mostly of hydrogen, sodium and chloride ions, with a pH of about pH 1–2 in the secreted juice. This fluid has a poor buffer capacity, and may be significantly diluted by water ingested with the dosage form. By contrast the fluid in the small intestine has a pH of about pH 6 and has a much higher buffer capacity due to the presence of bicarbonate. Dissolution tests run in water *in vitro* may not predict *in vivo* dissolution of ionizable drugs in the small intestine very well. This is especially likely if the drug has a low pK_a (in the case of a weak acid) and is at least sparingly soluble, because under these conditions dissolution of the drug at the surface buffers the boundary layer pH to a value near the drug's pK_a, considerably below the pH of the water in the bulk medium. The USP-simulated intestinal fluid test solution, while having a pH higher than usual intestinal pH, at least provides enough buffer strength to overcome pH effects induced locally in the boundary layer by the dissolving drug.

(b) Salt formation: the total solubilities of a drug and its salt form, in distilled water, may also differ. For example, if a weak acid drug is dissolved in distilled water, the final pH of the bulk solution will be lower than the pH which would result if a sodium salt of the acid was used.† Strictly speaking, salts do not provide higher solubility than the corresponding acids or bases at a given pH. However, because of the buffering capacity of the ionized form of the drug in the salt, the pH in the bulk solution will be affected (higher in the case of a sodium salt of a weak acid). Although under *in vivo* conditions, the amount of the administered drug is insufficient to regulate the pH of the GI contents,‡ many *in vivo* studies have demonstrated that the sodium or potassium salts of weak acids are absorbed more rapidly than the corresponding acids (e.g. salicylate, barbiturate, sulfonamide and penicillin salts). These results can be explained by the higher pH in the microenvironment of the solid particles during the dissolution of the salt in the stomach compared to the pH of the bulk solution. In addition, even if the non-ionized acid does precipitate in the stomach when the salt form is administered, the precipitate is likely to consist of the fine particles which can readily redissolve, as shown in Fig. 4.11.

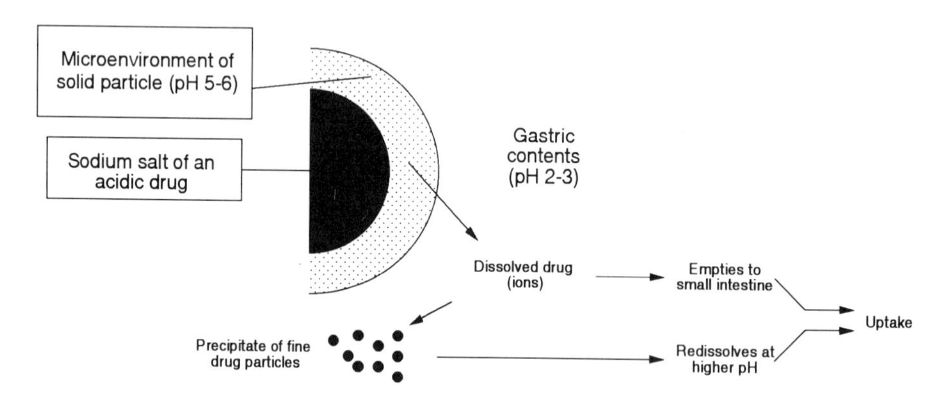

Fig. 4.11. Representation of the dissolution process of the sodium salt of a weak acid in the stomach.

† When a weak acid is dissolved in distilled water, the pH of the resulting solution can be roughly calculated by the equation, $pH = (pK_a - \log C)/2$, where C is the total concentration of the acid in the solution. Likewise the pH of a solution of a salt of an acid with a strong base can be roughly calculated from the equation, $pH = (pK_a + pK_w + \log C)/2$, where K_w is the ionization constant of water. The derivation of these equations are provided in the literature listed at the end of the chapter.

‡ This can be inferred by comparing the doses required for antacids to be effective, with usual doses of drugs.

(c) Solubilization: The term solubilization refers generally to the interaction of the drug with a compound or ion coexisting in solution. Different types of solubilization can take place, such as partitioning of the drug into the micelles of a surfactant, complexation of the drug with one or more substances or ions, or inclusion of the drug in the interior of another compound.

Solubilization of a drug in the micelles of a surfactant can significantly increase the total drug solubility. The oral administration of many surfactants in a quantity capable of exceeding the *critical micellar concentration* (CMC) would raise questions with respect to safety. However, there are physiological compounds in the small intestine with surfactant properties. The most important of these are the bile acids (Fig. 4.12), which are secreted by the gallbladder in large quantities during digestion (section 5.2). It is important to note that the concentrations of bile acids in the duodenum and the jejunum are higher than the CMC and that concentrations are higher during digestion than in the fasting state. Bile solubilization is thought to be at least partly responsible for increases in bioavailability that are often observed when extremely insoluble drugs are administered concurrently with food.

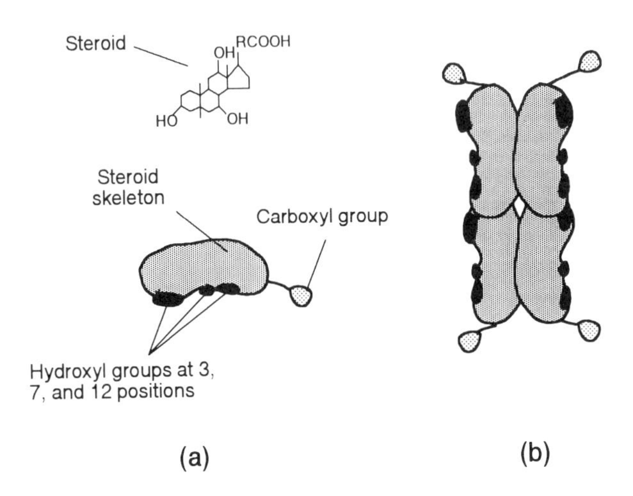

Fig. 4.12. (a) Bile acid structure and conformation. (b) Micelle of a bile acid.

The complexation of a drug can result in an increase of its total solubility†. Typical examples are the complexes of various drugs with caffeine. It must be noted that relatively high amounts of complexing agent are required to effect a significant increase in the total solubility of drug. However, with respect to the dissolution rate, the presence of small amounts of the complexing agent in the microenvironment of the drug's solid particles may result in dissolution rate enhancement. This has been explored *in vitro* using urea to enhance chloramphenicol dissolution. The solubility of the drug in water at

† Note that although an increase in solubility leads to a proportional increase of dissolution rate, this does not necessarily increase the uptake rate from the GI epithelium. Drug present in a large drug/solubilizing agent complex may be absorbed at slower rates and to a smaller extent than the uncomplexed drug.

37°C is doubled in the presence of 15% (w/w) urea. As would be predicted from equations (4.6) and (4.7), dissolution studies with physical chloramphenicol–urea mixtures at a 26:74 ratio show a parallel two-fold increase of the dissolution rate. Dissolution studies with solid dispersion formulations of chloramphenicol in urea, however, revealed a four-fold increase in the dissolution rate of chloramphenicol. This result is due to the formation of a *solid solution* and illustrates the importance of particle size (here drug particles versus molecular dispersion) as well as solubility, on the dissolution rate.

Finally, solubilization of the drug can be the result of its inclusion in the interior of another molecule in solution, e.g. cyclodextrins (Fig. 4.13). Cyclodextrins are products of the fermental decomposition of starch, and consist of six to eight glucose units connected by α-(1→4) glucosidic bonds. Depending on the number of their glucose molecules (six, seven or eight, they are called α-, β- or γ-cyclodextrins, respectively. Their toroidal shape permits the inclusion of non-polar molecules in their cavity. Hydrophobic interactions and van der Waals' forces stabilize the inclusion compound formed. The interaction results in an increase in the total solubility of the drug since both the free drug and inclusion compound contribute to the overall solubility. Cyclodextrins neither destroy nor penetrate to a significant degree the GI epithelium. For these reasons, it is believed that they would be useful for increasing the total solubility of drugs given orally. Increases in total solubility have been demonstrated for drugs such as digoxin, indomethacin, prostaglandins, naproxen, etc., and extensive studies are currently being performed to assess the use of hydroxypropyl-β-cyclodextrin (a semi-synthetic water-soluble analogue) as a solubility enhancer for oral and i.v. administration.

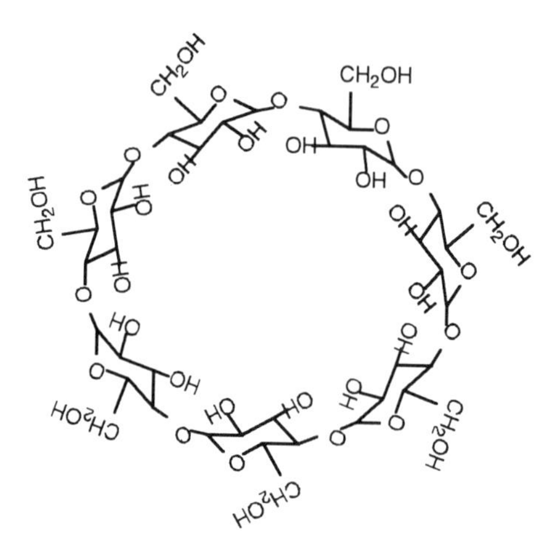

Fig. 4.13. Structure of β-cyclodextrin.

The concentration of free drug in the bulk solution can be maintained at low levels, provided that a process contributing to the 'removal' of free drug from the dissolution medium is operating. Such processes include partitioning into micelles and uptake across the GI mucosa. Another mechanism of decreasing the concentration of the drug in solution is the *adsorption* of the dissolved molecules on a solid material. Generally, the term 'adsorption' characterizes the process where molecules of a liquid (in our case: molecules of the dissolved drug) or a gas are deposited on the surface of a solid material (e.g. cholestyramine), and are bound by van der Waals' forces. Any increase in dissolution rate as a result of the adsorption of the dissolved drug on a solid material is unlikely to lead to increased (faster and/or more complete) absorption of the drug—quite the opposite. Activated charcoal, one of the most common adsorption agents, is used as a general antidote in cases of oral poisoning, exactly because it adsorbs the dissolved drug, preventing the uptake of the drug by the GI epithelium.

4.2.2.4 *Methods for describing the kinetics of dissolution of drugs administered orally in solid immediate-release formulations*

To develop a mathematical model for the dissolution of a drug from an immediate release dosage form, several characteristics of the formulation must be known, and some assumptions applied. These include:

— an estimate of the initial surface area of drug available for dissolution;
— the solubility of the drug in the medium in which dissolution occurs;
— the mechanism by which dissolution occurs;
— no change in particle shape occurs during dissolution; and
— the solubility does not vary with particle size.

To develop equations describing dissolution (see section 4.2.2.2), dissolution was assumed to occur from a non-disintegrating particle having a well-defined surface area. In practice, drug dissolution usually occurs from particles or granules whose surface area changes with time.

Dissolution of drug from suspensions and hard gelatin capsules

Here, dissolution occurs from drug particles with a range of surface areas.† The variability in surface area among particles can be taken into account by defining the initial particle size distribution for the system. This enables an estimation of the initial dissolution rate to be made. As small particles dissolve, there is a decrease in the number of particles, and the particle size distribution changes. Thus, polydispersity makes it more difficult to model the overall dissolution process.

Particle size distributions are usually skewed to the left with a right tail and only in exceptional cases is particle size normally distributed. In biopharmaceutics particle size distributions are often assumed to be log-normal, because manufacturing processes such as milling, precipitation and grinding usually produce size distributions which fit this functional form. For a log-normal distribution, if the particles are divided into i size groups ($i = 1, 2 \ldots$) and the frequency of the number of particles in each group is plotted versus the mean diameter on a logarithmic scale, a curve close to a normal (Gaussian) distribution will result. The mean diameter of such a distribution can be described according to a number of different definitions, the simplest of which is the arithmetic mean, d_a, as given by the following equation:

† Dissolution of the hard gelatin coating and deaggregation of particles assumed to be complete within a few minutes. If this is not the case, the dissolution process is analogous to that of immediate-release tablets.

$$d_a = \frac{\sum n_i d_i}{\sum n_i} \tag{4.19}$$

where d_i and n_i are the mean diameter and number of particles of the ith group, respectively. If calculation of the surface area or volume is needed, the mean diameter must instead be estimated from the appropriate equations:

Mean surface diameter

$$d_s = \left(\frac{\sum n_i d_i^2}{\sum n_i} \right)^{1/2} \tag{4.20}$$

Mean volume diameter

$$d_v = \left(\frac{\sum n_i d_i^3}{\sum n_i} \right)^{1/3} \tag{4.21}$$

Assuming that dissolution occurs from spherical particles with a monodisperse size distribution under sink conditions, and that the dissolution rate is limited by the route of diffusion across the boundary diffusion layer according to the diffusion layer model, Hixson and Crowell developed the following equation (the so-called cube root law) to describe the dissolution profile of drug from a sample of powder:

$$(W_0)^{1/3} - (W)^{1/3} = (\pi N \rho / 6)^{1/3} \left[(2DC_s)/(h_N \rho) \right] t \tag{4.22}$$

where W_0 and W are the total initial particle weight and the total particle weight at time t after the beginning of the process, respectively, N is the number of particles (which, since the powder is monodisperse, is considered to be constant through the whole process) and ρ is the particle density. According to equation (4.22), the plot of $[(W_0)^{1/3} - (W)^{1/3}]$ versus time will give a straight line with a slope of $(\pi N \rho/6)^{1/3}[(2DC_s)/(h_N \rho)]$. The value of the slope represents the cube root rate constant and can be used to characterize the dissolution process. Modifications of equation (4.22) have been proposed for use in cases where one or more of the assumptions in the Hixson–Crowell treatment do not apply. For example, when sink conditions do not apply, the following equation should be used instead of equation (4.22):

$$(W)^{-2/3} - (W_0)^{-2/3} = (\pi N/6)^{1/3} \left[(4D)/(h_N \rho^{2/3} V) \right] t \tag{4.23}$$

A restriction on using equation (4.23) is that the quantity of solid particles to be dissolved must be large enough that $W_0/V \geqslant C_s$ (where V is the volume of the bulk solution). Analytical derivation of equations (4.22) and (4.23) is beyond the scope of this book, but may be found in references listed at the end of this chapter.

Although the original Hixson–Crowell equation and its derivative forms are widely used in the study of powder dissolution, they have been criticized for the assumption that diffusion layer thickness does not vary with particle size. The diffusion layer thickness appears to depend somewhat on particle size. Thus, it is expected that the cube root rate constant will vary with particle size as well as stirring conditions.

Example 4.5: The following data were collected during an *in vitro* powder dissolution experiment and published in the *Journal of Pharmaceutical Sciences* **52**: 29–33 (1963):

Amount remaining to be dissolved (mg)	*Time (h)*
1830	0
1810	3.8
1790	7.5
1770	11.2
1735	15.0
1710	18.8
1690	22.5
1680	26.2
1655	30.0
1640	33.8
1610	37.5
1595	41.2
1585	45.0

If the particles are considered spherical with similar size and a mean diameter of 40 μm, have a density of 1.3 g/ml, and 1830 mg is the exact amount required to saturate the 750 ml dissolution medium, calculate the intrinsic dissolution rate constant.

Answer: The concentration of drug at the end of the experiment is $(1830 - 1585)/750 = 0.327$ mg/ml. Since the solubility is $1830/750 = 2.44$ mg/ml, and the final concentration is less than $0.20 \times 2.44 = 0.37$ mg/ml, it can be concluded that sink conditions prevail throughout the entire experiment. In addition, since the particles have similar size the cube root law can be applied.

First the data are transformed as follows:

$(W_0)^{1/3} - (W)^{1/3}$	Time (h)
0.043	3.8
0.088	7.5
0.134	11.2
0.214	15.0
0.272	18.8
0.319	22.5
0.342	26.2
0.401	30.0
0.437	33.8
0.510	37.5
0.546	41.2
0.571	45.0

Linear regression analysis based on equation (4.22) gives the following results (Fig. 4.14):

		Level of significance
Intercept (SE):	0.29×10^{-3} (0.98×10^{-2})	$p \gg 0.05$ (NS)
Slope (SE):	1.31×10^{-2} (0.04×10^{-2})	$p < 0.0004$
Correlation coefficient:	0.996	$p < 0.0004$

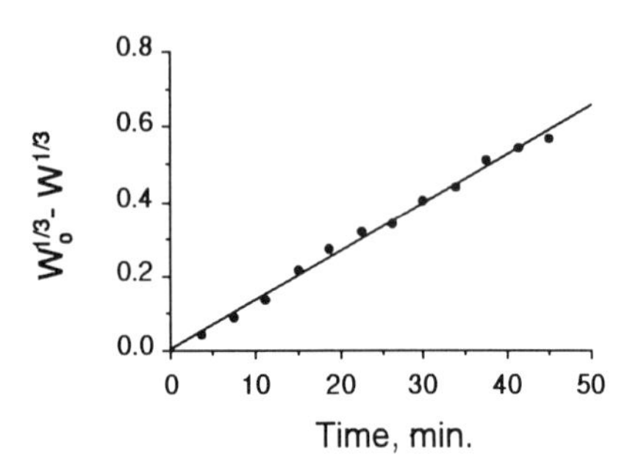

Fig. 4.14. Cube root law plot for the data of Example 4.5.

The weight of each particle is

$$\rho V = \left(1.30\ \text{g/cm}^3\right)\times(4/3)\times3.14\times(20.0\times10^{-4}\ \text{cm})^3 = 4.35\times10^{-5}\ \text{mg}.$$

Therefore the total number of particles is $1830/(4.35\times10^{-5}) = 4.20\times10^{7}$. From the slope of equation (4.22) and regression analysis one obtains

$$\left(\pi N\rho/6\right)^{1/3}\left[(2DC_s)/(h_N\rho)\right] = 1.31\times10^{-2}$$

and, therefore, the intrinsic dissolution rate constant is $k_N = D/h_N = 1.14\times10^{-2}$ cm/min.

Example 4.6: By repeating the experiment of Example 4.5 for a longer period of time, the following data were collected:

Amount remaining to be dissolved (mg)	*Time (h)*
1830	0
1733	15.0
1575	45.0
1440	75.0
1317	105
1224	125
1130	160

(a) Calculate the intrinsic dissolution rate constant from these data.
(b) Calculate the time for 50% and 75% dissolution.

Answer: In this case, after the third sample, sink conditions no longer prevail. Therefore, the equation of the cube root law cannot be used. However, since the amount to be dissolved exceeds $C_s V$, equation (4.23) can be applied.

(a) First the data are transformed as follows:

$\left[(W)^{-2/3} - (W_0)^{-2/3}\right]$, $\times 10^{-3}$	*Time (h)*
0.247	15.0
0.703	45.0
1.16	75.0
1.64	105
2.06	125
2.53	160

Linear regression analysis of data transformed according to equation (4.23) gives the following results (Fig. 4.15):

		Level of significance
Intercept (SE):	$-1.1\times10^{-5}(1.0\times10^{-5})$	$p \gg 0.05$ (NS)
Slope (SE):	$1.6\times10^{-5}(0.02\times10^{-5})$	$p<0.0004$
Correlation coefficient:	0.9991	$p<0.0004$

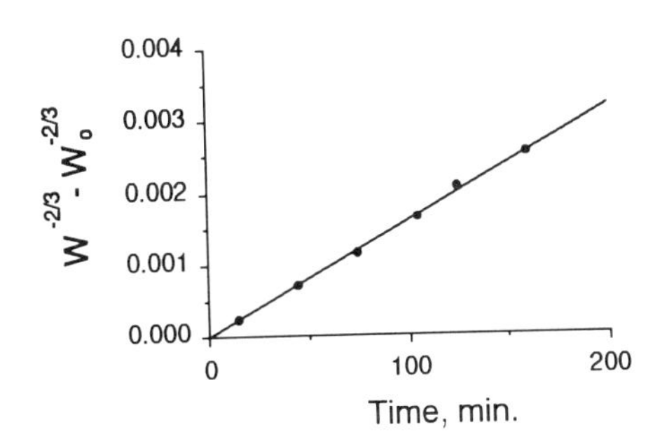

Fig. 4.15. Plot of the two-thirds power law for the data of Example 4.6.

Based on linear regression analysis, the number of particles (estimated in the previous example), and equation (4.23),

$$\left[4D/(h_N V\rho^{2/3})\right](N/6)^{1/3} = 1.6\times10^{-5}.$$

Therefore, the intrinsic dissolution rate is $k_N = D/h_N = 1.24 \times 10^{-3}$ cm/min. The value for k_N is slightly larger than the value calculated in the previous example because of rounding errors in the calculations.

(b) The time for 50% dissolution is the time at which the dissolved amount equals the amount remaining to be dissolved, i.e.

$$(W_0/2)^{-2/3} - (W_0)^{-2/3} = (\pi N/6)^{1/3}\left[(4D)/(h_N \rho^{2/3} V)\right]t$$

Therefore

$$915^{-2/3} - 1830^{-2/3} = (1.6 \times 10^{-5})t \quad \text{and} \quad t = 244 \text{ min}$$

Similarly, the time for 75% dissolution is the time at which the remaining amount to be dissolved equals $W_0/4$, i.e.

$$(W_0/4)^{-2/3} - (W_0)^{-2/3} = (\pi N/6)^{1/3}\left[(4D)/(h_n \rho^{2/3} V)\right]t$$

Therefore

$$458^{-2/3} - 1830^{-2/3} = (1.6 \times 10^{-5})t \quad \text{and} \quad t = 633 \text{ min}$$

It should be noted here that the calculations for both the time for 50% dissolution and 75% dissolution can only be done with equation (4.23). Using equation (4.22) would violate the assumption of sink conditions.

As mentioned earlier, in cases where the particle sizes are distributed in a polydisperse manner, a mathematical description of dissolution becomes much more complicated. Application of either the cube root law or the two-thirds law usually results in a biphasic plot, i.e. two straight lines are needed to fit the data (Fig. 4.16). As an approximation, the whole process is divided into an initial phase, during which dissolution of the smaller particles is completed, and a second phase, during which dissolution of larger particles is completed. The time required for the first phase to be completed is called the critical time. Although a detailed description of the equations which are used for polydisperse particle size distributions will not be given here, it is worth mentioning that calculation of the intrinsic dissolution rate constant requires the use of the geometric mean diameter† and its corresponding standard deviation.

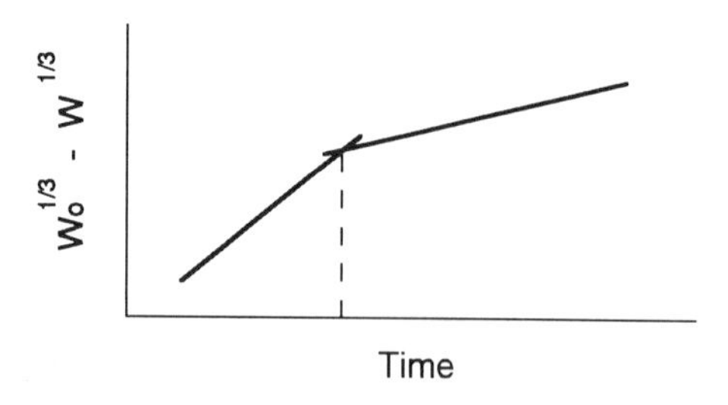

Fig. 4.16. The shape of the cube root plot when the dissolving powder is polydisperse. The two straight lines intersect at the time corresponding to complete dissolution of the smaller particles.

† The geometric mean diameter, d_g, corresponds to the arithmetic mean of a log-normal distribution and is estimated by the equation: $\log d_g = \Sigma(n_i \log d_i)/\Sigma n_i$.

Dissolution from immediate-release tablets

A typical profile of drug concentration in the bulk solution versus time for drug dissolution from an immediate-release tablet is shown in Fig. 4.17. Although the dissolution of solid drug particles is initiated as soon as the tablet is brought into an aqueous medium, dissolution proceeds more rapidly after disintegration is complete (Fig. 4.1). The disintegration time, τ, thus corresponds to the lag time prior to the beginning of the rapid phase of dissolution and can be approximated by the intercept of the extrapolated linear portion of the curve on the x axis (Fig. 4.17). Depending on the duration of the disintegration process the treatment of dissolution data varies.

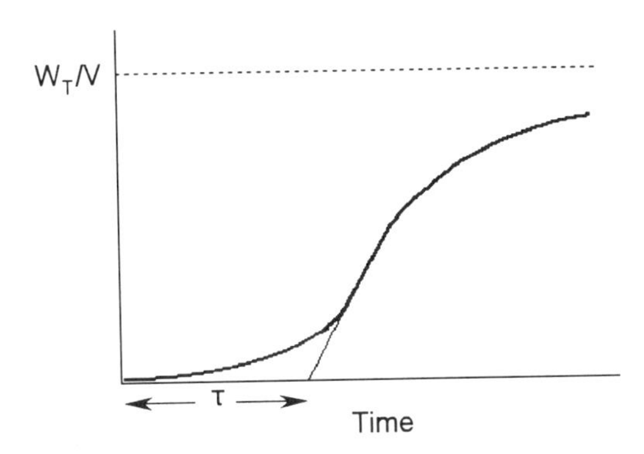

Fig. 4.17. Typical concentration versus time plot for the dissolution of an immediate-release tablet. Dissolution starts as soon as the tablet is introduced to the dissolution medium but proceeds much faster after disintegration is complete; τ is an estimate of the disintegration time.

When disintegration is fast, i.e. less than 5% of the time needed for dissolution to be completed, the treatment of the experimental data depends on the method by which the tablets were manufactured. If the tablet has been prepared by direct compression, dissolution can be modelled by equations (4.22) and (4.23), with the additional assumption that W equals W_0 for as long as disintegration lasts. For example, the cube root law becomes

$$W = W_0 \qquad \text{for} \quad t \leqslant \tau$$

$$(W_0)^{1/3} - (W)^{1/3} = (\pi N\rho/6)^{1/3}[(2DC_s)/(h_N\rho)](t-\tau) \qquad \text{for} \quad t > \tau \tag{4.24}$$

Note that if tablets are made by direct compression, one should consider the possibility that the mean particle diameter is reduced during compression. For treatment of such situations the reader is referred to relevant references at the end of this chapter.

When the tablet has been prepared by wet granulation, disintegration results in granules rather than drug particles. In this case, the liquid must first penetrate the pores of the granule for dissolution to take place—a process which makes it difficult to derive analytical equations to describe the overall dissolution. A simple way to overcome this difficulty is to use an empirical equation to describe the observed kinetics. One of the most frequently used equations assumes first order kinetics for the overall transfer of the drug molecules from the granule surface into the bulk solution, as follows:

$$C = \frac{W_0}{V}\left[1 - e^{-k_T(t-\tau)}\right] \tag{4.25}$$

where k_T is the overall first order dissolution rate constant which depends on the diffusion coefficient of the drug molecule and the geometrical characteristics of the granule. As with equation (4.24), equation (4.25) is valid only when $t > \tau$ (at $t \leqslant \tau$ no dissolution is assumed to take place). In addition, equation (4.25) can be logarithmically transformed to a linear form:

$$\ln\left(\frac{W_0}{V} - C\right) = \ln\left(\frac{W_0}{V}\right) - k_T(t-\tau) \tag{4.26}$$

When the disintegration time is greater than 5% of the total dissolution time, equations (4.24)–(4.26) are not appropriate for the study of dissolution. Three of the most frequently used methods are the Wagner method, the use of the Weibull distribution function and the use of statistical moments theory.

(a) *The Wagner method*: This method was proposed in the late 1960s. It basically suggests that, under sink conditions, the percentage dissolved at time t simply reflects the percentage surface area generated to time t. Further, the percentage dissolved–time data can best be described by a distribution function. Mathematically this can be written as follows:

$$\mathrm{d}C = \frac{k_i C_s}{V} A\,\mathrm{d}t \qquad \text{hence} \qquad \int_0^t \mathrm{d}C = (k_i C_s/V)\int_0^t A\,\mathrm{d}t$$

and

$$\%\text{ dissolved at time } t = \frac{C}{C_\infty} = \frac{\int_0^t A\,\mathrm{d}t}{\int_0^\infty A\,\mathrm{d}t} = \%\text{ of surface area generated to time } t$$

where C_∞ is the final concentration of the dissolved drug in the bulk solution. A plot of the cumulative generated surface area as a function of time will have the sigmoidal shape of Fig. 4.17. With such an approach, the parameters of the distribution function can be used to characterize the dissolution parameters. The parameters of a log-normal distribution can be estimated by plotting the cumulative data on a logarithmic scale so that the resulting profile will be a straight line. Some advantages associated with this technique include the requirement that sink conditions are extant, and the possibility that the surface area distribution is not log-normal.†

† The distribution of the surface area which is exposed for dissolution as a function of time is log-normal if the cumulative percentage dissolved plot is symmetrical around the point that has coordinates $[C_\infty/2, \log(t_{50\%})]$.

(b) *The Weibull distribution function*: In 1951, Weibull described a more general function which can be applied to all common types of dissolution curves, and especially to those where a lag time, τ, is observed prior to the beginning of the process. This function has been used in dissolution studies since early 1970s and it has the following form:

$$W_d/W_0 = 1 - \exp\left[-(t-\tau)^{\beta}/\alpha\right] \tag{4.27}$$

where W_d is the cumulative amount dissolved, W_0 is the total amount that can be eventually dissolved, and α and β are constants. The *scale parameter*, α, defines the time scale of the process. The *shape parameter*, β, characterizes the shape of the curve. The curve may be exponential ($\beta = 1$), sigmoidal ($\beta > 1$) or have a steeper initial slope than the exponential shape ($\beta < 1$). These relationships are illustrated in Fig. 4.18. Both the initial lag time and the constants can be estimated by either non-linear fit of equation (4.27) to the (W_{di}/W_0, t_i) data, or by linear regression analysis after linearization of equation (4.27), i.e.

$$\log\left[-\ln\left(1 - W_d/W_0\right)\right] = -\log\alpha + \beta\log(t-\tau) \tag{4.28}$$

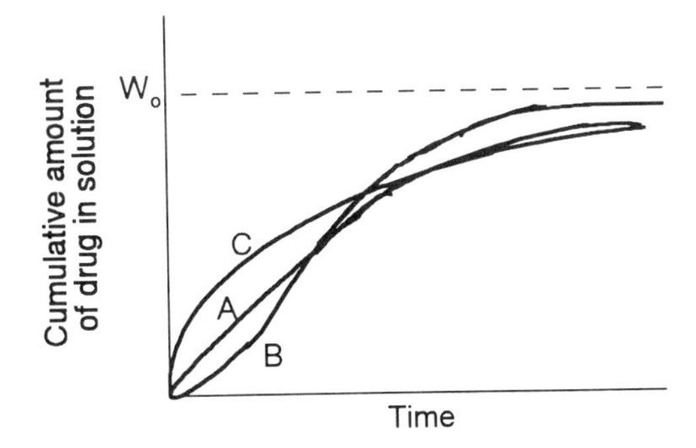

Fig. 4.18. Graphical representation of the Weibull distribution function for various values of the parameter β. (A) $\beta = 1$; (B) $\beta > 1$; (C) $\beta < 1$.

Equation (4.28) (which was first proposed by Langebucher in 1972) is initially fitted to the data assuming $\tau = 0$. If the lag time happens to be significant, the early data points show a concave downwards curvature. Whenever this occurs it is possible to straighten the curve by shifting all data points horizontally by the same time interval. The time shift required to give the best linearization can be found by a trial-and-error technique, and represents the lag time, τ.† The shape parameter, β, is obtained from the slope of the line which results if the data are plotted as $[-\ln(1 - W_d/W_0)]$ versus $[t - \tau]$ on a log–log scale. Similarly, the scale parameter, α, is estimated from the negative antilog of the

† Sometimes curvature is also observed in the upper tail of the plot. This happens when the data do not asymptotically approach the final plateau ($W_d/W_0 = 1$). This may happen in cases where the drug decomposes in the dissolution medium, and can be overcome by estimating the correct plateau value and adjusting all percentages accordingly.

intercept of the regression line. It should be noted that the scale parameter is often replaced by the more informative *dissolution time*, t_d. The relationship between α and t_d is

$$\alpha = (t_d)^\beta$$

The dissolution time can be read from the x axis of the $[-\ln(1 - W_d/W_0)]$ versus $[t - \tau]$ plot on a log–log scale as the time which corresponds to an ordinate value of *one*, i.e.

$$-\ln\left(1 - W_d/W_0\right) = 1$$

At t_d, $(1 - W_d/W_0) = e^{-1}$ and $W_d/W_0 = 0.632$, so the dissolution time actually represents the time required for 63.2% of the drug to be dissolved (assuming that the amount of drug added to the dissolution medium does not exceed its solubility limit).

Example 4.7: The following data were collected during an *in vitro* dissolution study of nitrofurantoin tablets, in which the volume of the dissolution medium was 800 ml:

C(mg/l):	10.5	34.0	56.4	75.6	90.2	104	114	122	124
t(min):	10	20	30	40	50	60	70	90	110

Analyse the data using the Weibull distribution, assuming that each tablet contains 100 mg of active ingredient.

Answer: First, the percentage of nitrofurantoin remaining to be dissolved at the corresponding time points is calculated:

$1 - W_d/W_0$:	0.916	0.728	0.549	0.395	0.278	0.168	0.088	0.024	0.008
t:	10	20	30	40	50	60	70	90	110

Then the log $(-\ln(1 - W_d/W_0))$ versus log (t) values are calculated:

log $[-\ln(1 - W_d/W_0)]$:	−1.057	−0.498	−0.222	−0.032	0.107	0.251	0.386	0.572	0.684
log (t):	1.00	1.30	1.48	1.60	1.70	1.78	1.85	1.95	2.04

Linear regression analysis according to equation (4.28), and assuming $\tau = 0$, results in (Fig. 4.19A) the following parameters:

		Level of significance
Intercept (SE):	−2.698 (0.048)	$p < 0.0004$
Slope (SE):	1.665 (0.024)	$p < 0.0004$
Correlation coefficient:	0.9990	$p < 0.0004$

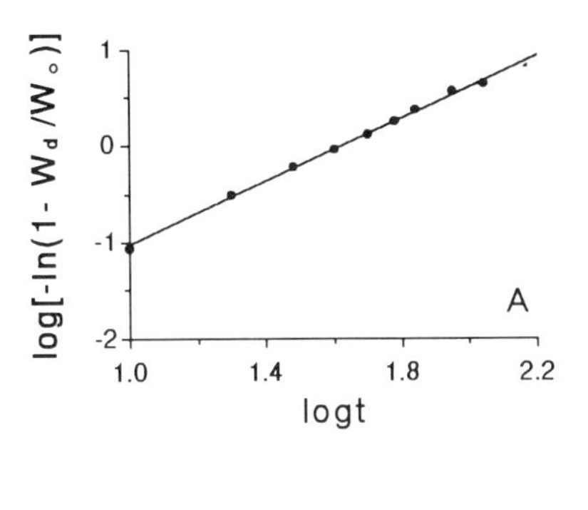

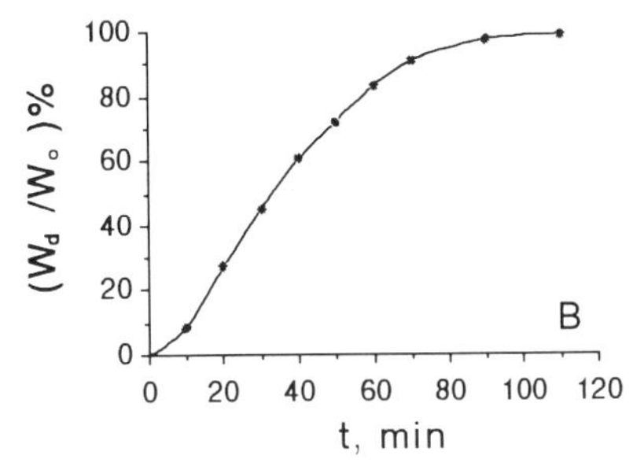

Fig. 4.19. (A) Plot of data from Example 4.8 according to equation (4.28) and assuming instant disintegration, i.e. $\tau = 0$; (B) plot of the percentage of drug dissolved versus time.

The high correlation coefficient indicates that, compared to dissolution, disintegration is rapidly completed. However, the fact that $\beta > 1$ indicates that the profile of the percentage dissolved as a function of time is sigmoid (this can be also confirmed by Fig. 4.19B). Thus, in the early stages of the dissolution process there is a lag time which may be due to the disintegration process. Using the trial-and-error method, it can be found that when $0 < \tau < 2$ the value of the correlation coefficient is higher. For example, by assuming $\tau = 1$ min, and, therefore, changing the values on the time axis to

$\log(t - \tau)$:	0.95	1.28	1.46	1.59	1.69	1.77	1.84	1.95	2.04

the results of the regression analysis are:

		Level of significance
Intercept (SE):	–2.564 (0.032)	$p < 0.0004$
Slope (SE):	1.597 (0.019)	$p < 0.0004$
Correlation coefficient:	0.9996	$p < 0.0004$

It should be mentioned that the curvature in this case could not be identified visually (Fig. 4.19A) because disintegration time was small and the linearized form of the Weibull function with $\tau = 0$ was well fitted to the data. To identify curvature in such cases, a *plot of residuals* (section 10.2.3) must be used.

Based on equation (4.28) and the linear regression analysis with $\tau = 1.0$ min, it is concluded that

$$-\log\alpha = -2.564 \quad \text{therefore} \quad \alpha = 366$$

$$\beta = 1.60, \quad \text{and}$$

$$t_d = (\alpha)^{1/\beta} = 366^{1/1.60} = 40.0 \text{ min}$$

(c) *Statistical moments*: Statistical moment theory can be applied to practically any type of dissolution data. This method is useful especially in cases where a correlation of *in vitro* with *in vivo* parameters is desired. It has a stochastic character (section 2.2.2) in so far as the time during which the drug remains undissolved is considered to be a statistically random variable. As dissolution proceeds, the number of molecules in the bulk solution increases and the cumulative amount of drug dissolved as a function of time is considered to be a cumulative density distribution of the random variable 'time'. Based on the cumulative amount dissolved versus time plot, the first moment represents the mean dissolution time, MDT, which can be estimated by the following equation:

$$\text{MDT} = \frac{\int_0^\infty t W_d(t)\,dt}{\int_0^\infty W_d(t)\,dt} = \frac{\text{ABC}}{W_0} \tag{4.29}$$

where ABC (area between curves) is the shaded area in Fig. 4.20 and W_0 here is the actual (as opposed to labelled) quantity of drug which is available for dissolution. ABC can be estimated algebraically (if the function which describes the process is known) or arithmetically.† In either case, estimation of MDT requires a knowledge of the time at which the dissolution process is complete.

Example 4.8: If the dissolution of drug from an immediate-release formulation is assumed to follow first order kinetics, without a lag time, and the cumulative amount dissolved as function of time is given by the following equation:

$$W_d = 0.625\,(1 - e^{-0.200t})$$

what is the mean dissolution time?

Answer: By assuming that the process is complete after a period of five half-lives (section 2.2.1) the time at which the dissolution process is complete is calculated to be

$$5(\ln 2/0.200) = 17.3$$

† Arithmetic estimation of ABC is usually made using the *trapezoidal rule*. This technique involves division of the shaded area of Fig. 4.44 into small trapezoids by drawing lines parallel to the abscissa until they intersect the dissolution curve, starting from each experimental point on the ordinate axis. The sum of the areas of the deprived trapezoids is the ABC.

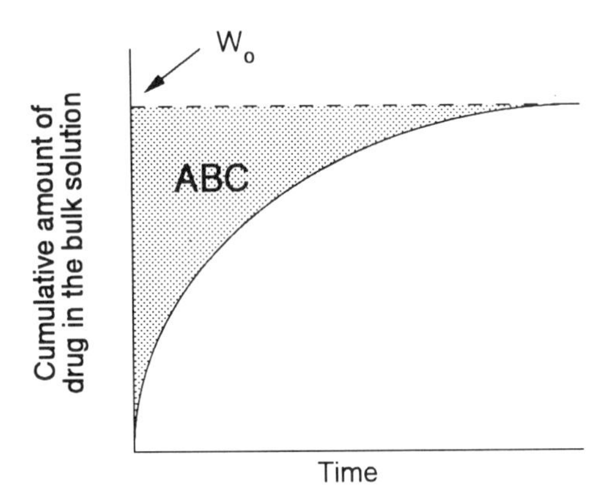

Fig. 4.20. Graphical presentation of the parameters used to estimate the mean dissolution time. W_0 is the actual quantity of drug which is available for dissolution, and ABC is the shaded area.

Therefore†

$$\mathrm{ABC} = 17.33 \times 0.625 - \int_0^{17.3} 0.625(1 - e^{-0.200t})\,\mathrm{d}t = 3.03$$

and

$$\mathrm{MDT} = 3.03/0.625 = 4.85$$

The mean dissolution time represents a useful parameter not only for *in vitro–in vivo correlations* but also whenever dissolution data from different *in vitro* apparatus (section 4.4.2.2) are correlated. Provided that the total amount dissolved is the same, two dissolution curves obtained from different *in vitro* apparatus can be correlated by shifting one of the two horizontally so that it overlaps the other. The procedure for this shifting involves the use of the mean dissolution time and a detailed description can be found in the references at the end of this chapter.

Treatment of dissolution data by either one of the latter two methods (i.e. Weibull distribution or statistical moments) requires minimal assumptions, which makes them extremely useful in a practical setting. A possible source of confusion between these two methods can arise from the definition of the *dissolution time* (Weibull distribution) and the *mean dissolution time* (statistical moments). Although the *mean dissolution time* has a different derivation and definition than the *dissolution time*, the two times become identical when

(1) the dissolution process follows first order kinetics; and
(2) has no lag time.

† As mentioned in section 2.2.2, the mean time of a first order process is the inverse of the rate constant. In this example the dissolution rate constant is 0.200 and, therefore, $\mathrm{MDT} = 1/0.200 = 5.00$. This is slightly different than 4.85 due to the rounding error.

4.3 DRUG RELEASE FROM AN EXTENDED-RELEASE SYSTEM

4.3.1 The need to modify the rate of release from the dosage form

Immediate release of the active ingredient with resulting fast absorption rate may not always be desirable. If the drug has narrow therapeutic index, fast and complete absorption may result in plasma concentrations that correspond to toxic levels. This sort of problem becomes more significant in cases where frequent administration is required because of fast elimination of drug from the body. In Table 4.4 the most important reasons for developing dosage forms with modified release rates are presented.

Table 4.4. Some rationales for modifying the release kinetics of the drug from the dosage form

1.	To sustain the pharmacological effect
2.	To achieve a 'flatter' blood level curve, thus avoiding toxic *peak* levels and subtherapeutic *valley* levels of drug
3.	To increase the extent of absorption, e.g. (i) to avoid stability problems in specific regions of the GI tract (as with erythromycin which degrades in the stomach's acidic environment), or (ii) when uptake occurs in only a limited region in the GI tract (as with vitamin B_{12})
4.	To programme release of the active ingredient, for example, to delay pharmacological action (as desired in treatment of morning stiffness in arthritis)
5.	To avoid a direct or adverse pharmacological action in the GI tract, e.g. irritation of gastric mucosa by ferrous ions
6.	To achieve a local and specific pharmacological action in the GI tract, e.g. administration of non-steroidal anti-inflammatory drugs

Extended-release systems were introduced into the pharmaceutical market in the early 1950s when Smith Kline & French made an orally administered formulation of dextroamphetamine sulphate by incorporating the drug in pellets coated with wax. For some years after that there was little additional progress in extended-release formulations, mostly because they lacked reproducibility in terms of the release rate. However, since the late 1970s, when more reliable technologies were developed, the number of new extended-release formulations has increased exponentially. Specific reasons for this progress include the development of new materials, methods for manufacturing and analytical techniques, and better understanding of the influence of the physiology on the performance of dosage forms.

The release kinetics of drugs administered orally in solid extended-release formulations are described below. However, for other information related to the design and the technology of manufacture of such systems (both of which are also of great importance for efficient *in vivo* performance)† the reader can refer to some of the references at the end of this chapter.

4.3.2 Kinetics of the release of drugs administered orally in solid extended-release formulations

An extended-release system should release the active ingredient at a rate which is not only predetermined by the manufacturer but also unaffected by variations in GI conditions. The mechanism by which drug is released from the dosage form is an important factor in determining whether both of these objectives can be achieved. Table 4.5 shows the various mechanisms of release from systems which were commercially available at the end of the 1980s. Among these, the kinetics of diffusion through an inert matrix or a membrane and the release due to osmotic effects are well described, hence *a priori* prediction of the release rate from dosage forms releasing drug by these mechanisms can be made.

Table 4.5. Some mechanisms of drug release from extended-release systems

Diffusion through an inert matrix
Diffusion through a hydrogel
Diffusion with erosion of the formulating material
Diffusion through a membrane
Release due to osmotic pressure differences
Release due to ion exchange

Release kinetics for most types of extended-release dosage forms are usually described by empirical relationships between the amount of drug in solution and time. In general, the release process may occur at a rate which continuously decreases with time, at a constant rate or, in more sophisticated situations, at a variable but controlled rate (Fig. 4.21).

4.3.2.1 Release at a continuously decreasing rate

Release at a continuously decreasing rate is usually observed when the mechanism of the release is diffusion through an inert matrix or across a membrane. In the first case, the cumulative amount released is usually linearly related to the square root of time. In the second case the amount released is usually related to time by first-order kinetics.

Diffusion through an inert matrix is a linear function of the square root of time. When the drug is homogeneously distributed in the matrix, the matrix keeps its shape and size during the release process, and the medium into which drug is released acts essentially as a perfect sink. Typical examples of inert matrices which release drug linearly with the

† Proper design is essential for reproducible *in vivo* performance because shape, size and manufacturing material determine the system's GI residence time. Several factors related to manufacturing, which directly or indirectly affect the use of an extended-release system, include *in vivo* compatibility, mechanism of release and cost of preparation.

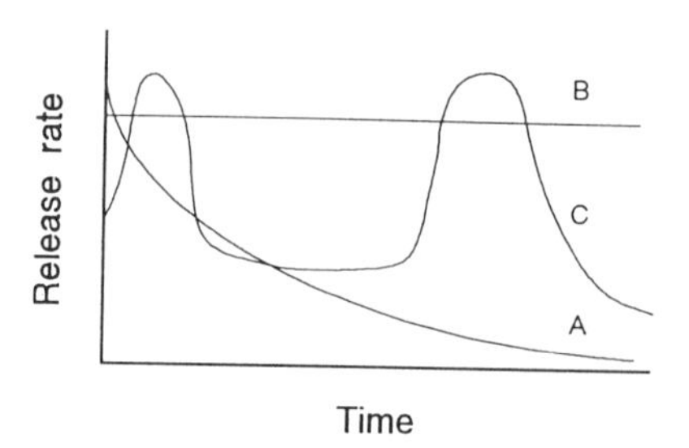

Fig. 4.21. Profiles of release rate as a function of time for three hypothetical extended release systems. (A) Continuously decreasing; (B) constant; (C) bimodal.

square root of time include certain types of waxes and plastic polymers. The equation used to describe the kinetics varies according to the geometry of the dosage form.

If the release is considered from a planar matrix in which the drug is homogeneously dispersed, the amount of drug released into the bulk solution under sink conditions is determined by the following relationship:

$$W_r' = \left[D_m\left(2W_0/V_m - C_m\right)C_m t\right]^{1/2} \tag{4.30}$$

where W_r' is the amount of drug released after time t per unit exposed area, D_m is the diffusion coefficient of the drug in the homogeneous matrix medium, W_0 is the total amount of drug loaded into the matrix, V_m is the total volume of the matrix, and C_m is the solubility of the drug in the matrix substance. This equation was derived by Higuchi in the early 1960s (the original article is cited at the end of this chapter). Initially this equation was introduced for drug release from an ointment base but it is also often used to describe release from extended-action matrices.

If a planar system comprised of granular matrix is considered, the release mechanism occurs via diffusion across intergranular openings. For this type of system the following equation is used to describe the release kinetics:

$$W_r' = \left[\left(D\varepsilon/\tau_\tau\right)\left(2W_0/V_m - \varepsilon C_s\right)C_s t\right]^{1/2} \tag{4.31}$$

where D here is the diffusion coefficient of the drug in the permeating fluid, τ_τ is the tortuosity factor of the capillary system (which is usually considered equal to 3), ε is the porosity of the matrix, and C_s is the solubility of the drug in the permeating fluid. In cases where the initial porosity is very small or where the fraction of the matrix volume occupied by the drug is relatively large, the value of ε can be estimated by the following equation:

$$\varepsilon = \left(W_0/V_m\right)\rho$$

where ρ is the density of the drug. It should also be mentioned that both equation (4.30) and equation (4.31) are valid for systems in which W_0/V_m is greater than C_m and εC_s, respectively, by a factor of three or four. Note that if W_0/V_m is less than C_m or εC_s, the drug is no longer present as a solid, and a different equation would apply.

From rearrangement of equation (4.30) or (4.31) it can be concluded that, as long as the surface area of release remains constant throughout the process, a plot of the cumulative amount of drug released, W_r, versus the square root of time will yield a straight line passing through the origin:

$$W_r = AW_r' = Ak_{1/2}t^{1/2} \tag{4.32}$$

Depending on how the drug is dispersed in a planar matrix, the half-order rate constant, $k_{1/2}$, is equal to

$$\left[D_m(2W_0/V_m - C_m)C_m\right]^{1/2} \quad \text{or} \quad \left[(D\varepsilon/\tau_\tau)\,(2W_0/V_m - \varepsilon C_s)\, C_s\right]^{1/2}$$

It should be mentioned at this point that data which give a straight line if plotted as W_r versus $t^{1/2}$ may also give a straight line when plotted according to first-order kinetics, i.e.

$$dW_r/dt = k_1(W_0 - W_r) \quad \text{and} \quad \ln(W_0 - W_r) = \ln W_0 - k_1 t \tag{4.33}$$

To distinguish between the half and first order release kinetics, the corresponding rate equations can be used. Taking the derivative of equation (4.32), one obtains

$$dW_r/dt = k_{1/2}^2 A^2/2W_r \tag{4.34}$$

If the cumulative amount released is linearly related to the square root of time, the release rate is inversely proportional to the released amount and independent from the initial amount of drug in the matrix. In this case a plot of dW_r/dt versus $1/W_r$ yields a straight line. If first order kinetics prevail,† this plot is not linear.

Equations corresponding to (4.30) and (4.31) have been also derived for the case where the matrix, homogeneous or granular, is a spherical pellet (see citations at the end of this chapter).

Another case in which the release rate continuously decreases is when release occurs via diffusion through a continuous polymeric membrane. In this case first-order kinetics apply and the release rate is given by the following equation:

$$\frac{dW_r}{dt} = \frac{AD_m P_{m/aq}}{h_m}(C_m - C) \tag{4.35}$$

where $P_{m/aq}$ is the partition coefficient between the membrane and the aqueous phase, and h_m is the membrane thickness.

Many extended-release systems which release the active ingredient with accurately defined first or half order kinetics have been developed. Due to their design, however, these systems cannot succeed in maintaining constant plasma drug levels. For this reason, much of the focus in recent years has been directed toward developing dosage forms which can release drug at a constant rate.

4.3.2.2 Release at a constant rate

An effective way to reduce the fluctuation of plasma blood levels is to deliver the drug in a dosage form which results in zero order absorption kinetics. Assuming that the release

† In practice, values for dW_r/dt can be approximated by the slopes of the W_r versus t curve.

rate is the rate-limiting step for drug arrival at the systemic circulation, the kinetics of the release process should be of zero order. During the last 10–20 years, this hypothesis has constituted the basis for the design of more effective extended-release systems. Mechanisms of release that usually result in zero-order kinetics include diffusion through a porous membrane and release driven by osmotic pressure differences. Zero-order kinetics can also be achieved using inert matrices discussed in section 4.3.2.1, but in which the active ingredient is concentrated in the centre of the matrix rather than being homogeneously distributed. Among all these mechanisms, release due to osmotic phenomena is probably most appropriate since it is least likely to be affected by the variability in luminal conditions. In the osmotically driven system, water permeates through the semi-permeable membrane and dissolves the core interior to generate osmotic pressure, which forces the drug solution out at zero order rate as long as there is solid osmotic agent in the tablet. The release with this mechanism is usually programmed according to the following equation:

$$\frac{dW_r}{dt} = \frac{AC_m \pi P_{mem}}{h_m} \tag{4.36}$$

where P_{mem} is the permeability coefficient of the membrane, A is the surface area of the tablet and $\pi = 3.416$. The corresponding equation for the release kinetics when the mechanism involves diffusion through a porous membrane has the following form:

$$\frac{dW_r}{dt} = \frac{ADC_s}{h_m} \tag{4.37}$$

Finally, zero-order release from a planar system having non-homogeneous matrix (drug distribution is more dense in the centre of the system) is usually followed with equation (4.38):

$$W_r = \frac{D_m C_m A \varphi}{2\tau_\tau \rho} t \tag{4.38}$$

where φ is a proportionality constant.

4.3.2.3 Release at a variable rate

Although the manufacture of reliable zero-order extended-release systems was a major breakthrough in the pharmaceutical field the last 15 years, it can be argued that zero-order release rate will only result in less fluctuation of plasma levels if uptake of the drug:

— occurs at the same rate in all parts of the GI tract in which drug is released; and
— is at least as high as the release rate in all these regions.

Unfortunately this is not always the case. For example, many drugs are taken up from the gastric and/or the colonic mucosa at a much slower rate than from the small intestine (section 5.2). The ultimate extended-release system would take such variations into account, as shown in Fig. 4.23, curve C. The increased release rate in the beginning and at the end of the duration of the release process corresponds to the gastric and colonic residence times whereas the intermediate, lower, release rate corresponds to the period of residence in the small intestine.

Attempts to manufacture systems which would release the active ingredient at variable rates depending on their location in the GI tract started in the 1980s. However, such systems are still at the experimental stage. A potential problem associated with variable-release systems is the high inter- and intra-subject variability of transit times through the GI tract, which may lead to mismatches in release versus transit rates in some individuals.

4.4 ASSESSING DRUG DISSOLUTION AND RELEASE *IN VITRO*

The ability of the active ingredient to dissolve in the gastrointestinal fluids and thus be available for uptake is usually tested in two stages. The inherent ability of the solid drug to dissolve in aqueous media is tested in pre-formulation studies. During development, the ability of potential formulations to release† the drug into aqueous media forms part of the basis for selection of the final dosage form. At both stages, dissolution data are collected almost exclusively from *in vitro* experiments.

4.4.1 Assessing dissolution properties of non-formulated drugs

Pre-formulation studies of the dissolution characteristics of drugs usually aim at establishing the mechanism of the dissolution process and may also study the influence of various components of the dissolution medium on the dissolution rate. A frequently used *in vitro* apparatus is the *rotating disk apparatus*. This was first introduced in the early 1960s and consists of (Fig. 4.22):

— a stainless-steel die system in which solid drug is compressed (at pressures up to about 5000 lb/inch^2);
— a drive shaft (usually made of plexiglass or stainless steel);
— a motor (capable of rotational speeds in the 5–500 rmp range); and
— a thermostated vessel in which dissolution takes place (made of glass or other inert material, and usually having a capacity of about 200 ml).

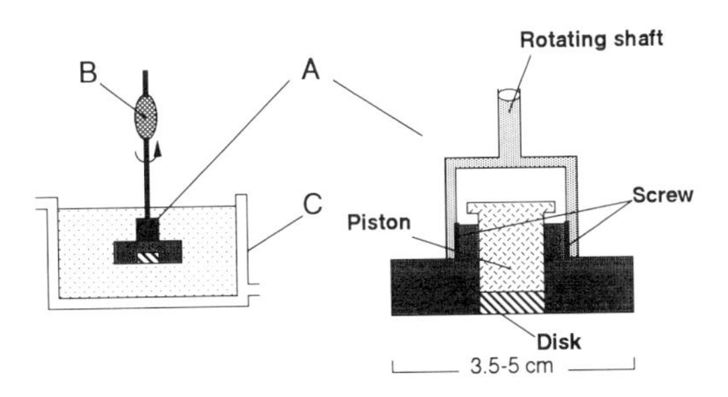

Fig. 4.22. The rotating disk apparatus used to study dissolution characteristics of the pure (non-formulated) drug substances. (A) The die system; (B) the drive shaft and motor; (C) the thermostated glass vessel.

† In this last section of chapter 4, the term *release* is used in its broadened meaning as it includes both *dissolution* from immediate-release dosage forms and *release* from extended-release formulations.

This apparatus is used because it allows for accurate definition of most of the parameters that affect dissolution process (section 4.2.2.3), especially the effective surface area and the hydrodynamic conditions. The surface area of the dissolving drug substance (or, the surface area which is in contact with the dissolution medium) is planar (any deviations from planarity are assumed to be insignificant) and dictated by the geometry of the die. Most importantly, it remains constant and equal to πr^2 (where r is the radius of the die, if circular) during the whole process. As far as the hydrodynamic conditions are concerned, the effective diffusion layer (section 4.2.2.1) is defined over the whole surface area of the disk. The mathematics that apply to such a system have been described by Levich (some of the equations are presented in section 4.2). Briefly, if the mechanism of the process is convection/diffusion, the stirring conditions do not produce turbulent flow, and the diffusion coefficient can be considered constant, the dissolution rate is given by the following equation:

$$\mathrm{d}m/\mathrm{d}t = 0.62\, AD^{2/3}\eta_k^{-1/6}\,\omega^{1/2}(C_s - C) \tag{4.39}$$

where $A = \pi r^2$ and ω is the angular velocity of the disk (usually in rad/s).† Comparison of equations (4.39) and (4.3) shows that the intrinsic dissolution rate constant, k_i, is equal to $0.62 D^{2/3}\eta_k^{-1/6}\omega^{1/2}$. If during the dissolution process sink conditions also prevail and A is substituted by πr^2, equation (4.39) becomes

$$\mathrm{d}m/\mathrm{d}t = 1.95 D^{2/3}\,\eta_k^{-1/6} r^2 C_s \omega^{1/2} \tag{4.40}$$

and finally

$$m = 1.95 D^{2/3}\eta_k^{-1/6}\omega^{1/2} r^2 C_s t \tag{4.41}$$

Equation (4.41) suggests that, in cases where sink conditions prevail and the mechanism for dissolution is convection-diffusion, the plot of the amount of drug dissolved versus time will be a straight line passing through the origin. Similar, but more complex, equations have been derived under turbulent flow or when the diffusion coefficient is not constant (e.g. when the drug is extremely soluble or when the viscosity changes during dissolution). Deviations from linearity in plots employing equation (4.41) should be considered as an indication that dissolution does not occur purely by a convection-diffusion mechanism.

4.4.2 Assessing the release of drugs from solid dosage forms

4.4.2.1 Advantages and disadvantages of in vitro *testing*

In principle, prediction of the *in vivo* performance of a solid dosage form with *in vitro* experiment(s) is limited by a number of disadvantages, which can be divided into two categories:

† 1 rad corresponds to a turn of $360/2\pi = 57.3°$.

Failure to simulate composition of the GI contents: An approximation of the composition of the luminal contents can be made by controlling the pH and the ionic strength as well as by incorporating surfactant(s), enzymes or other physiological substances in the aqueous medium. However, the high variation between subjects (due to disease state, administration of other drugs, etc.) and within the same subject (e.g. between the fed and the fasted state) limits the ability to accurately represent either the quality or the quantity of the GI contents. In the past, various media have been suggested to simulate the luminal contents after a meal intake. These include low fat milk, diluted emulsions used in parenteral feeding, etc. Although the release profiles in those media sometimes give better correlations with *in vivo* data, problems associated with drug assay in such complex media have prevented their widespread use. For this reason, the choice of a suitable aqueous medium for *in vitro* release testing is usually the result of a compromise between the accuracy of simulation of *in vivo* conditions and the need to establish experimental conditions which can give reproducible results.

Failure to simulate the luminal hydrodynamics: Upper GI motility is complex (section 5.2) and it varies with time even when no external stimuli are applied (e.g. administration of food). There is currently no simple accepted description of the hydrodynamics (effective stirring rate and flow patterns) in the GI tract. As a result, the type and the intensity of agitation used in the *in vitro* apparatus are tailored more toward giving reproducible test results than toward simulating the hydrodynamics in the GI tract.

Despite the aforementioned problems, *in vitro* testing of the release characteristics *can* be of great value and, compared to *in vivo* studies, it possesses certain advantages. Specifically:

(a) *In vitro* tests can provide useful information about consistency in the manufacturing process for the dosage form. This becomes extremely important when sparingly soluble drugs or modified-release formulations are considered. An idea of the significance of the *in vitro* test as a quality test can be taken from the number of monographs in the United States Pharmacopeia (USP), where this test is mandatory (Table 4.6). Based on the last edition of the USP (edition XXII, 1990) the only dosage forms for which

Table 4.6. Number of monographs in the US Pharmacopeia and the National Formulary which require dissolution or release tests

Edition/year	Monographs for immediate release dosage forms	Monographs for modified-release dosage forms	
		Extended	Delayed
USP XX-NF XV/1980	60	—	—
USP XXI-NF XVI/1985	400	1	—
USP XXII-NF XVII/1990	462	18	5

dissolution data are not required are chewable tablets and some immediate-release multivitamin and mineral dosage forms.

(b) Although the luminal conditions can only be approximated, the *in vitro* release profile may, under certain conditions, be closely correlated to the *in vivo* performance. Such correlations tend to be most successful when the overall absorption process is limited by the release rate and in these cases the *in vitro* release profile can be used as an indirect absorption indicator. Two examples include immediate-release formulations of sparingly soluble drugs, and extended-release systems.

(c) *In vivo* methods used to assess the release characteristics of dosage forms are more expensive, labour intensive and time consuming than *in vitro* methods.

4.4.2.2 Apparatus used to study drug release from orally administered solid formulations

Selection of an apparatus to study the release characteristics of a pharmaceutical dosage form is usually based on two criteria: the degree of inter- and intra-laboratory variability of the data and the strength of *in vitro–in vivo correlations*. Among several devices proposed during the last 30 years, two have been shown to fulfil these criteria more consistently and have thus become official for *in vitro* testing in most of the national pharmacopeias (Fig. 4.23). Their widespread use and efficient performance are based on the ability to develop strong *in vitro–in vivo correlations*, well-controlled hydrodynamics, ease of sampling, ability to automate, ease of calibration and low cost.

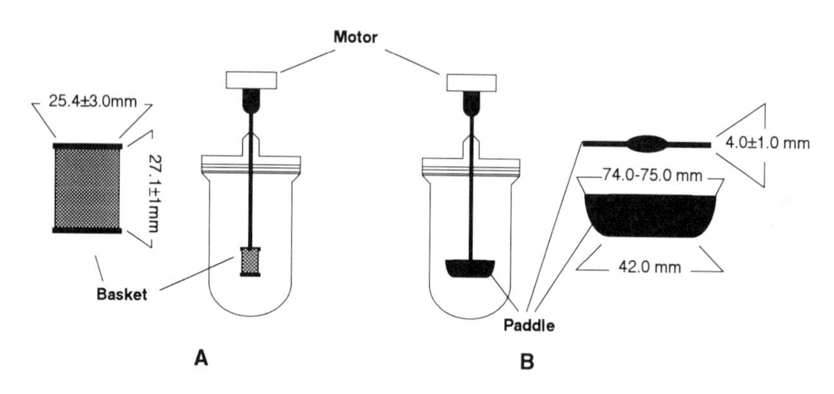

Fig. 4.23. The two most frequently used apparatus for the study of the release of the drug from orally administered solid dosage forms. (A) The rotating basket apparatus (apparatus I); and (B) the rotating paddle apparatus (apparatus II). The numbers for the basket size indicate internal dimensions.

The *rotating basket apparatus* (usually referred to as type I apparatus) consists of a covered cylindrical vessel made of an inert transparent material (usually glass), a motor, a metallic rotating shaft and a cylindrical basket (Fig. 4.23A). The vessel is cylindrical, with a hemispherical bottom, has a nominal capacity of 1000 ml, and is immersed in a water bath to maintain the temperature of the aqueous medium inside the vessel at 37 ± 0.5°C. The large capacity facilitates maintenance of sink conditions and, thus, better simulation of the *in vivo* conditions throughout the entire experiment. Both the shaft and the basket are of stainless steel and they rotate at speeds usually in the range 50–150 rpm. At the beginning of each experiment the dosage form is placed in a 40-mesh dry basket, and the basket is lowered into the medium until it reaches a distance of about 25 mm from the inside bottom of the vessel. Samples are withdrawn from the medium during the course of the experiment without interruption of the rotation of the basket.

The *rotating paddle apparatus* (usually referred to as type II apparatus) is similar to apparatus I described above. The major difference lies in the stirring element, which consists of a blade instead of a basket (Fig. 4.23B). At the beginning of the experiment, the dosage form is allowed to sink to the bottom of the vessel, then the blade rotation is started. If the dosage form has a low density and hence a tendency to float, a few loose turns of wire helix of an inert material are attached to force it to sink. The paddle apparatus is also used for research purposes, especially in cases where an interaction between the drug and a solute in the dissolution medium occurs. For example, the relative contributions of wetting and solubilization effects due to the presence of a surfactant can be assessed by comparing data obtained with this apparatus and results obtained using the rotating disk apparatus.

At this point it is useful to briefly describe the criteria on which the pharmacopeias base the acceptance of the release characteristics of an orally administered dosage form. The decision is usually based on the percentage of active ingredient released under certain conditions (i.e. type of apparatus, rotating speed, etc., are all clearly specified) within a specified time period. According to most pharmacopeial guidelines, the test should be performed on six units of the dosage form and the requirements are met if the percentage of active ingredient released conforms to a specific acceptance table. An acceptance table from the USP Pharmacopeia is presented in Table 4.7.

Table 4.7. The acceptance table of the US Pharmacopeia XXII (1990) for immediate-release dosage forms which are administered orally. The requirements are met if the quantities of active ingredient dissolved from the units tested conform to this table. Testing is continued through the three stages unless the results conform at either stage S_1 or S_2

Stage	Number tested	Acceptance criteria
S_1	6	Each unit is not less than $Q^a + 5\%$
S_2	6	Average of 12 units ($S_1 + S_2$) is equal to or greater than Q, and no unit is less than $Q - 15\%$
S_3	12	Average of 24 units ($S_1 + S_2 + S_3$) is equal to or greater than Q, not more than 2 units are less than $Q - 15\%$, and no unit is less than $Q - 25\%$

[a] Q is the amount of dissolved active ingredient specified in the individual monograph and is expressed as a percentage of the labelled content.

Example 4.9: According to the relevant monograph in the XXII USP, the immediate-release tablets of hydrochlorothiazide should release at least 60% of their content within 30 min. The results for the first two stages corresponding to the instructions of Table 4.7 were as follows:

S_1	62	68	54	58	70	72
S_2	66	55	74	54	78	73

Is the third stage necessary for deciding whether the tablets from this particular batch conform to the XXII USP standards?

Answer: According to the directions of Table 4.7 all values from stage 1 should be higher than $60 + 5 = 65\%$. Since this criterion is not met the second stage was performed. The average of all the 12 tests should now be at least 60 and all individual values higher than $60 - 15 = 45\%$. Since the average of the above data is 65 and no value is lower than 45 it can be concluded that the tablets meet the XXII USP specifications and that stage 3 testing is not necessary.

Although empirical testing according to tables like Table 4.7 is reliable in terms of assessing manufacturing quality, attempts to determine the mechanism of release require the use of other methods, such as those described earlier in sections 4.2.2.4 and 4.3.2. Furthermore, specific tests must be developed to determine whether release from extended-release systems is affected by the changing luminal conditions as the system travels down the GI tract. Although extended-release dosage forms are usually designed to have release characteristics which are independent of luminal conditions, this does not always prove to be the case. One parameter that changes dramatically with position in the GI tract, and which may strongly influence the rate of release, is the luminal pH. Fig. 4.24 shows two hypothetical cases of release profiles of the same drug from two different extended-release systems as a function of pH. It is obvious that system B, unlike system A, releases its drug content evenly over the entire pH range tested and, therefore, it is more appropriate for use than system A.

As well as the officially sanctioned *in vitro* apparatus for studying release rate, in some cases other devices may be used. Unofficial apparatus are often used when the release of a sparingly soluble drug needs to be studied. In this case the official devices may be problematic either because one dose cannot be dissolved in 1000 ml of the aqueous medium or, more frequently, because sink conditions cannot be maintained. Although one could increase the total solubility by using a mixture of organic and aqueous solvents as the release medium, a physiologically more realistic way of maintaining sink conditions is to keep the aqueous release medium and use a different device, e.g. the so-called *flow-through system*.† With these systems (Fig. 4.25) the effective volume of the release medium is drastically increased and solubility problems or maintenance of sink conditions are overcome. Furthermore, it is possible (by following a procedure based on the mean dissolution time, described in the reference at the end of

† This became official in the US Pharmacopeia in September 1991, 5th Supplement.

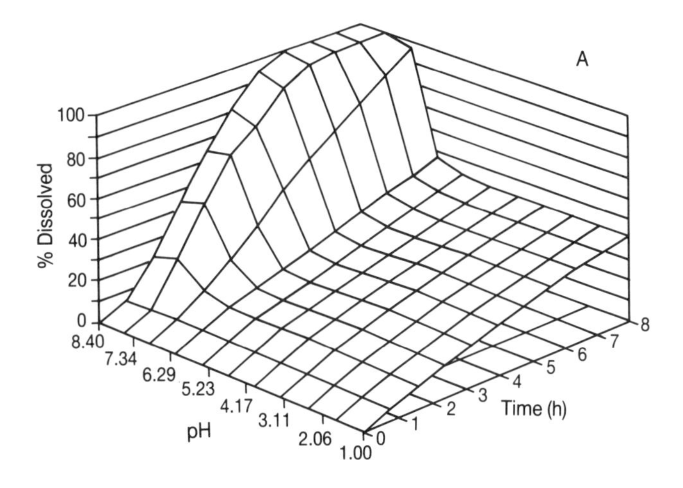

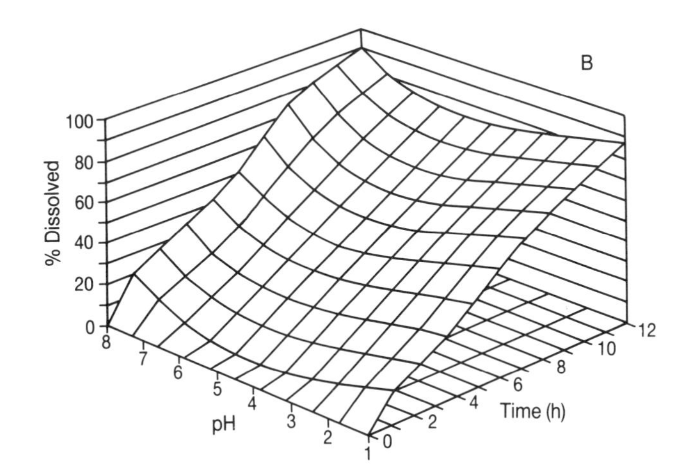

Fig. 4.24. Examples of topographical plots of drug release from extended-release systems. (A) Release is greatly affected by the pH value of the medium; (B) the release profile is practically independent of the pH value of the medium.

this chapter) to compare two release curves obtained with two different *in vitro* devices. The most important disadvantages of the flow-through systems include cost and difficulty in keeping uniform flow pattern throughout the experiment.

FURTHER READING

Ashby LJ, Beezer AE and Buckton G. In vitro Dissolution Testing of Oral Controlled Release Preparations in the Presence of Artificial Foodstuffs. I. Exploration of Alternative Methodology: Microcalorimetry. *Int. J. Pharmacol.* **51**: 245–251 (1989).

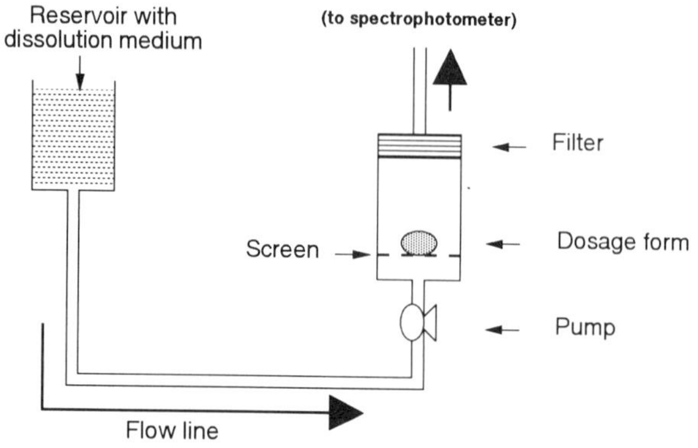

Fig. 4.25. Schematic of a flow-through system used in drug release studies.

Brockmeier D and von Hattinberg HM. In Vitro–In Vivo Correlation. A Time Scaling Problem? Basic Considerations on In Vitro Dissolution Testing. *Arzneim.-Forsch/Drug Res.* **32**: 248–251 (1982).

Brockmeier D, Voegele D and von Hattinberg HM. In Vitro–In Vivo Correlation. A Time Scaling Problem? Basic Techniques for Testing Equivalence. *Arzneim.-Forsch/Drug Res.* **33**: 598–601 (1983).

Cohen JL, Hubert BB, Leeson LJ, Rhodes CT, Robinson JR, Roseman TJ and Shefter E. The Development of USP Dissolution and Drug Release Standards. *Pharm. Res.* **7**: 983–987 (1990).

Goldsmith JA, Randall N and Ross SD. On Methods of Expressing Dissolution Rate Data. *J. Pharm. Pharmacol.* **30**: 347–349 (1978).

Grijseels H, Crommelin DJA and de Blaey CJ. Hydrodynamic Approach to Dissolution Rate. *Pharm. Weekbl.* **3**: 129–144 (1981).

Hanson WA. *Handbook of Dissolution Testing*, 2nd edn, Aster Publishing, Eugine, OR (1991).

Hattinberg HM von and Brockmeier DA. A Method for In Vivo–In Vitro Correlation Using the Additivity of Mean Times in Biopharmaceutical Models. In: *Methods in Clinical Pharmacology* (Proceedings of an International Symposium, Frankfurt, May 1979), pp. 85–93, Woodcock BG and Neuhaus G (eds), Vieweg, Braunschweig/Wiesbaden (1980).

Higuchi T. Rate of Release of Medicaments from Ointment Bases Containing Drugs in Suspension. *J. Pharm. Sci.* **50**: 874–875 (1961).

Higuchi T. Mechanism of Sustained-Action Medication. Theoretical Analysis of Rate of Release of Solid Drugs Dispersed in Solid Matrices. *J. Pharm. Sci.* **52**: 1145–1149 (1963).

Higuchi W. Diffusional Models Useful in Biopharmaceutics. Drug Release Rate Processes. *J. Pharm. Sci.* **56**: 315–324 (1967).

Langenbucher F. Linearization of Dissolution Rate Curves by the Weibull Distribution. *J. Pharm. Pharmacol.* **24**: 979–981 (1972).

Leeson LJ and Carstensen JT (eds). *Dissolution Technology*, Industrial Pharmaceutical Technology Section of the Academy of Pharmaceutical Sciences, Washington, DC (1974).

Levich VG. *Physicochemical Hydrodynamics*, pp. 60–72, Prentice Hall, Englewood Cliffs, NJ (1962).

Lu ATK, Frisella ME and Johnson KC. Dissolution Modelling: Factors Affecting the Dissolution Rates of Polydisperse Powders. *Pharm. Res.* **10**: 1308–1314 (1993).

Macheras P, Koupparis M and Antimissiaris S. An In vitro Model for Exploring Controlled Release Theophylline–Milk Fat Interactions. *Int. J. Pharmacol.* **54**: 123–130 (1989).

Martin AN, Swabrick J and Cammarata A. (eds). Physical Pharmacy (3rd edn), p. 223 (Buffers and buffered isotonic systems), Lea & Febiger, Philadelphia (1983).

Neervannan S, Reinert JD, Stella VJ and Southard MZ. A Numerical Convective-Diffusion Model for Dissolution of Neutral Compounds under Laminar Flow Conditions. *Int. J. Pharmacol.* **96**: 167–174 (1993).

Schwartz JB, Simonelli AP and Higuchi WI. Drug Release from Wax Matrices. I. Analysis of Data with First-Order Kinetics and with the Diffusion-Controlled Model. *J. Pharm. Sci.* **57**: 274–277 (1968).

Scott DC and Hollenbeck RG. Design and Manufacture of a Zero-Order Sustained-Release Pellet Dosage Form through Nonuniform Drug Distribution in a Diffusional Matrix. *Pharm. Res.* **8**: 156–161 (1991).

Yacobi A and Halperin-Walega E (eds). *Oral Sustained Release Formulations. Design and Evaluation*, Chapters 1, 2, 3, 7, Pergamon Press, New York (1988).

5

Delivery of the drug to and removal of drug from uptake sites

Objectives
The reader will be able to identify:

—*The characteristics of processes which lead to the approach of the drug molecule to uptake sites*
—*The characteristics of the processes which lead to the removal of the drug molecule from uptake sites*
—*Elements of the structure and the physiology of the gastrointestinal tract essential for the understanding of the disposition of the drug in the gastrointestinal tract*
—*Methods of studying gastrointestinal transit of dosage forms*

Delivery of a drug molecule into the general circulation requires its ability to be present and chemically stable in areas of the gastrointestinal (GI) lumen where uptake is facile. This will depend not only on the dosage form design and drug properties, but also on the physiological conditions existing in the GI tract following the administration of the drug.

The anatomical and physiological factors which lead to delivery of the drug to and removal from the uptake sites are presented schematically in Fig. 5.1.

5.1 PROCESSES INVOLVED IN THE DELIVERY OF DRUG TO AND REMOVAL OF DRUG FROM UPTAKE SITES

5.1.1 Processes which favour absorption

Apart from the release process (which was discussed in chapter 4) there are two additional processes which favour approach of the drug/dosage form to uptake sites (Fig. 5.1):

(1) gastric emptying; and
(2) in cases where the drug is presented as a prodrug, conversion of the prodrug to the active form.

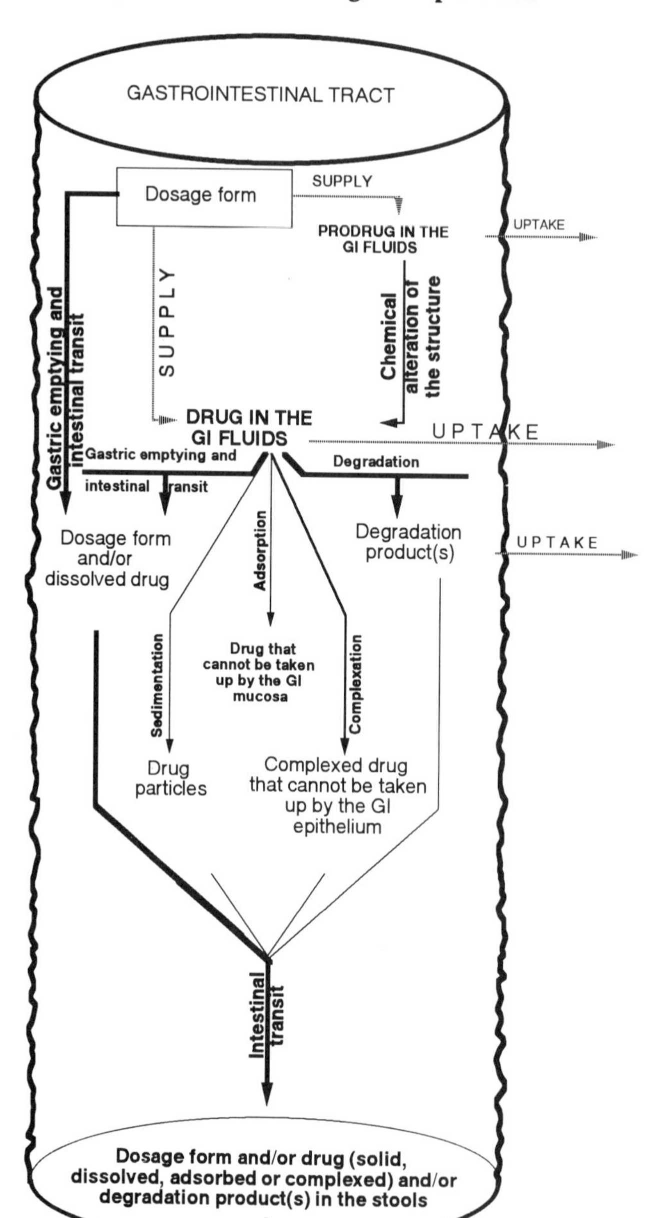

Fig. 5.1. Schematic description of processes which may affect the delivery of the drug molecule to and the removal from the uptake sites. Bold arrows indicate the most important processes, and dotted arrows correspond to other processes which, in conjunction with the delivery of the drug to and the removal from the uptake sites, control absorption.

5.1.1.1 Gastric emptying

As discussed in detail in section 6.1, the site with greatest potential for drug uptake in the GI tract is the small intestine. In most circumstances, the dosage form is delivered through the oesophagus to the stomach quickly and without difficulty. The time required to reach the primary absorptive sites is therefore mainly controlled by gastric emptying. If there are no solubility limitations and its uptake in the small intestine is rapid, the overall absorption process is primarily controlled by gastric emptying (Table 5.1). This is especially important when immediate pharmacological effect is needed. For example, when analgesics or antihistamines are administered, the absorption process should be completed as fast as possible, and it is desirable that gastric emptying does not present a limitation. Fig. 5.2 shows that for acetaminophen gastric emptying controls the overall absorption process.

Table 5.1. GI absorption of these drugs can be affected by the gastric emptying process

Acetaminophen	Furosemide	Pentobarbitone
Amoxicillin	Griseofulvin	Phenobarbitone
Ampicillin	Isoniazid	Phenylbutazone
Aspirin	Lidocaine	Quinine
Digoxin	L-Dopa	Riboflavin
Ethionamide	Penicillin	Tetracycline

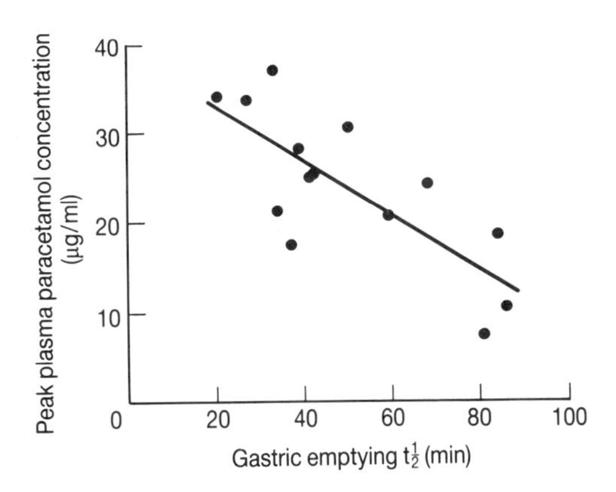

Fig. 5.2. Correlation between the maximum plasma acetaminophen concentration and the half-life for gastric emptying. The study was performed using 14 volunteers. Plasma concentration measurements were obtained following the per os administration of three 500 mg tablets with 50 ml water. Gastric emptying was measured in another series of experiments following the administration of a standard meal to the subjects ($R = -0.77$, $p < 0.005$). (From the *British Journal of Pharmacology* **47**: 415–421 (1973) with permission.)

One of the earlier references to the importance of gastric emptying rate on drug absorption can be found in an Agatha Christie novel *The Mysterious Affair at Styles* (1920), in which Hercule Poirot was informed that narcotic pain relievers delay the absorption of lethal strychnine doses, apparently as a result of delayed gastric emptying. In general, gastric emptying rate of the dosage form and/or the drug molecule dissolved in the gastric contents can affect the absorption process if:

(1) The drug is, regardless of the pH of the solution, sparingly soluble in the GI environment (such as griseofulvin or digoxin, Table 5.1). In this case, increasing the gastric residence time increases the percentage of drug that can dissolve before it passes potential uptake locations.
(2) The drug is only soluble at low (gastric) pH, e.g. ketoconazole and dipyridamole.
(3) An enteric coated dosage form is administered. In this case gastric emptying is the predominant requirement for absorption. Pancreatic enzyme replacement therapy formulated as enteric coated products fits this category. The enzymes are delivered specifically to the upper small intestine when the enteric coating dissolves. Gastric emptying concomitant with the meal will optimize the efficacy of the formulation.
(4) The drug molecule is not stable in the gastric environment. Gastric emptying will play a significant role in drug absorption only if both rates, i.e. gastric emptying and degradation, are of similar magnitude. For example, erythromycin is extremely unstable in the stomach, with a degradation half-life of less than 1 min. Since gastric emptying usually takes several minutes to hours, physiological variations in gastric emptying rate are not likely to be of practical importance to erythromycin bioavailability as it will be completely degraded in the stomach under almost any dosing circumstances. By contrast, hydrocortisone has a half-life of about 1 h in acid and in this case the gastric emptying rate may be quite critical to bioavailability.

5.1.1.2 Conversion of prodrugs to the active form

One way of improving dissolution or mucosal uptake properties is to make a prodrug. The prodrug should be converted to the active, parent form during or after the absorption process, but before it reaches the intended site of action.

An example of this approach to improving drug absorption is the synthesis of prodrugs by reaction with an amino acid if the drug possesses a free hydroxyl, amino, and/or carboxyl group. Depending on the polarity of the amino acid used, the production of esters or amides with desired physicochemical properties (e.g. increased solubility) is possible. These prodrugs are degraded *in vivo* by hydrolases such as carboxypeptidase in the lumen or aminopeptidases on the brush border (see section 6.1). Another example is the esterification of the free carboxyl groups of the drug molecule with dextrans, glucose, galactose or cellobiose. The glycosidic linkages escape small bowel digestion and are cleaved only by colonic bacteria. Thus the prodrug arrives intact and, after cleavage to its parent form, is absorbed from the colon. This strategy is used in cases where local treatment of large bowel disease is desired or when the parent drug is not stable under upper GI tract conditions but possesses satisfactory colonic absorption characteristics.

Examples of such drugs include anti-inflammatory agents like hydrocortisone, prednisolone naproxen (Fig. 5.3), etc.

Sulfasalazine, another drug used in the treatment of inflammatory bowel disease is composed of the antibacterial sulfapyridine, linked to the anti-inflammatory 5-aminosalicylic acid (section 3.2.1) by an azo bond. Sulfasalazine is a prodrug which carries the active 5-aminosalicylic acid to the colon, where bacterial azo reduction splits it, releasing the anti-inflammatory agent directly to its site of action.

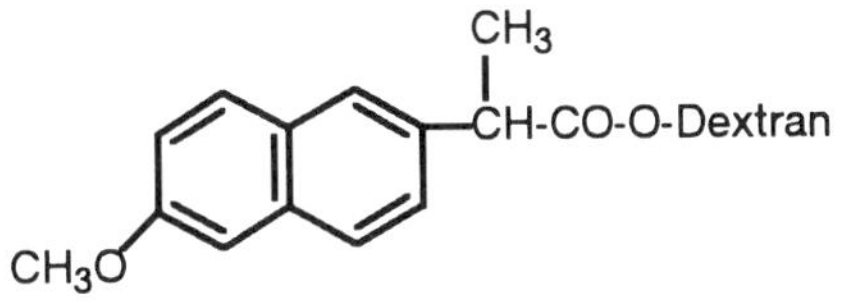

CH_3
CH-CO-O-Dextran
CH_3O

Fig. 5.3. Prodrug of naproxen specifically designed to reach the large intestine.

Chemical modification during the uptake process

Biotransformation of the administered prodrug molecule to the parent compound by the brush border enzymes (section 6.1) may be of practical importance whenever the parent drug is sparingly soluble in the GI fluids, or its transport through the GI mucosa is not favourable. For example, pivampicillin (the pivaloyl-oxy-methyl ester of ampicillin), the lysine ester of oestrone and the phosphate ester of hydrocortisone are more hydrophilic than ampicillin, oestrone and hydrocortisone, respectively. Similarly, the relative lack of permeability of the GI epithelium to α-methyldopa can be overcome by administration of a dipeptide prodrug such as phenylalanyl-α-methyldopa. In all cases the hydrolysis of the linkage between promoiety and parent compound is mediated by enzymes in the brush border.

5.1.2 Processes which reduce absorption

The processes which decrease drug concentration at the uptake sites include (Fig. 5.1) sedimentation of the drug in the GI fluids, adsorption onto luminal solid particles, formation of a non-absorbable complex, chemical or enzymatic degradation of the drug, and transit past the uptake sites.

5.1.2.1 Sedimentation

As described in chapter 4, drugs which are weak bases usually do not present dissolution problems in the acidic gastric environment. From equilibrium considerations, these compounds may precipitate in the considerably higher pH environment of the small intestine (equation (4.18). However, the fast dispersion of the drug along the small intestine and the greater (compared to the stomach) ability of the small intestine to absorb the drug tend to counteract the unfavourable pH conditions. For this reason, precipitation due to pH changes along the upper GI tract becomes a potential mechanism for reduced uptake only in cases of very poorly soluble weak bases with pK_as well below 7.

5.1.2.2 Adsorption

Although adsorption may increase dissolution rate by removing the dissolved drug from solution and thus maintaining sink conditions, drug uptake may be reduced if significant adsorption to luminal contents occurs. The main sources of adsorbents are foodstuffs and co-administered drugs. Cholestyramine and cholestipol, two anion-exchange resins which adsorb bile salts, preventing their reabsorption and thereby exerting a hypocholesterolemic action, may also adsorb other compounds. The adsorption of ketoconazole by sucralfate and subsequent reduced ketoconazole bioavailability provides a further example of drug/drug adsorption interactions.

5.1.2.3 Complexation

Owing to the high number of exogenous and physiological constituents of the GI fluids, it can be difficult to identify the source of a complexation reaction which results in decreased absorption. The example of complexation of tetracyclines with certain minerals, which results in reduced tetracycline absorption, is typical. Specifically, administration of declomycin, minocyclin, demeclomycin or tetracycline with multivitamin products which contain ferrum, aluminium hydroxide gels, milk or (more generally) dairy products reduces the incidence of nausea and emesis. This is due to the production of chelate complexes between drugs and ferrum, aluminium and/or calcium ions. As a result, the absorbable (free) drug concentration in the GI tract is reduced, leading to a decrease in the absorption of the tetracycline by as much as 80% (Fig. 5.4).

5.1.2.4 Degradation

Chemical reactions which lead to degradation of the administered drug in the GI tract can include hydrolyses, oxidations and reductions and are catalysed by the pH conditions and/or enzymes in the small intestine, or the bacterial flora of the lower intestinal tract.

A typical example is the gastric hydrolysis of certain penicillins and erythromycin. Penicillins are not stable in a strong acidic environment and, depending on their substituent on the amide group (position 6, Fig. 5.5), the degradation half-life ranges from 2 to 700 min. Similarly, erythromycin (a macrolide antibiotic) is a weak base not stable at pH below 4. Its hydrolysis in the stomach may be prevented by using either enteric coated dosage forms or prodrugs. Examples include certain esters which are hydrolysed after they arrive in the general circulation. Administration of the sodium lauryl sulfate salt of erythromycin 2-propionate (erythromycin estolate) results in increased plasma erythromycin concentrations (Fig. 5.6) for two reasons: first, the administered prodrug is stable at acidic pH; and second it has higher partition coefficient and lower pK_a (pK_a = 6.9) than erythromycin base (pK_a = 8.8). As a consequence, uptake by the intestinal epithelium becomes more favourable.

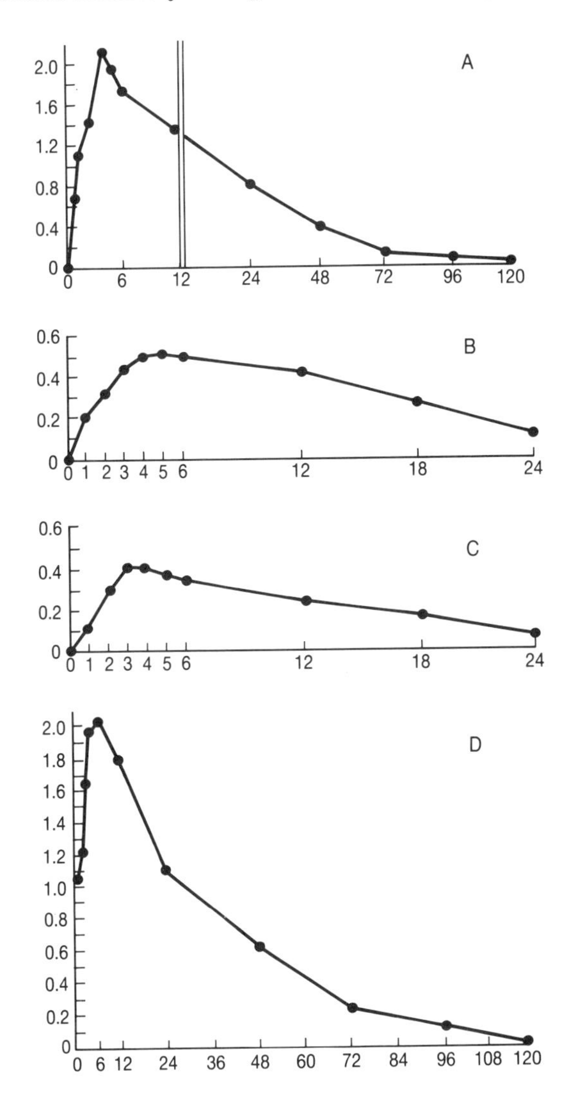

Fig. 5.4. Average serum concentration of 7-chloro-dimethyl-tetracycline (declomycin) to four to six subjects following a single oral dose of 300 mg with (A) water 60 ml, (B) Amphojel (aluminium hydroxide) 20 ml, (C) whole milk 236 ml, and (D) non-dairy meal. (From *Surgery, Gynecology and Obstetrics* **114**: 9–14 (1962) with permission.)

Compared to gastric degradation, intestinal stability problems are not easily overcome because the small intestine is the main region where uptake occurs. Many peptides have stability problems in the small intestine due to degradation by pancreatic enzymes. Instability in the small intestine calls for approaches such as chemical modification of the peptide, synthesis of a more stable prodrug, a specifically designed dosage form which

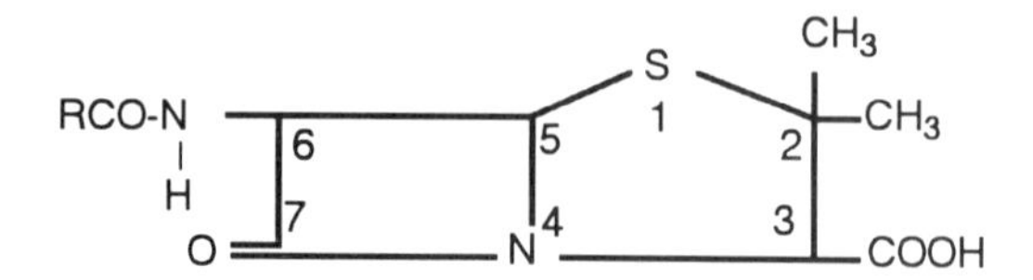

Fig. 5.5. The structure of penicillins. Penicillins are 6-acyl-amino-penicillinic acids and differ in their alcyl or aryl-alcyl substituent.

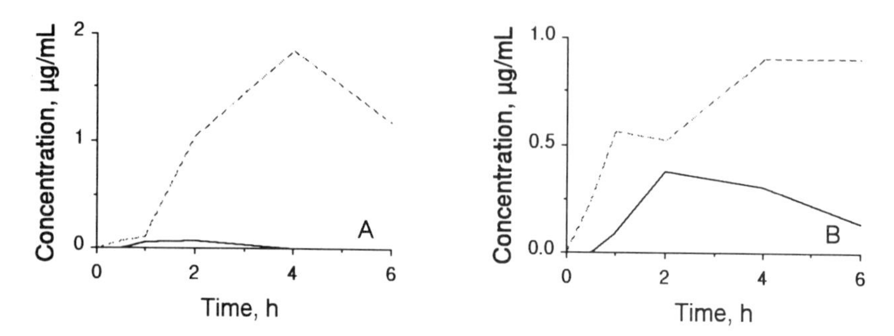

Fig. 5.6. Average blood erythromycin concentration following administration of 250 mg of (—) erythromycin stearate (which in the elevated small intestinal pH is converted to erythromycin base), and of (- - -) erythromycin estolate (which is stable in the small intestine) to 12 subjects. (A) Administration under fasting conditions; (B) administration under fed conditions. These plots were constructed according to data published in the *American Journal of Medical Sciences* **247**: 69–74 (1964).

releases the drug to the colon (provided that colonic uptake is satisfactory for the drug), or, as a last resort, parenteral administration.

Colonic degradation is important only in cases where drug absorption is not completed in the small intestine. Examples of compounds which present decreased stability in the lower intestine due the bacterial flora are shown in Table 5.2.

Table 5.2. Drugs that are biotransformed by the large intestinal flora

Atropine	Lactulose
Chloramphenicol	L-Dopa
Cyclamate	Morphine
Drugs with nitro or azo groups	Phenacetin
Digoxin	Sulfasalazine
Indomethacin	Sulfinpyrazone

5.1.2.5 Intestinal transit

Although in certain circumstances degradation and/or complexation of the drug in the GI tract are important limitations to bioavailability, the most common mechanism that leads to a reduction in drug concentration at the uptake sites is the movement of the luminal contents along the intestinal tract. As discussed later in more detail, transit through the small intestine is less variable than gastric emptying. Small intestinal transit time represents 10–25% of the total GI residence time and usually takes between 2 and 5 h. Transit through the large intestine takes longer and may vary considerably. Large intestinal transit time may therefore be important to drug absorption since, in contrast to what was believed in the past, colonic uptake is significant for a number of drugs. Table 5.3 shows some drugs for which intestinal transit represents a significant contribution to absorption.

Table 5.3. The GI absorption of these drugs can depend on small intestinal transit

Acyclovir	Ketoprofen
Diltiazem	Naproxen
Ibuprofen	Nifedipine
Indomethacin	Theophylline

Intestinal transit time is an important factor in drug absorption in the following situations:

(1) When the drug penetrates the mucosa very slowly. This is the case for acyclovir in the small intestine and with many drugs in the colon. In this case the extent of absorption is limited by the residence time at the uptake sites.
(2) When the ratio of dose to solubility is high (as in the case of chlorothiazide) and/or dissolution rate is slow.
(3) When the drug is taken up selectively at a specific location of the intestine (sometimes referred to as an *absorption window*). In this case, timely release of the drug is crucial for efficient absorption. An example is lithium carbonate, which is taken by the small intestine but not by the colon.
(4) When an extended-release system is administered. Any release of drug from the dosage form that occurs beyond the uptake sites is useless since no uptake can take place. It should be noted, however, for drugs that can be absorbed from the colon, colonic residence time of the extended-release dosage form becomes much more important than that of the small intestine. Fig. 5.7 shows an example with exprenolol. The longer the formulation remains in the colon the higher are the plasma concentration levels achieved.

5.1.3 Overall effect of processes that affect drug concentration at uptake sites

From the 'rate' point of view the most important processes that affect delivery of drug to and removal from the uptake sites are gastric emptying of the dosage form and/or the drug, complexation, degradation and intestinal transit. In many cases, degradation and complexation can be circumvented, or at least minimized, by chemical or formulation

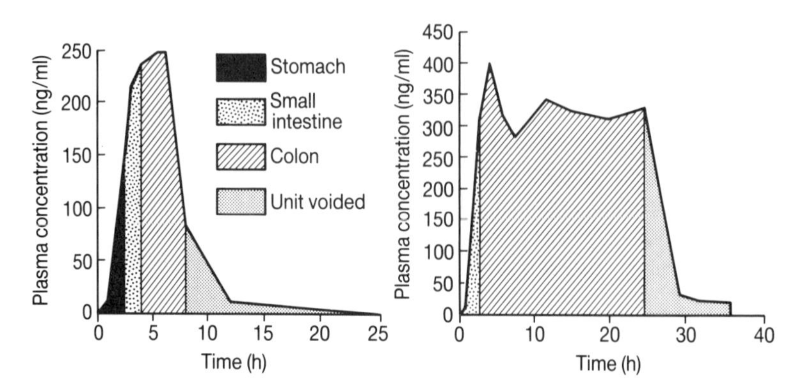

Fig. 5.7. Relationship between the transit of a sustained-release formulation of oxprenolol and the plasma concentration of the drug in two volunteers who exhibited different colonic transit times. (From the *British Journal of Clinical Pharmacology* **26**: 435–443 (1988) with permission.)

approaches so that they do not present a limitation to drug uptake. In contrast, gastric emptying and intestinal transit cannot be avoided since they are inherent in the GI physiology. Assuming that degradation and complexation do not occur, the processes that affect delivery to or removal from the uptake sites (Fig. 5.1) may be schematically summarized as in Fig. 5.8.

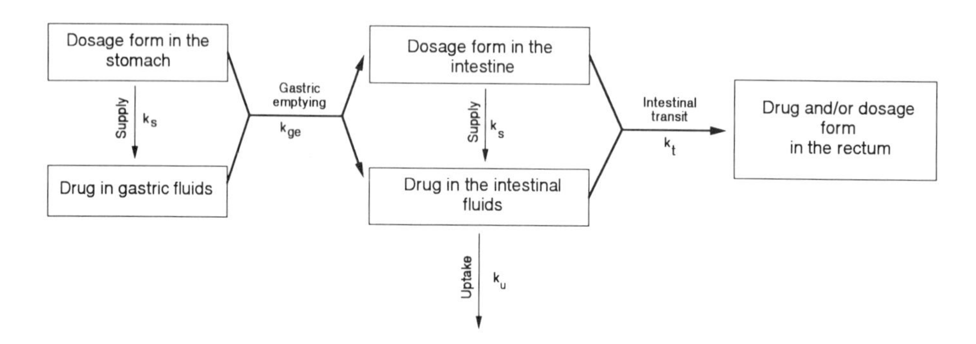

Fig. 5.8. Simplified model for the description of the major processes that affect the delivery of drug to and removal from the uptake sites.

The effect of a process which leads to delivery towards the uptake site(s) has from the kinetic point of view a different impact from a process which leads to removal of drug from the uptake site: processes that effect delivery occur in series with uptake and they must be completed for the uptake to take place (section 2.3.1.2). In contrast, processes that lead to removal from the uptake sites occur in parallel with uptake and compete with the arrival of the drug at the general circulation (section 2.3.1.1). Consider, for example, gastric emptying. The sequence of events required for absorption is as follows:

gastric emptying $\rightarrow$ drug in solution in intestine $\rightarrow$ drug uptake

If $R_{0,ge} \ll R_{0,s}$ and $R_{0,ge} \ll R_{0,u}$, then overall rate of uptake will be dictated by the slowest step, gastric emptying. If we assume that gastric emptying is a first-order process, i.e.

$$R_{0,ge} = k_{1,ge} C_0 V_\phi$$

then $R_{0,a}$, the rate of absorption, can be written as

$$R_{0,a} = k_{1,ge} C_0 V$$

where $R_{0,ge}$, $R_{0,s}$ $R_{0,u}$ and $R_{0,a}$ are the initial rates of gastric emptying, supply of GI fluids with drug, uptake and absorption, respectively, $k_{1,ge}$ is the first-order gastric emptying rate constant, C_0 is the initial drug concentration in the GI fluids and V is the volume of the GI fluids. It is obvious that whenever the drug does not present release or uptake limitations then the absorption rate is controlled by gastric emptying rate.

Parameters that may affect the GI transit of drugs and dosage forms include the presence of nutrients, pathological changes and the coadministration of other drugs. Therefore the essentials of the GI physiology and the GI transit characteristics as well as methods of study will be discussed next.

5.2 REVIEW OF THE ANATOMY AND PHYSIOLOGY OF THE GASTROINTESTINAL TRACT

Since most problems associated with per os administration occur usually after the dosage form arrives in the stomach, the following review focuses on GI rather than oesophageal physiology.

5.2.1 Review of the anatomy of the gastrointestinal tract

A schematic of the GI tract is shown in Fig. 5.9 and its basic anatomical and physiological characteristics are presented in Table 5.4.

Each part of the GI tract has been anatomically designed to accomplish specific goals. In general, the oesophagus serves simply as a conduit between the mouth and the stomach. The environmental and anatomical conditions of the stomach result in reduction in bacterial count of ingested material, liquefaction of solid food and, for many dosage forms, are conductive to disintegration and drug dissolution. The small intestine represents the primary area for digestion and absorption of food constituents and uptake of drugs. Although absorption may take place in the large intestine, the physiologically important events are the exchange (uptake or secretion) of minerals and water.

The anatomical characteristics important to drug absorption are presented next.

The stomach

For oral dosage forms the stomach may be considered as a reception area. Although the gastric mucosa is folded into ruggae which, to a limited extent, increase the epithelial surface area, the stomach is not the principal region for uptake because:

Table 5.4. Summary of GI physiology and anatomy in normal adults

Region of the GI tract			Characteristic
			Length (cm)[a]
Entire GI tract			500–700
Small intestine	Duodenum		20–30
	Jejunum		150–250
	Ileum		200–350
Large intestine	Caecum		≈7
	Colon		90–150
	Rectum		11–16
			Surface area (cm^2)
Entire GI tract			2×10^6
			Internal diameter (cm)
Small intestine			3–4[b]
Large intestine			6
			pH
Stomach	Fasted state		1.5–3
	Fed state		2–5
Small intestine	Duodenum	fasted state	≈6.1
		fed state	≈5.4
	Ileum		≈7[c]
Large intestine	Caecum and colon		5.5–7
	Rectum		≈7
			Volume (ml)
Stomach	Fasted state		25–50
	Capacity		1000–1600

a These numbers have been obtained from autopsy and hence may be somewhat elongated as compared to living tissue. For example, the small intestinal length of a live adult is estimated to be approximately 3.5 m.
b Decreases gradually from duodenum to ileum.
c pH may be as high as 8 at the terminal part of the ileum.

(a) the total mucosal area is small;
(b) the epithelium is dominated by surface mucosal cells rather than absorptive cells; and
(c) the gastric residence time is limited. In fact, the time required for drug release may exceed the residence time, in which case there will be little or no opportunity for gastric uptake of drug.

Anatomically the stomach may be divided into four areas (Fig. 5.10): the cardia, the fundus, the body and the antrum. In the absence of food, the stomach resembles a

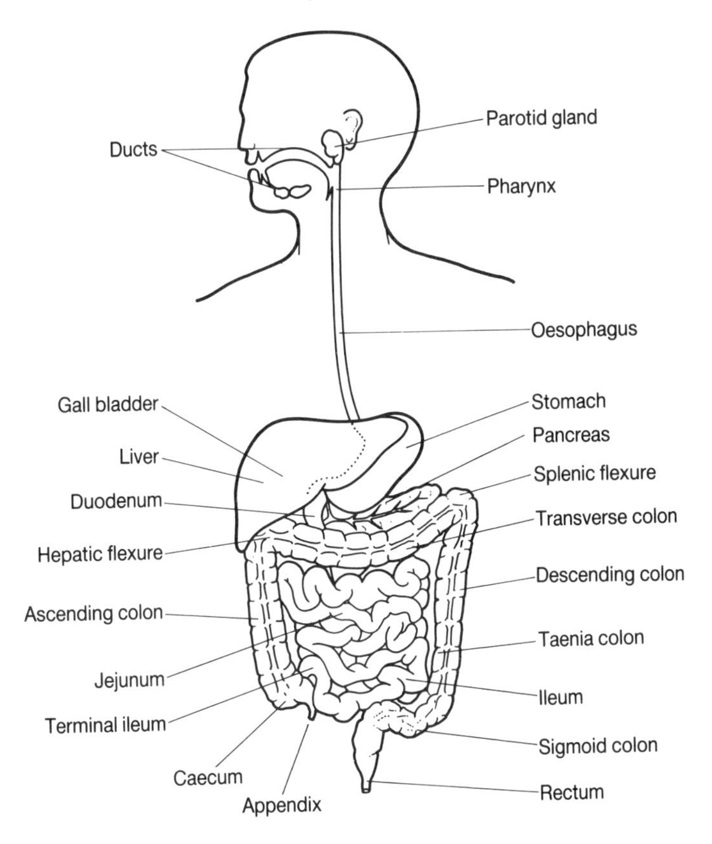

Fig. 5.9. Schematic representation of the gastrointestinal tract. (Reprinted with permission from *Oral Sustained Release Formulations. Design and Evaluation*, A. Yacobi and E. Halperin-Walega (eds), p. 127, Pergamon Press, Oxford, 1988.)

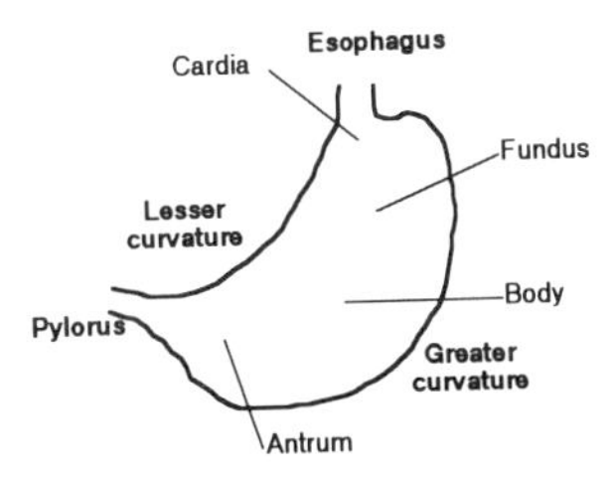

Fig. 5.10. Schematic representation of the stomach.

crumpled paper bag, with small quantities of chyme in the fundus. After meal ingestion, the bulk of the food remains in the fundus and the body, while in the antrum particle size is reduced and initial stages of digestion occur.

The small intestine

The small intestine can be divided into three areas (Fig. 5.9): the duodenum, the jejunum and the ileum. Like the stomach and most of the large intestine it is covered by a membranoid tissue, the mesentery, which contains arteries, veins, nerves and lymphatics. Bile and pancreatic fluid are secreted via the common bile duct (Fig. 9.25) and the greater pancreatic duct, which enter the duodenum 9–10 cm below the pylorus. Due to the huge amplification of surface area, the duodenum and jejunum are the main regions for drug uptake (section 6.1).

The large intestine

The large intestine is morphologically divided into three parts (Fig. 5.9):

— the caecum with the appendix, which are located just distal to the ileum;
— the colon, which is further divided anatomically into the ascending (≈15 cm), transverse (50 cm), descending (≈20–25 cm) and sigmoid colon (≈40 cm); and
— the rectum, which is the last part of the intestine and is contiguous with the anus.

The walls of caecum and ascending colon are usually folded into sacs, or haustra. Haustra are not fixed structures but are formed by contraction of the circular muscle. The main absorptive process of the large intestine is the active uptake of Na^+ and, consequently, water. As the chyme moves through the colon and water is reabsorbed, it becomes more viscous. Orally administered drugs may be absorbed from the large intestine, with the proximal colon being the most efficient site. A list of drugs which are absorbed in the colon is given in Table 5.5. The uptake rate is usually slower in the colon than in the small intestine, partly because the effective surface area is lower due to the lack of villi, and perhaps because of the increased viscosity of the colonic contents. Another potential limitation to colonic drug uptake is the biotransformation of the drug molecule by the bacterial flora.

Table 5.5. These drugs can be completely absorbed from the colon

Brompheniramine	Nifedipine
Diclofenac	Oxprenolol
Ibuprofen	Pseudoephedrine
Isosorbite dinitrate	Theophylline
Metoprolol	

The gastrointestinal wall

The wall of the stomach, the small intestine and the colon consists of four layers (Fig. 5.11): the serosa, the muscularis, the submucosa and the mucosa. The oesophagus and the distal part of the rectum lack a serosal layer and a mesentery. The muscle layer is divided into two layers: the longitudinal (external) and the circular (internal). The circular muscle layer controls the peristaltic movements of the GI tract. It is the dominant muscle layer in the pylorus, the caecum and colon. The submucosa consists of loose connective tissue,

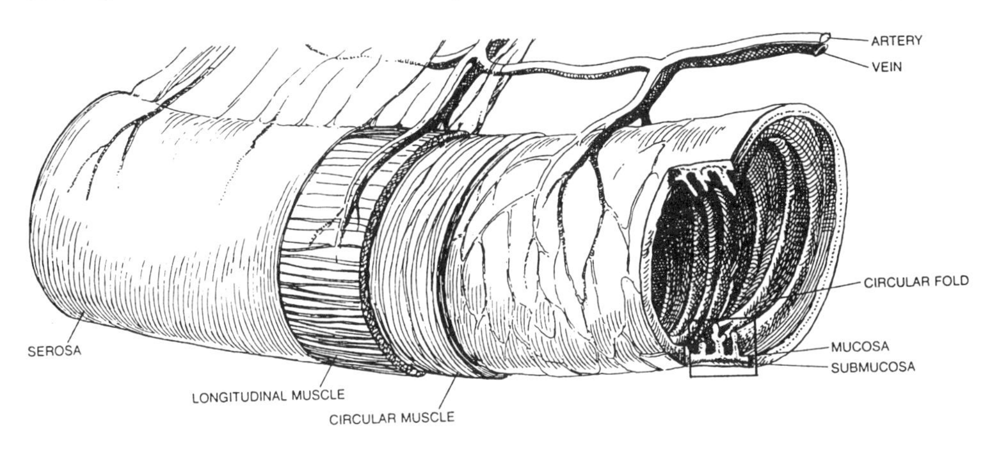

Fig. 5.11. Structure of the gastrointestinal wall.

and the mucosa consists of a muscle layer (usually longitudinal), glands, subepithelial connective tissue and a single layer of columnar epithelium. Between layers there is a network of blood vessels which is more dense in the internal than in the external layers. Because of the close proximity of blood vessels to the mucosa, the epithelium presents the major obstacle to arrival of the drug in the blood capillaries. The structure of the mucosa and its underlying capillary network is described in more detail in chapter 6, where the uptake mechanisms of drugs are discussed.

5.2.2 Review of the physiology of the gastrointestinal tract

This review addresses only those issues which are important to the delivery of the drug to and the removal from the uptake sites of the GI tract under normal physiological conditions. For issues related to nutrient absorption, water and electrolyte homeostasis, immunoreactivity mechanisms and the process of defaecation, the reader is referred to a general physiology text (see bibliography at the end of this chapter).

5.2.2.1 Composition of the luminal contents

Secretions of the mucosa of the entire gastrointestinal tract

Mucus is secreted throughout the entire GI tract. This is a viscous, slippery, aqueous fluid which covers the internal area of the GI lumen and consists mainly (up to 95%) of an aqueous electrolyte solution. Approximately 5% consists of a complex mixture of glycoproteins which impart viscosity to the mucus. The remainder consists of micro-organisms, intracellular organelles, macromolecules and plasma components. The ability of mucus to protect the sensitive epithelial cells is attributed to the glycoproteins, which are usually called mucins. Although the structure, the size and the contents of mucins vary with the region of the GI lumen, a common feature is the high carbohydrate content (more than 50% w/w) which imparts viscoelastic properties. The type, molecular weight and concentration of polysaccharides determine the ability of mucus to protect the epithelial cells. Intestinal mucins consist of glycoproteins which vary in size (from 2.5×10^5 to

2×10^6 Da) and in the structure of the carbohydrate. The most common amino acids are threonine, serine, proline, glycine and glutaminic acid. The most common carbohydrates are fucose (an aldose-pentose), galactose and *N*-acetylglucosamine. Functions of the mucous layer include:

(a) coating of particles present in the GI lumen (bacteria, destroyed cells, inert non-digestible particles, food residues, etc.) so that they can move along the GI tract without injuring the membrane of the epithelial cells. The hydrophilic properties and the viscoelasticity of the mucin make it an efficient biological lubricant;
(b) protection of the gastric mucosa from the destructive effects of acids, alcohol, and other ingested irritants, and of the small intestinal mucosa from proteolytic pancreatic enzymes;
(c) protection of the GI epithelium from invasion by microorganisms which may be ingested with food or which colonize the lower part of the GI tract;
(d) maintaining the mucosa in a hydrated condition via the ability of the mucins to hold water and ions.

Secretions of the gastric mucosa

Apart from mucus, the gastric mucosa secretes pepsinogen, hydrochloric acid and ions (mainly Na^+ and K^+). Urease and lipase are also secreted but their participation in digestion are of limited significance. Gastric secretion is stimulated by the presence of food, but even in the fasted state there is usually approximately 20 ml of secretion in the stomach.

Pepsinogen is a proenzyme which, in the presence of acid, is converted to pepsin (a proteolytic enzyme, active in solutions of pH 3 or less). It is secreted in significant quantities only in the presence of food and its secretion is regulated by the hormone secretin.

From the physiological point of view, the most important constituent of gastric chyme is hydrochloric acid because it acts as an antiseptic to the gastric contents and controls activation of pepsin. The acid concentration in the gastric contents varies between the fasted and fed state. When the stomach is emptied of food, stimuli for secretion, apart from those occurring intermittently during the interdigestive migrating motility complex (section 5.2.2.2), die out. Upon food intake, gastric secretion is stimulated through the cephalic, gastric and intestinal phases. During the cephalic phase, secretion occurs in response to stimulation of afferent nerves in the central nervous system. The gastric phase begins when food enters the stomach, with the major stimuli being the distension of the stomach and digestion of food (chiefly of protein). Finally, the intestinal phase accounts for the secretion stimulated by the presence of chyme in the duodenum and/or jejunum.

The duration of gastric secretion depends on the protein content in the ingested food and also on the serum gastrin levels. Proteins have high buffering capacity and their digestion products are the major stimulus for gastrin release. Owing to the buffering capacity of proteins the intragastric pH is significantly increased immediately after the ingestion of food rich in proteins. Gradually, the secreted acid reduces the pH of the stomach contents until the gastrin secretion is interrupted, with consequent interruption of acid secretion. Thus, following meal consumption, hydrochloric acid is secreted for a period which is partly determined by the meal's buffering capacity.

Secretions of the small intestinal mucosa

Duodenal secretions include mucus, enzymes and isotonic fluid. The amount of mucin that is secreted by the duodenum represents only about 0.5% of the secretions of the glands and crypts.

The most important enzyme that is secreted from the duodenal mucosa is enterokinase, an enzyme necessary for the activation of peptidases. Amylase and various other peptidases are also secreted in small quantities. Most of these enzymes are actually constituents of the brush border (section 6.1). The continuous exfoliation of the epithelial cells releases the enzymes into the lumen (every day about 17 billion cells are sloughed off into the lumen).

The aqueous part of the secretions of the small intestine contains Na^+, Cl^-, K^+ and mainly HCO_3^-. As in the stomach, the secretion rate in the duodenum increases with food intake. In the case of the jejunal mucosa, secretions are observed only during digestion.

Secretions of the large intestine mucosa

The secretions of the large intestine consist mainly of mucus and alkaline solution which contains HCO_3^-, Na^+ and K^+. Lysozyme (a hydrolase responsible for balancing the bacterial content of the colonic flora) is also secreted.

Other physiological constituents of the intestine

Apart from the mucosal secretions, there are several other sources of luminal constituents.

Pancreatic secretions: Pancreatic secretions (200–800 ml/d) are discharged to the duodenum during the digestion process. They constitute of two fractions: an isotonic alkaline (rich in HCO_3^-) aqueous solution, and a secretion rich in enzymes. The HCO_3^- ions increase the pH of the gastric chyme that enters the duodenum and their concentration in the pancreatic fluid increases with increase in the secretion rate, in a manner analogous to hydrochloric acid secretion in the stomach. Increased HCO_3^- concentration is accompanied by a decrease in the concentration of other anions (such as Cl^-) so that the ratio between cations (K^+, Na^+) and anions (Cl^-, HCO_3^-) is held constant. Pancreatic fluid contains three types of enzymes (in terms of their ability to digest carbohydrates, lipids and proteins), the total concentration of which is 0.1–10%. Specifically, pancreatic fluid contains amylase, at least three lipolytic enzymes, and the proteolytic enzymes trypsin, chymotrypsin and carboxypeptidase.

Gallbladder secretions: The gallbladder is continuously supplied with bile from the liver. However, maximal contraction of the gallbladder and emptying to the duodenum occurs only in response to the consumption of a meal (section 9.3.3.2). Bile consists of two fractions: an alkaline fraction resembling that of the pancreatic fluid, i.e. it contains ions (HCO_3^-, Cl^-, Na^+ and K^+), bilirubin (an aliphatic tetrapyrole compound, produced by catabolism of haem, which imparts a yellow colour to the bile) as glucuronic conjugate, enzymes and some metal ions; and a lipophilic fraction which contains mainly bile acids, lecithin (a phospholipid) and cholesterol (a steroid).

Bile has five major constituents: water, lecithin, bile acids, cholesterol and bilirubin. Lecithin forms mixed micelles with bile acids, thus providing a means of solubilizing cholesterol (which otherwise would not be in solution, Fig. 5.12). The most important constituents of the bile in terms of their effect to drug absorption are the bile acids, the most common of which are shown in Fig. 5.13. The primary bile acids, synthesized in the liver from cholesterol, include trihydroxycholic acid and dihydroxychenodeoxycholic acid. In the intestine those molecules are dehydroxylated to form the secondary bile acids, deoxycholic and lithocholic acids. Both the primary and the secondary bile acids are always present as the salt form of amino acid conjugates. In the intestine the bile salts can be reabsorbed, by passive mechanisms in the duodenum and the jejunum or by active processes in the ileum. Absorption is highly efficient and more than 95% of the bile salts entering the small intestine is reabsorbed there. Most of the reabsorbed bile salts are transported through the portal blood to the liver and then recycled to the gallbladder (enterohepatic circulation, section 9.3.3.2). Because enterohepatic cycling is so frequent, about 25% of the bile acid pool escapes into the colon each day. Some of those bile acids are absorbed in the colon by passive diffusion. The rest (about 500 mg/d) is excreted in the stools after bacterial cleavage of the peptide linkage and dehydroxylation.

The role of bile salts in drug absorption is related to their surfactant properties and their ability to form micelles (an example is given in Fig. 5.12). At concentrations lower than the critical micellar concentration (CMC) bile salts exert wetting effects on drug particles and consequently increase the effective surface area for dissolution (section

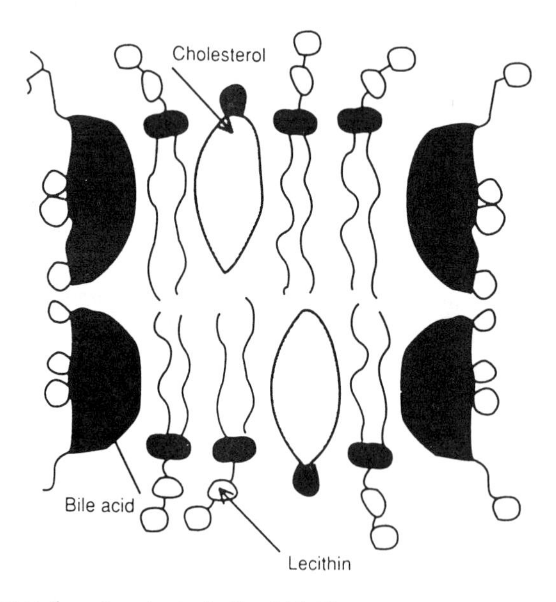

Fig. 5.12. Cross-section of a mixed micelle which illustrates the relationship of bile salts and lecithin to cholesterol. This is the structure of the micelles immediately after their discharge from the gall bladder. During digestion monoglycerides are also present. (From the *Journal of Clinical Gastroenterology* **10** (Suppl. 2): S12–S13 (1988) with permission.)

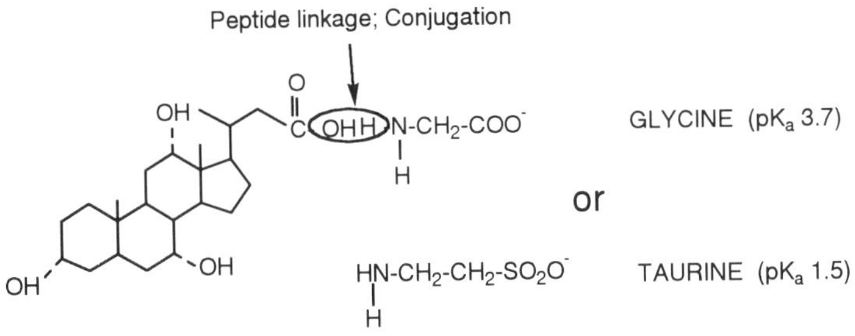

Cholic acid (Primary Bile Acid)
All -OH in α configuration

-OH on 3 and 7, not on 12: Chenodeoxycholic Acid - Primary
-OH on 7 and 12, not on 7: Deoxycholic Acid - Secondary
-OH on 3, not on 7 and 12: Lithocholic Acid - Secondary
-OH on 3 sulfated : Sulfolithocholic Acid
-OH on 3α, -OH on 7β : Ursodeoxycholic Acid - Tertiary

Fig. 5.13. Structure of the most common bile acids. Cholic acid is bound by a peptide linkage to glycine or taurine. At the right-hand side of the figure, the ionization constants of glycocholic acid and of taurocholic acid are shown.

4.2.2.3). At concentrations higher than the CMC, the interior of the bile salt micelle offers a more lipophilic (compared to the rest of the GI fluids) environment which enhances solubility of some sparingly water-soluble drugs. Gallbladder emptying after meal intake leads to high bile salt concentrations in the duodenum (usually 10–20 mM) which in all cases is at least equal to the CMC (≤1 mM in the presence of lecithin). Therefore, administration of a sparingly soluble drug with a meal may facilitate its solution process since the bile salts will act as both solubilizing and wetting agents. By contrast, bile salt concentration in the fasted state at the duodenum is usually 0–5 mM and in this concentration range they act primarily as wetting agents.†

Secretions of the appendix: Like the Peyer's patches (section 6.1), the lymphoid tissue of the appendix is one of the regions where antibodies are produced. Unless drainage is obstructed by the intestinal movements and/or the relative anatomical position of the intestine, the appendix secretes a fluid rich in antibodies into the caecum. By the time that the luminal contents reach the caecum, absorption of nutrients and drugs is usually complete, so the physiological significance of the fluid of the appendix is minimal.

The intestinal flora: Towards the ileo-caecal valve a significant increase in the number of microorganisms can be observed. In the colon, 60% of the weight of the liquid contents is accounted for by anaerobic bacteria, the most common of which are *Bifidobacterium*, *Lactobacillus* and *Bacteroides*. The bacterial content of the colon can be 10^8 colony-forming units per millilitre of wet sample (Table 5.6) or even higher. The main activity of

† Although information on the mechanism is limited, certain bile salts may also increase the mucosal permeability of the drug, acting as penetration enhancers (section 6.3).

the gut flora is the digestion of the plant cell walls and other macromolecular compounds which are not digested in the upper GI tract. Digestion of these materials is achieved mainly with reductions or hydrolytic reactions.

Table 5.6. Distribution of the gut flora in humans[a]

Region of the GI tract	Viable count/gram of wet sample
Stomach	$0–10^6$
Initial part of the small intestine	$0–10^6$
Terminal part of the small intestine	$10^6–10^7$
Large intestine	$10^7–10^8$
Rectum/faeces	$10^{10}–10^{11}$

[a] The oral cavity contains approximately $10^5–10^7$ bacteria per gram of wet sample.

5.2.2.2 *Motility of the gastrointestinal tract*

Patterns of contractions in the upper gastrointestinal tract
As in many other animals that consume food on a discrete basis, two patterns of upper GI motility are observed in humans:

(1) the interdigestive motility pattern; and
(2) the digestive motility pattern.

The interdigestive pattern dominates in the fasted state. The primary function of this pattern is to periodically clean the residual content of the upper GI tract in the fasted state and therefore it is organized into alternating phases of activity and quiescence. Each cycle lasts approximately 2 h (90–120 min) and consists of four phases. The duration of each phase is controlled by the concentration of the hormone *motilin* in blood. A pictorial representation of the four interdigestive motility phases (relative intensity and frequency) is given in fig. 5.14. Phase I corresponds to 40–50% of the cycle duration, phase II to 20–30%, phase III to 10–15% and phase IV to 0–5%. During phase I a relatively limited number of weak-intensity contractions are observed. Phase II is initially characterized by irregular contractions of medium amplitude. However, the amplitude is gradually increased and it is at the end of this phase that the onset of the discharge of gastric contents occurs. Phase III corresponds to the period during which a maximum in the amplitude and frequency of contractions is observed. The basic characteristic of this phase is the high amplitude and the regularity of the contractions (three to four contractions per minute). Discharge of cellular debris, mucus and particles is complete during this phase. The transitional phase IV period (Fig. 5.14) corresponds to a reduction in intensity and frequency of contractions. However, the transition between phase III and phase I is sometimes quite abrupt.

This cyclic pattern can be interrupted during any phase by the administration of food. It is also important to point out that each phase is not observed at the same time throughout the upper GI tract. Each phase is initiated in the lower oesophageal sphincter or at the

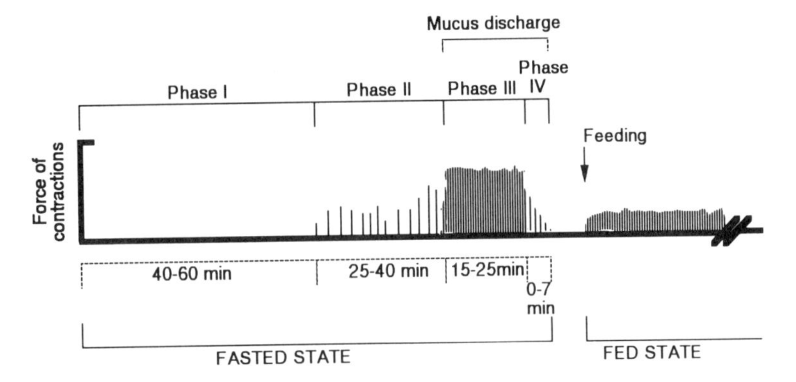

Fig. 5.14. Schematic of the two motility patterns (interdigestive and digestive) of the upper GI tract. (Reprinted with permission from *Oral Sustained Release Formulations. Design and Evaluation*, A. Yacobi and E. Halperin-Walega (eds), p. 130, Pergamon Press, Oxford 1988.)

gastric pacemaker, then propagates over the entire stomach, the duodenum, the jejunum and ileum, where it finishes. The time required for a phase to pass through the upper GI is approximately equal to the duration of a cycle (90–120 min). In other words, when a phase III contraction ends at the ileum, the phase III of the next cycle is starting in the proximal stomach. The coordination of activity at adjacent and distant sites involves reflexes in the intrinsic and/or the extrinsic nerves and humoral agents. The continuously cycling pattern of contractions led to the name *interdigestive migrating motility complex* (IMMC) to characterize the interdigestive motility pattern. Finally it should be mentioned, that propagation of the GI contents does not occur during all phases of the fasted state motility pattern. Only during phase III are complete gastric emptying and rapid transit of the intestinal contents observed.

The second motility pattern, the digestive or fed motility pattern, is observed in response to meal ingestion. As for the regulation of the interdigestive motility pattern, regulation of the fed pattern may involve humoral substances (such as gastrin, cholecystokynin, glucagon, insulin, etc.), extrinsic nerves and intrinsic nerves. In the stomach, the pattern of contractions is such that solid food is reduced to particles of less than 1 mm in diameter and emptied through the pylorus as a suspension at a rate which is controlled by feedback mechanisms in the small intestine. The fed state pattern aims at the propagation of the luminal contents along the intestine at a rate slow enough to ensure satisfactory nutrient absorption. It is characterized by regular and frequent contractions (four to five contractions per minute) of an amplitude similar to that of phase II (Fig. 5.14). Although chyme transit during this pattern is continual, it occurs at a slower rate than that of phase III in the fasted state.

The type of contractions in the small intestine may differ significantly in terms of their intensity, the length of the segment that they travel over (usually a few centimetres), and the duration of activity (from a few seconds to several minutes). Depending on the activity of adjacent loci, the mode of contractions generally consist of either:

(1) rhythmic segmentation, i.e. temporary concentric or eccentric contractions at one locus. These may be phasal (with distinctive beginning and ending) or tonic (indefinite beginning or ending and of longer duration than phasal contractions); or
(2) peristaltic contractions: this type of contraction leads to transit of chyme and, therefore, occurs at adjacent loci in an oral to aboral sequence.

The duration of the fed state depends basically on the physicochemical characteristics of the ingested meal and to a lesser extent on the volume and/or quantity of food. For example, 400 ml of saline do not interrupt the IMMC, whereas 400 ml of milk induce the fed state for 3–4 h. In general, a meal of 450 kcal will interrupt the fasted state motility for about 3–4 h.

Patterns of contractions in the lower gastrointestinal tract
Usually nutrient and drug absorption is completed before the chyme arrives at the ileocaecal valve. However, in certain cases drugs (Table 5.2) and nutrients (usually polysaccharides not digested in the small intestine) can be digested and absorbed in the colon.

In the fasted state, colonic motility has no cyclic or migrating character. Weak tonic contractions lead to formation of sacculations known as haustra (section 6.1). In the presence of food some peristaltic contractions are observed; however, these are weak and possess minimal propagating ability (the mean propagation rate is approximately 5 cm/h). It is worth mentioning that food residues may be retained in the large intestine for up to 3–5 days. This high residence time may offset the limited surface area and the increased intra-colonic viscosity, resulting in an additional absorption site for drugs.

5.3 TRANSIT OF THE DOSAGE FORM AND THE DRUG THROUGH THE GASTROINTESTINAL TRACT

Transit along the GI lumen is a complex process which is affected by both the anatomy and the motility characteristics of the various parts of the GI tract.

Since the patterns of oesophageal, gastric or colonic transit differentiate between solids and liquids, the discussion of transit will be addressed separately for solids and liquids in these regions. In contrast, transit along the small intestine is basically similar for liquids and solids and will be discussed at the same time.

5.3.1 Oesophageal transit

5.3.1.1 Transit of liquid dosage forms
Liquids pass along the oesophagus faster than solids. The transit time of 10 ml in a healthy adult in the supine position is about 20 s and even less if the subject is in the standing position. Even so, some liquid dosage forms may be irritating for the oesophageal mucosa, especially if they are formulated at low pH. Examples include solutions of tetracyclines, ferrous salts and quinidine.

5.3.1.2 Transit of non-digestible solids (solid dosage forms and/or drug particles)

In adults with normal oesophageal function, the transit of solids is usually accomplished without difficulty and regardless of the motility pattern is completed in under 2 min. In general, bigger and spherical dosage forms may pass slower than those which are small and elliptical. In addition, transit is facilitated if the dosage form is administered in the standing rather than the supine position, and if it is accompanied by some water (about 100 ml). If the dosage form is hydrated very quickly and adheres to the oesophageal mucosa, this may cause problems in terms of both delay in drug absorption and topical irritation of the oesophagus. Acetaminophen and antipyrine have been shown to exhibit delayed absorption due to altered oesophageal transit depending on the dosage form and the administration procedure.

5.3.2 Gastric emptying

In contrast to the oesophageal transit where both longitudinal and circular muscles are involved in propagation, gastric emptying is governed entirely by the contractions of the circular muscle. Therefore, gastric emptying is totally controlled by the two motility patterns. Table 5.7 gives an idea of the variability of the gastric emptying rates as a function of the type of dosage form and the motility state.

Table 5.7. Representative gastric residence times (expressed as half-lives of gastric emptying) for several types of dosage forms[a]

Dosage form	Fasted state or after light meal	Fed state
Aqueous solution	8, 18 (4)	40 (14)
Suspension (microspheres)	46 (32–87)	58 (34–75)
Pellets (<2 mm)	99 (7), 70 (60–150)	285 (45), 119 (15)
Tablets (indigestible)	45 (15–120)	180–780
Monolithic dosage form	183 (77)	>550

[a] These representative data have been collected from studies done in the 1980s. The variability is shown in parentheses as standard error of the mean or as range.

5.3.2.1 Gastric emptying of liquid dosage forms

Gastric emptying of non-nutrient liquids (fasted state)

The emptying process of liquids with volume of less than 50 ml is controlled by the IMMC. During phase I gastric emptying is negligible, whereas it reaches its maximum during phase III. The bigger the volume the less dependent is gastric emptying on the IMMC.

First order kinetics apply when volumes are about 200 ml or larger. The half-life of gastric emptying of 400 ml saline is typically 5–10 min. In this volume range, the rate of gastric emptying is controlled by feedback mechanisms. There are two types of small intestinal receptors which may affect the gastric emptying of non-nutrient liquids. One is activated by H^+ and the other by the osmolality of the gastric chyme that reaches the small intestine. The lower the pH and the further from isoosmotic the liquid is, the slower will be its rate of emptying.

Using the canine model it has been shown that volumes bigger than 300 ml induce the fed state (i.e. disruption of one cycle is observed). However, if the viscosity of the liquid is elevated this induction happens at lower volumes.

Gastric emptying of nutrient liquids (fed state)

Nutrient liquids with volumes more than 200 ml empty slower than non-nutrient liquids of identical volume. Kinetics are approximately zero order. The energy content of the liquid appears to be the most important determinant of the rate of emptying. A high energy content decreases the rate of gastric emptying. For example, if glucose is added to 400 ml of saline at concentrations of 0.2 kcal/ml or 1 kcal/ml then the half-life for gastric emptying becomes 10 min and 70 min, respectively (compared to approximately 8 min in the absence of nutrient). The delay in gastric emptying resulting from ingestion of proteins, lipids or carbohydrates is similar provided that the energy content is the same, with an emptying rate of about 2 kcal/min. The calories per gram of the basic food categories are given in Table 5.8.

Table 5.8. Energy content per gram (kcal/g) of various foodstuff categories

Carbohydrates	4
Lipids	9
Proteins	4
Alcohol	7

Other factors that affect the gastric emptying of liquids

Apart from the presence of nutrients, gastric emptying of liquids is affected by other factors such as viscosity and disease states.

Liquids with elevated viscosity empty slower from the stomach. However, under some circumstances it is the lag time prior to the onset of emptying that changes rather than the actual emptying rate. In addition, if the colonic content of the liquid is such that feedback mechanisms are fully activated, elevation of the viscosity will have practically no further effect on gastric emptying.

5.3.2.2 *Gastric emptying of non-digestible solids (solid dosage forms and drug particles)*

Fasted state

Solid dosage forms arrive initially in the fundus (Fig. 5.10). If administration is accompanied by less than 50 ml of water, both the water and the dosage form leave the stomach in a manner that depends on the phase of the IMMC. Substantial transport to the duodenum occurs only during phase III.

If administration is accompanied by more than 50 ml of water, gastric emptying will depend on the physical characteristics of the solids. If gelatin capsules or immediate-release tablets are administered, drug particles or granules may disperse over the intragastric area. Particles with size less than 0.5 mm may become trapped in the mucus and empty only when mucus discharge occurs in conjunction with phase III contractions (Fig. 5.15). Particles of ≤1 mm size and about 1 g/ml density will empty the stomach first with the water according to the pattern of emptying described above (*Gastric emptying of non-nutrient liquids*). Gastric emptying of the rest of the particles and granules will be contingent on the phase of the IMMC. In general, 2–6 mm particles empty only during phase III. Gastric emptying of non-disintegrating dosage forms with a diameter more than 6 mm (monolithic dosage forms) occurs only during phase III contractions, which may be any time from a few minutes up to several hours following administration. Depending on the shape and the flexibility of the dosage form it is possible for the gastric residence time to be delayed up to 24 h. In fact, the intra-subject variability in the gastric emptying times of monolithic dosage forms (with consequent variability in bioavailability) has led to their gradual replacement by multiparticulate dosage forms.

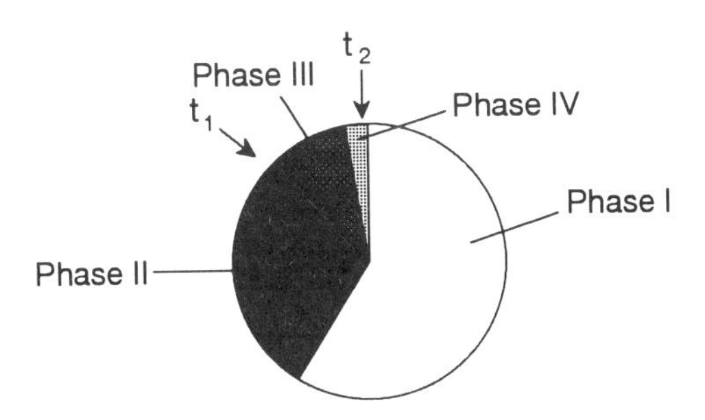

Fig. 5.15. Importance of the relative duration of the interdigestive motility phases in the stomach on the gastric emptying of particles or granules with diameter smaller than 0.5 mm or larger than 1 mm. If disintegration and deaggregation are not rate limiting, then administration at time $t = t_1$ would result in immediate gastric emptying. In contrast, administration at $t = t_2$ would retard gastric emptying until next phase III of the IMMC.

A significant consequence of the non-uniform pattern of gastric emptying of solids is the observation of two peaks in plots of drug concentration in serum as a function of time in the absorptive phase (Fig. 5.16). Apparently, between two consecutive phase III periods little gastric emptying (and, consequently, uptake) occurs whereas during phase III delivery to the absorptive sites in the small intestine becomes maximal.†

Fed state

The gastric emptying of non-digestible solids in the fed state is controlled by intragastric hydrodynamics. Important variables to consider include the size and the density of the

† Double peak phenomenon in the absorptive phase of concentration versus time plots can be seen with solutions, too.

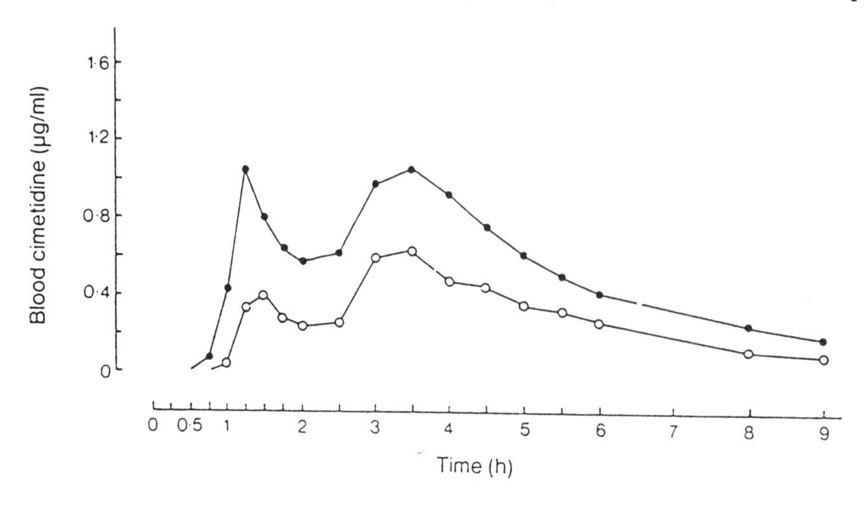

Fig. 5.16. Administration of 200 mg (○) or 400 mg (●) cimetidine on a fasting stomach in one patient results in two peaks due to non-uniform gastric emptying. (From the *British Journal of Clinical Pharmacology* 7: 23–31 (1979) with permission.)

solids, as well as the viscosity and emptying rate of the liquid fraction of the gastric contents.

In general, particles with diameter of less than about 1 mm empty with the liquid fraction of the meal (see above, *Gastric emptying of nutrient liquids*). Particles of bigger size show a lag time prior to the onset of emptying. If the diameter is 2–5 mm and density is about 1 g/ml the particles enter the duodenum with rate inversely proportional to their size according to a pattern similar to that followed by the liquid fraction of the meal. In this size range density can play a significant role. Significant deviations in dosage form density from that of the liquid food result in a delay in gastric emptying. If the size is bigger than 5 mm, particles remain in the stomach until the digestive motility pattern is replaced with the fasting pattern and phase III contractions occur.

Other factors that affect gastric emptying of solids

Apart from food, GI motility is affected by additional factors such as gender, age, emotional status, certain diseases, and administration of other drugs which can therefore indirectly affect the gastric emptying of solids.

In young men the gastric residence time of big particles (of about 7 mm diameter and greater) is significantly shorter than in older people. Aggression and stress accelerate gastric emptying whereas depression and vigorous exercise reduce the rate of gastric emptying. Gastric trauma or pain, migraines, gastric ulcer, coeliac disease and diabetes tend to decrease the gastric emptying of solids. Likewise, narcotic analgesics (such as morphine and meperidine), anticholinergics (such as atropine and propantheline), beta agonists (such as isoproterenol and salbutamol), certain hormones (such as somatostatin), and L-dopa all decrease the rate of appearance of solids in the duodenum. In contrast, a duodenal ulcer, and beta blockers such as propranolol and metoclopramide, are associated with an acceleration in gastric emptying.

To close the discussion of gastric emptying, an example indicative of the significance of this process to drug absorption is presented.

Example 5.1: For a drug A administered orally as an immediate-release tablet with 250 ml of water, the values of the first-order duodenal uptake rate constant (which is calculated using one of the methods described in section 6.4.2.2), the first order dissolution rate constants at pH 1.2 and at pH 6.0 (which are determined *in vitro* as described in section 4.4), and the first-order gastric emptying rate constant (which was estimated using one of the techniques described below in this chapter) are 11.9 h^{-1}, 0.00140 min^{-1} and 0.090 min^{-1} and 5.45 h^{-1}, respectively. What is the rate-limiting step for absorption?

Answer: Based on the values of the rate constants the mean times (which in the case of first-order kinetics are the inverse of the rate constants, section 2.2) of each process are calculated to be

Process	*Mean time (min)*
Duodenal uptake	5.04
Dissolution at pH 1.2	714
Dissolution at pH 6.0	11.1
Gastric emptying	11.0

Based on these numbers, dissolution is minimal during gastric residence and, consequently, uptake from the gastric mucosa is negligible. Dissolution in duodenum and gastric emptying occur at similar rates and both will most likely affect the absorption, since they occur more slowly than uptake.

5.3.3 Small intestinal transit

Small intestinal transit does not differ much between solids and liquids and is independent of meal intake (provided that viscosity is not altered significantly) (Fig. 5.17). Also, pathological situations such as those which affect gastric emptying or large intestine physiology such as diarrhoea, constipation or ulcerative colitis do not significantly affect transit through the small intestine. For solids, specifically, transit time is independent of density (for densities lower than 3 g/ml) and size (for sizes smaller than 25 × 9 mm, Fig. 5.17). The different transit behaviour between the stomach and small intestine may be attributed, apart from physiological differences, to some key anatomical differences between these two parts of the GI tract, such as:

— The stomach is more fixed in position than the small intestine, which is suspended in the abdominal area by the mesentery.
— In the stomach, the pylorus is located above the stomach curvature (Fig. 5.10), which makes emptying from this region difficult. In contrast, the small intestine lacks variations in its internal diameter (the ileo-caecal junction does not constitute significant problems since it is a normal continuation of the ileal wall).
— The internal diameter of the small intestine is much smaller and the effects of the contractions in the mixing and the velocity of the chyme are more significant.

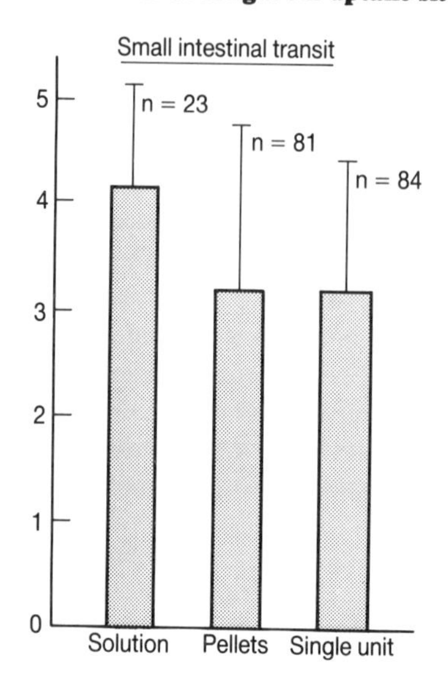

Fig. 5.17. Small intestinal times (mean + SD) of various dosage forms. The size of the pellets was approximately 0.3–1.2 mm and the size of the monolithic dosage forms varied from 2.5 mm (diameter) to 25 × 9 mm. Each column includes data from subjects who ingested the test dosage forms under fasting or fed conditions; *n* is the number of subjects. (From *Gut* **27**: 886–892 (1986) with permission.)

Generally, the time between administration and arrival at the ileo-caecal valve is approximately 4–8 h in the fasted state and 8–12 h in the fed state. This difference may be attributed almost entirely to differences in gastric emptying and not in small intestinal transit. Under most conditions small intestinal transit takes 3–4 h (range: 1–6 h).

5.3.4 Large intestinal transit

The time for arrival of a drug into the colon may range from 3 to 20 h. In contrast to the small intestine, in the large intestine dispersion of the drug may occur and colonic transit varies considerably.

In general, particles with size bigger than 6 mm (e.g. monolithic dosage forms) pass through the large intestine faster than solutions or smaller particles. Dosage forms which have approximately the size of a capsule or a tablet pass through the colon in 15–30 h (range: 1–60 h) regardless of their density. In contrast, solutions and small particles remain in the colon for 25–40 h (range: 6–50 h).

Colonic transit varies with gender (1.5 times slower in women) and certain pathological situations (for example, in the presence of diarrhoea the transit time is halved and in Crohn's disease is increased). In contrast, inflammatory bowel disease and irritable bowel syndrome have little effect on transit times.

5.3.5 Methods for increasing gastrointestinal residence time

Since the small intestine represents the most favourable area for uptake, the objective in the majority of cases is to increase the residence of the dosage form and/or the drug molecules in regions above the ileo-caecal valve. However, since the small intestine transit is limited to 3–4 h and difficult to manipulate, the modification of the upper GI transit is usually endeavoured by increasing the gastric residence time.

An increase in the transit time through the upper GI tract is especially desired when:

— modified-release formulations are administered;
— the drug is taken up by the GI epithelium very slowly;
— absorption is dissolution rate limited; and/or
— absorption from the colon is minimal.

Delay of gastric emptying may be achieved by adjusting the dosing conditions (for example by coadministering the drug with food) in conjunction with the physical characteristics of the administered formulation (size, density, etc.). Another way may be to use materials which adhere to the gastric mucosa and therefore do not empty with the rest of the contents.

5.3.5.1 Adjustment of dosing conditions

The ability to alter gastric emptying by changing the conditions of administration conditions has been discussed previously in this chapter. For drugs which are not satisfactorily absorbed from the colon, twice-a-day administration (the usual dosing regimen of extended-release dosage forms) requires approximately 10 h of residence time of the drug in the upper GI tract. Since the transit from the small intestine is completed within 3–4 h, it is necessary that the dosage form be retained in the stomach for at least 5 h. This goal may be more easily achieved if the dosage form is coadministered with food.

5.3.5.2 Dosage form strategies

The use of gastric retention devices is one way of increasing gastric residence time. The concept is to form *in situ* a device of dimensions too great to empty under normal motility conditions. Often this is achieved by unfolding or swelling. Sometimes during the swelling process they trap air bubbles, reducing the density and consequently floating on the top of the gastric fluids. This results in a further delay in emptying. Such dosage forms may be retained in the stomach (or eventually accumulated in the colon) for very long periods. The variability in retention is the main reason this type of device has not been widely employed. Recently, the use of bioerodible materials to ensure more reproducible transit behaviour has gained much interest but this approach is still in the research phase.

5.3.5.3 Bioadhesives

The use of polymers with adhesive properties in oral dosage formulations was one of the most popular topics in pharmaceutics research in the 1980s and continues to be of interest. The concept of using mucosal adhesives has its origin in the 1960s when dentists first used such materials to improve the fit and stability of artificial dentures in the oral cavity.

The most frequently studied material with bioadhesive properties in the GI is polycarbophil (polyacrylic acid cross-linked with divinyl alcohol). Although the most important factors that affect the extent of bioadhesion have been elucidated (i.e. ionization, density, hydrophobicity and polymer's hydration rate), the practical applicability of this approach is yet to be determined. Two potential limitations are that:

— the ingested dosage form may adhere to the oesophageal wall; and more importantly,
— the physiological mucus turnover in the upper GI tract limits the adhesion period.

5.3.6 Methods for studying gastrointestinal transit

GI transit of a dosage form and/or the drug can be performed directly in humans. Important information may also be collected from animal experiments provided that the GI tract of the animal resembles both anatomically and physiologically the human GI tract. The canine model is the most frequently used. Also, provided that careful justification of the importance of a specific study has been made, the use of animals allows the application of invasive techniques which give information that is extremely difficult or impossible to collect from experiments in humans.

Among the methods which have been used in humans, the most popular include intubation, radiotelemetry, hydrogen breath test, and gamma-scintigraphy. Each of these methods possesses certain advantages and the selection of the technique is based on the type of the information that needs to be collected.

5.3.6.1 Intubation

This technique was first introduced in the 1930s. It is a useful way of studying the GI transit of non-viscous liquids but it can be also applied to drug absorption from various regions of the GI tract (section 6.4.2.2).

The transit and uptake characteristics of water, ions and nutrients were determined with this method. For its application, a flexible multi-channel tube (i.e. two to four tubes one into the other with different lengths and no access between them) is inserted via the nasal (or oral) cavity down to the appropriate region of the GI tract. The solution is infused via the shortest tube to the desired area of the GI. The GI contents are then aspirated at predetermined time intervals via another opening (one of the internal tubes) from the desired region(s) (Fig. 5.18).

The difference between the drug concentration infused and recovered combined with the flow rate, permit calculation of drug uptake with time. Any biotransformation in the lumen must be taken into consideration, as must changes of net water flux across the gut wall (and therefore the possibility of collecting non-reliable data). This is monitored by the coadministration of a non-absorbable marker (such as polyethylene glycol 4000). Interpretation of results is facilitated if the blood levels are simultaneously monitored.

Intubation is the only method that can be used in humans to analyse the GI contents directly.

5.3.6.2 Radiotelemetry

Radiotelemetric capsules, such as the Heidelberg® capsule, are high-radiofrequency transmitters (about 2 MHz) encased in an inert (usually polyacrylate) indigestible shell. The frequencies transmitted reflect pH changes of the medium in which the capsule is placed. The power required to operate the transmitter is provided by a built-in battery. For the Heidelberg® capsule specifically, one of the two battery electrodes also serves as the reference electrode for the pH measuring system. The battery comprises a zinc and a silver chloride electrode and a physiological solution as the electrolyte. The electrolyte is

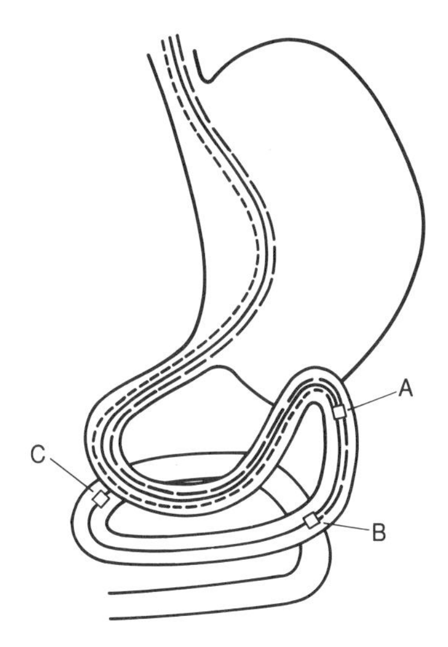

Fig. 5.18. Intubation with a triple-lumen tube. The length of each lumen varies. One ends at the duodenum (A), one at the beginning of the jejunum (B), and the third at the end of the jejunum (C).

introduced into the battery immediately prior to use and is bound with an absorbent filling. The pH measuring system comprises an external ring electrode made of antimony and the silver chloride electrode of the battery. The potential difference which develops between the two electrodes and is dependent upon the pH is applied to a transistor as a frequency-determining measuring voltage. The radio signals are picked up by a belt antenna of the receiver are reconverted to pH, displayed on a pH-meter and simultaneously records them on a strip-chart recorder.

This technique was initiated in the 1970s for the measurement of the pH of GI fluids. Based on the pH changes one is also able to assess the small intestinal transit or the gastric emptying (Fig. 5.19). This method can be more easily applied than the intubation and no radioactive materials are used. If necessary, fluoroscopy can be used to verify position since the metal components of the capsule are radio-opaque. The size and shape of the capsule are similar to those of monolithic dosage forms (approx. 7 mm diameter, 20 mm length and 1.5 g/cm^3 density). Due to their relatively large size, the radiotelemetric capsule may be retained at the ileo-caecal valve or in the stomach for a long time, so that the upper gasto-intestinal transit time may be longer than for dosage forms of smaller dimensions.

5.3.6.3 Hydrogen breath technique

The mouth to caecum transit time may be determined with the hydrogen breath test. This test is based on the biotransformation of carbohydrates, resistant to amylase attack, by the intestinal flora, which is significant below the ileo-caecal valve (Table 5.6). Lactulose, (1,4-galactosido-fructose) is most commonly used. Volatile metabolites of these compounds (hydrogen in the case of lactulose) are detectable in the exhaled air and the

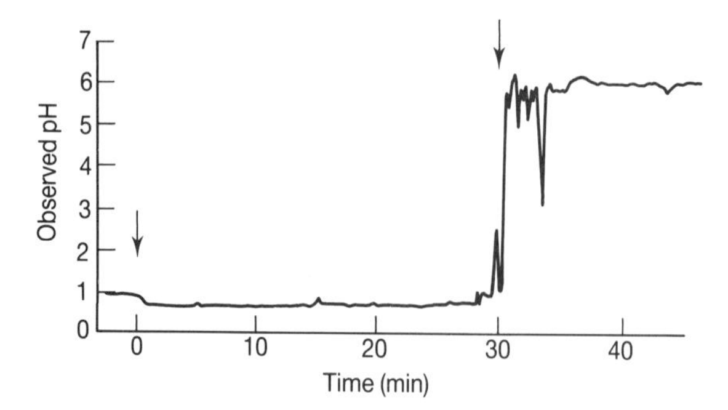

Fig. 5.19. Plot of pH as a function of time, following the administration of a Heidelberg® capsule in one volunteer under fasting conditions. Gastric emptying is noted by the abrupt increase in pH (arrow) and in this case was observed 30 min after administration. (From *Pharmaceutical Research* **8**: 97–100 (1991) with permission.)

estimation of the time of arrival in the colon is therefore possible. When interpreting hydrogen breath test results, it should be remembered that the initial rise in H_2 levels corresponds to arrival of the leading front of the chyme into the colon, not the mean transit time.

A potential source of error using this method is related to osmotic effects that the model compound may induce, with consequent alteration of the upper intestinal transit time. Moreover, antibiotic administration contraindicates the application of this method since the concentration of the colonic flora may be decreased and the metabolites in the exhaled air may not be detectable. Finally, in some cases intestinal flora is significant in the ileum, resulting in underestimation of the small intestinal transit time. It is therefore advisable that this method is used in conjunction with other methods (Fig. 5.20).

5.3.6.4 Gamma scintigraphy

This is non-invasive and probably the most accurate and easiest method for studying GI transit. However, the expensive equipment required makes it less accessible for formulation research. In this method, the dosage form is labelled with a radionuclide which emits gamma scintigraphy (usually ^{99m}Tc or ^{111m}In) and the transit is followed by a gamma camera (Fig. 5.21).

For monolithic dosage forms the transit time is estimated by the difference between gastric emptying and arrival at the ileo-caecal valve. For multiparticulate systems, where gastric emptying is not uniform, small intestinal transit time is estimated from the gastric emptying half-life and the half-life for colonic filling.

One disadvantage of this method is that the drug itself cannot usually be labelled because carbon, nitrogen and oxygen radionuclides are positron emitters with very small half-lives and high radiation burdens. A further limitation to this technique is that it cannot distinguish between a radionuclide present as a solid and that present in solution. This difficulty may be overcome by the use of perturbed angular correlation studies. Radionuclides which decay by emitting two gamma rays in cascade, such as ^{111m}In, emit

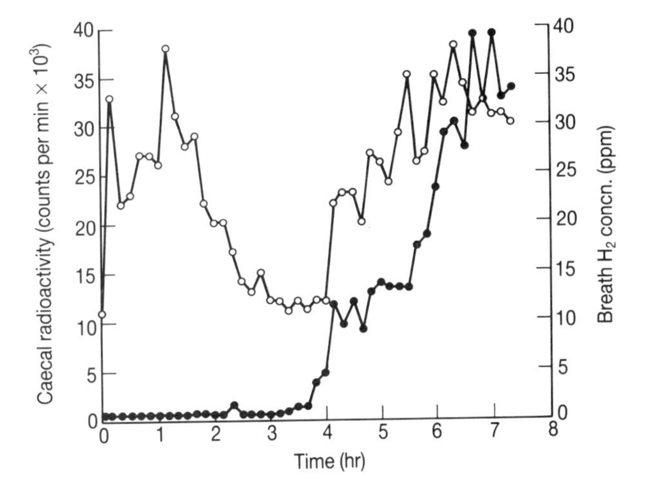

Fig. 5.20. Hydrogen concentration in exhaled air, following the administration of a radiolabelled meal as a function of time (○) and the radioactivity which was monitored simultaneously at cecum (●). The first peak on the hydrogen concentration versus time plot corresponds to the arrival of previous food residues in the colon. (Reprinted with permission from Drug Delivery to the Gastrointestinal Tract, p. 11, Ellis Horwood Series in Pharmaceutical Technology, Chichester, 1989.)

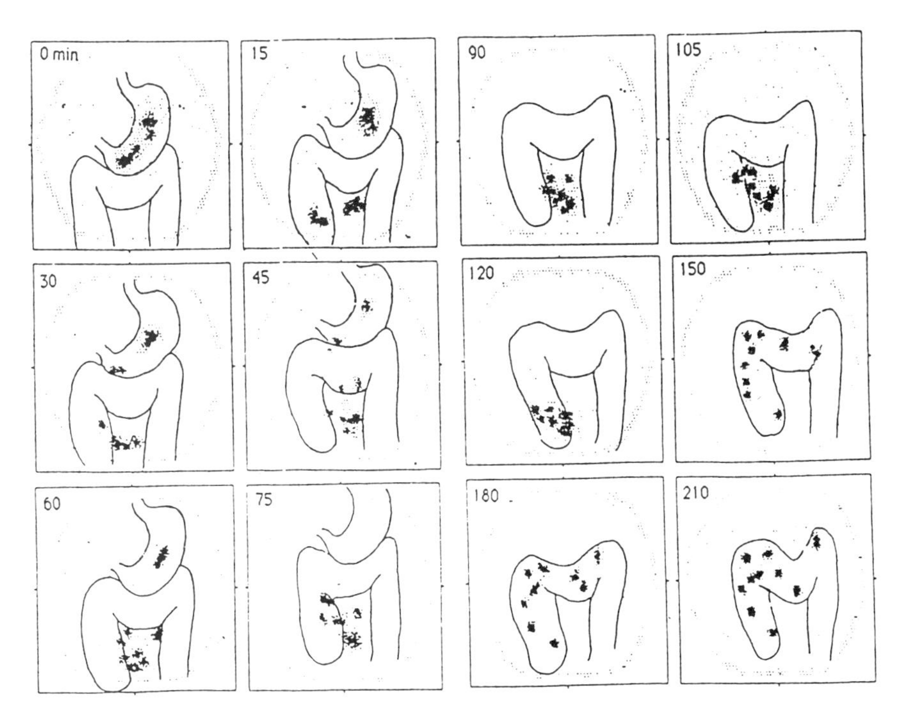

Fig. 5.21. Example of the GI transit profile of tablets 4 × 10 mm administered in one subject with a light breakfast as observed by gamma scintigraphy. (From the *International Journal of Pharmaceutics* **53**: 107–117(1989) with permission.)

the rays with a certain angular correlation between them. This can be perturbed if the physical environment of the nucleus changes, for example, by dissolution.

5.3.6.5 Other methods

One of the very first innovations (1920s) in the study of GI transit was the use of non-digestible non-absorbed materials (such as glass beads, carmine and other dyes, pieces of rubber, etc.). The evaluation of the total GI transit time was based on the time elapsed from the administration until the excretion of these markers with faeces. Later this method was improved with the use of radioactive materials and repeated administration to collect data on intra- and inter-subject variability. Nevertheless this method is time consuming, gives quantitative information only for the transit of solids, and is problematic in terms of volunteer compliance.

Two other methods are *applied potential tomography* and *impedance epigastrography*. Both detect the changes in gastric electrical impedance that takes place when a meal, which is either more conductive or less conductive than normal abdominal contents, empties from the stomach. Measurements are performed by means of 4–16 electrodes which are positioned on the surface of the body and in the area where the stomach is located. In general, impedance is increased after a meal is administered and then is gradually decreased as gastric contents are transported to the duodenum. These methods do not require any radioactive materials and may therefore be used in sensitive groups of subjects such as children and pregnant women. However, a disadvantage may be the difficulty associated with exact determination of the stomach position and also the fact that gastric secretions may interfere with the measured electrical impedance.

FURTHER READING

Davenport HW. *Physiology of the Digestive Tract. An Introductory Text* (5th edn), Year Book Medical Publishers, London (1982).

Digenis GA. The Utilization of Short-lived Radionuclides in the Assessment of Formulation and In Vivo Disposition of Drugs, in: *Radionuclide Imaging in Drug Research*, chapter 9, Wilson CG, Hardy JG, Davis SS and Frier M (eds), Croom Helm, London (1982).

Friend DR, Phillips S and Tozer TN. Colon-Specific Drug Delivery from a Glucoside Prodrug in the Guinea-Pig. Efficacy Study. *J. Controlled Rel.* **15**: 47–54 (1991).

Hardy JG, Davis SS and Wilson CG (eds). *Drug Delivery to the Gastrointestinal Tract*, Ellis Horwood, Hemel Hempstead (1989).

Harris D, Fell JT, Sharma HL and Taylor DC. GI Transit of Potential Bioadhesive Formulations in Man: A Scintigraphic Study. *J. Controlled Rel.* **12**: 45-53 (1990).

Hoelzel F. The Rate of Passage of Inert Materials through the Digestive Tract. *Am. J. Physiol.* **92**: 466–497 (1930).

Hunt JN and Stubbs DF. The Volume and Energy Content of Meals as Determinants of Gastric Emptying. *J. Physiol.* (London) **245**: 209–225 (1975).

Karr WG and Abbott WO. Intubation Studies of the Human Small Intestine. IV. Chemical Characteristics of the Intestinal Contents in the Fasting State and as Influenced by the Administration of Acids, of Alkalies and of Water. *J. Clin. Invest.* **14**: 893–900 (1935).

Macheras P, Reppas C and Dressman JB. Estimate of Volume/Flow Ratio of Gastrointestinal (GI) Fluids in Humans Using Pharmacokinetic Data. *Pharm. Res.* **7**: 518–522 (1990).

Meeroff JC, Go VLW and Phillips SF. Control of Gastric Emptying by Osmolality of Duodenal Contents in Man. *Gastroenterology* **68**: 1144–1151 (1975).

Meyer JH and Doty JE. GI Transit and Absorption of Solid Food: Multiple Effects of Guar. *Am. J. Clin. Nutr.* **48**: 267–273 (1988).

Minami H and McCallum RW. The Physiology and Pathophysiology of Gastric Emptying in Humans. *Gastroenterology* **86**: 1592–1610 (1984).

Nimmo WS. Drugs, Diseases and Altered Gastric Emptying. *Clin. Pharmacokinet.* **1**: 189–203 (1976).

Oberle RL and Amidon GL. The Influence of Variable Gastric Emptying and Intestinal Transit Rates on the Plasma Level Curve of Cimetidine: An Explanation of the Double Peak Phenomenon. *J. Pharmacokinet. Biopharm.* **15**: 529–543 (1987).

Peppas NA. Biomaterials: Interfacial Phenomena and Applications, in: *Structure, Testing and Applications of Biomaterials*, Cooper SL and Peppas NA (eds), Advances in Chemistry series, vol. 199, American Chemical Society, Washington, DC (1982).

Rubinstein A. Microbially Controlled Drug Delivery to the Colon. *Biopharm. Drug Dispos.* **11**: 465–475 (1990).

Yacobi A and Halperin-Walega E. *Oral Sustained Release Formulations. Design and Evaluation*, Ch. 6, Pergamon Press, Oxford (1988).

6

Uptake of the drug by the gastrointestinal mucosa

Objectives

The reader will be able to identify:

— *Which factors regulate the uptake of the drugs from the gastrointestinal (GI) mucosa*
— *The properties of drug transport from the GI fluids to the vessels of the mucosa*
— *Methods for increasing the uptake of drugs and techniques for studying the uptake of drugs from the GI mucosa*

As defined previously (chapter 3), the term *uptake* includes all the individual processes that lead to the transport of drugs from the lumen of the gastrointestinal (GI) tract to the blood capillaries and (to a lesser degree) to the lymph vessels, and finally to the general circulation.

Prerequisite to the transport of a drug from the GI tract to the general circulation is its presence at locations where absorption is possible, in a form which can cross the various barriers to its uptake. The extent of each barrier's resistance depends on the physicochemical characteristics of the drug and on the characteristics of the GI mucosa. The barriers are mainly physical (i.e. those which prevent immediate access of the drug to the vessels) but may also be metabolic (i.e. those which lead to biotransformation of the drug during permeation and consequently to reduction of the fraction of the drug that reaches the general circulation). In this chapter only phenomena associated with the penetration through the gut wall will be discussed. The metabolic properties of the GI mucosa will be discussed in chapter 9 as part of the first-pass effect.

In order to reach the blood and lymph vessels from the GI fluids, the drug molecule must pass through two major barriers which possess quite different properties:

— the stagnant aqueous layer, adjacent to the epithelial cells of the GI tract; and
— the mucosa, which comprises a single layer of columnar epithelial cells and intracellular fluid.

As shown in Fig. 6.1, there is a concentration gradient for the drug across each of these two barriers. This situation, is due to the fact that the transport of the drug from one area to another is not instantaneous and it depends, as will be discussed in more detail, on the following factors:

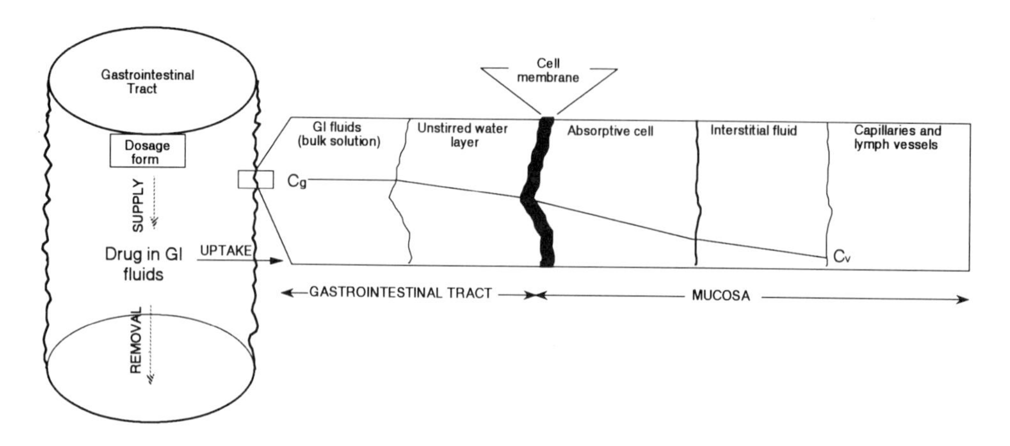

Fig. 6.1. Barriers to drug uptake from the GI fluids to the blood capillaries and the lymph vessels. C_g and C_v are the concentrations of the drug in the GI fluids and the vessels, respectively. The dotted lines symbolize the other two processes ('supply' and 'removal'), which together with 'uptake' regulate the absorption of xenobiotics.

- —Diffusion through the stagnant aqueous layer. Compounds which present problems at this stage either have poor aqueous solubility or are of high molecular weight.
- —Transport through the mucosa. This step can be problematic for compounds with poor lipophilicity. Some examples of drugs that have difficulty penetrating this barrier include acyclovir, 6-carboxyfluorescein, certain antibiotics of the β-lactam category like ceftizoxime and cefoxitine, phenol red and polypeptides.
- —Binding of the drug molecule with components of the stagnant aqueous layer and/or the mucosa.
- —Blood flow rate in the capillaries, for drugs which cross both the stagnant layer and the mucosa very rapidly.
- —Entrance of the drug to the lymph vessels (depends on the presence of fats and chylomicron formation).

Lack of ability of the drug to cross the stagnant aqueous layer and the epithelium will result in uptake becoming the rate-limiting step to absorption.

Assuming that the small intestine is the main region of drug uptake (section 6.1), if the uptake rate is slower than both the GI transit and release from the dosage form, and if transit is slower than release, then the process of the arrival of the drug in the vessels will be limited by the uptake rate. Considering that all the processes follow first-order kinetics and that uptake and transit are parallel processes, while supply and uptake are in series, the following relationship exists:

$$R_{0,u} < R_{0,t} < R_{0,s}$$

where $R_{0,t}$ is the initial transit rate, $R_{0,u}$ is the initial uptake rate and $R_{0,s}$ is the initial supply rate. Therefore, the initial rate of absorption, $R_{0,a}$, depends in this case on the uptake of the drug, i.e.

$$R_{0,a} = k_u C_{g0} V$$

where k_u is the uptake rate constant, C_{g0} is the initial drug concentration in the GI fluids and V is the volume of the GI contents.

6.1 TRANSFER OF THE DRUG FROM THE GASTROINTESTINAL FLUIDS TO THE INTERIOR OF THE EPITHELIAL CELL

6.1.1 Transfer of the drug from the gastrointestinal fluids to the surface of the epithelial cell

The surface of the epithelial cells is covered by an aqueous matrix, which is poorly mixed (stagnant aqueous layer or unstirred water layer, Fig. 6.1) and consists mainly of water and mucus (section 5.2).

If one accepts the simplifying analogy that flow through the small intestine resembles flow through a pipe, only the part of the layer which is in contact with the epithelial cell is stagnant, with the stirring intensity increasing gradually with distance away from the surface of the mucosa towards the centre of the GI tract. The hydrodynamics can be approximated by a film layer model, consisting of a liquid layer (having thickness h_{aq}) in contact with the GI membrane, which is not stirred and through which drug molecules are transported by simple diffusion. Further away from the epithelial surface (i.e. distances beyond h_{aq}), stirring is considered to be complete and uniform. The thickness of the unstirred water layer depends on the morphology of the mucosal surface, the viscosity of the luminal contents, and the flow rate of the luminal contents. Recent studies in dogs and humans have shown that, in contrast to what was previously suggested, the stagnant layer in the intestine has an apparent thickness of about 40 μm.

Transport through the aqueous layer may be a significant limitation to drug uptake. Assuming that the drug does not accumulate at the interface between the aqueous layer and the cell membrane, permeation follows the principles of non-reversible passive diffusion (section 2.3.1) and the flux of the drug, J_1, through the aqueous layer is described by the following equation:

$$J_1 = \left(D_{aq}/h_{aq}\right) C_g = P_{aq} C_g \quad (6.1)$$

where C_g is the concentration of the drug in GI fluids, D_{aq} is the diffusion coefficient through the layer, h_{aq} the thickness of the stagnant aqueous layer and P_{aq} the *permeability coefficient* in the aqueous layer.

Generally, diffusion through the stagnant layer becomes problematic and consequently affects drug uptake in the following situations:

— When the drug molecule is extremely lipophilic. The uptake of drugs with $\log P \geqslant 2.5$ (in an n-octanol/water system) is considered to be greatly dependent on the transport through the stagnant aqueous layer. Long-chain fatty acids represent typical examples.
— When the drug has a high molecular weight (slow diffusivity). Typical examples include proteins and steroidal hormones.
— When the drug complexes with the components of the aqueous layer. Such a situation may be significant in certain diseases, such as cystic fibrosis, where increased quantities of mucus are observed, and binding with mucin can lead to a reduction in drug diffusion towards the surface of the mucosa. Binding to mucin has been observed for compounds such as tetracyclines, salicylates, quaternary ammonium salts and phenylbutazone.
— When the viscosity of GI fluids is increased. In such cases, h_{aq} increases and/or D_{aq} decreases (equation (6.1)).
— When luminal stirring varies (for example, with the different motility patterns during the interdigestive migrating motility complex).

The pH in the aqueous stagnant layer
The relationship between the pH inside and the pH outside of the stagnant layer depends on the region of the GI tract and the GI contents. It has been confirmed, for example, that protection of the gastroduodenal mucosa from the highly acidic pH is achieved by retardation of the hydrogen cation diffusion through the stagnant aqueous layer, as well as by secretion of bicarbonate from epithelial cells. Generally, the pH of the membrane surface is closer to neutral than the pH of the bulk GI fluids. Therefore, when the pH effect on drug uptake is discussed, the pH in the microclimate next to the lining mucosa is frequently mentioned.

6.1.2 Transfer of the drug from the surface of the mucosa into the interior of the epithelial cells

Throughout the GI tract the mucosa comprises epithelial cells (secretory and absorptive), intercellular liquid and vessels (blood capillaries and the central lymphatic lacteal). However, there are macroscopic differences between regions which may affect the ability of the drug molecules to reach the blood and/or lymph vessels.

As discussed in previous chapters, drug uptake mainly takes place in the small intestine. This occurs because of its specialized morphology which is optimized for absorption.

6.1.2.1 The gastrointestinal mucosa

The mucosa of the stomach
The surface of the stomach mucosa is covered by a single layer of, mainly mucus-secreting, epithelial cells punctuated by gastric 'pits'. There are approximately 100 pits/mm^2, so they occupy almost half of the stomach surface. The distance between the centres of the pits is approximately 0.1 mm. Three to seven glands open into each pit. Three types of tubular secretory glands can be specified.

The first type constitutes the glands which are found in the fundus and the body of the stomach and contain three kinds of secretory cells: the mucosal cells, which are found at the gland neck and secrete mucus, alkaline liquid and pepsinogen (section 5.2); the parietal (oxyntic) cells, which are found directly beneath and secrete hydrochloric acid; and finally, the chief cells, which are found at the gland base and secrete pepsinogen.

The second gland type is situated at the antrum and mainly consists of gastrin cells which secrete gastrin (section 5.2).

The third type of gland occurs in the pyloric and cardiac regions and secretes mainly mucus.

The stomach mucosa is differentiated morphologically from the small intestinal mucosa in that:

(1) it has little augmentation of available surface area; and
(2) the surface mucosa are mainly mucus-secreting cells rather than absorptive cells.

From a physiological point of view, administration of certain substances may cause significant damage to both the structure and the function of the gastric epithelial cells. Such a situation occurs when aliphatic acids (acetic, propionic, butyric, etc.), surfactants (natural, such as bile acids and lysolecithin, or synthetic) or certain drugs are administered. Obviously, if part of the mucosa is destroyed, then the rate of drug uptake may be increased locally. Aspirin represents a typical compound which can destroy the gastric mucosa. Administration of acetylsalicylate under fasting conditions (i.e. when the stomach pH is very low) results in fast conversion to the free acid form and consequently fast uptake (Fig. 6.2) (see below for the uptake of ionized and non-ionized molecules). The almost instantaneous uptake destroys the cells, resulting in the exfoliation and regional destruction of the gastric mucosa. Under fed conditions the absorption mechanism is the same (Fig. 6.2), but because the stomach pH is higher, the drug molecule is partly ionized and the slower uptake rate results in less injury to the surface of the mucosa.

Briefly, quantitative drug uptake is limited by the relatively low mucosal surface area of the stomach, and the low percentage of absorptive cells on what surface area is

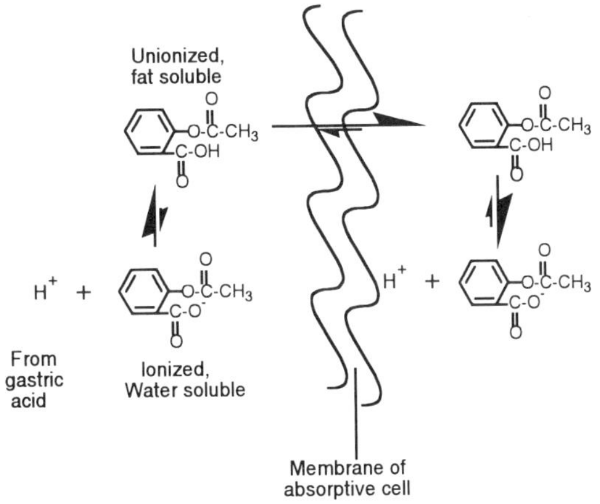

Fig. 6.2. Absorption of aspirin from the stomach, when administered in the form of acetylsalicylate.

available. Thus, despite the fact that from the physicochemical point of view there may exist ideal conditions for drug absorption, substance exchanges in the stomach consist mainly of the secretion of water and certain ions.

The small intestinal mucosa

The major characteristic of the small intestinal mucosa is its enormous surface area compared to the limited volume that it occupies. This is due to the fact that the mucosa of the small intestine is distinguished by three groups of projections: circular folds, villi and microvilli.

The circular folds (Fig. 6.3A), 8–10 mm long, are thicker in the region of the jejunum and succeed in tripling the inner small intestinal surface area. Out of these folds the villi are projected (Fig. 6.3B). Villus height ranges between 0.5 and 1.5 mm, and their density is 10–40/mm^2. Inside every villus there is a thick network of capillaries and the central lacteal, while on the outside each is covered by a layer of epithelial cells, mainly absorptive but also containing some mucus-secreting goblet cells (Fig. 6.3C).

The absorptive cells are elongated (Fig. 6.4A) and closely connected by the tight junctions, which limit direct communication between the contents of the GI tract and the intercellular space. The most distinctive feature of the absorptive cells is a striated end

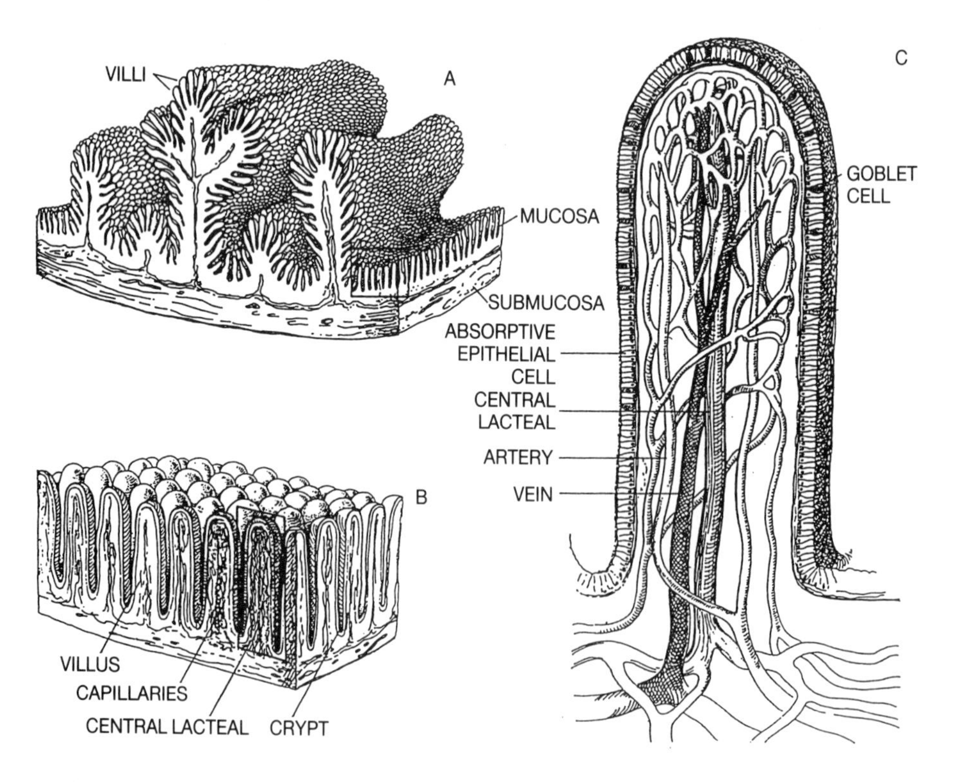

Fig. 6.3. Schematic representation of the small intestinal mucosa. (A) Circular folds with villi, (B) villi, (C) structure of villus.

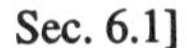

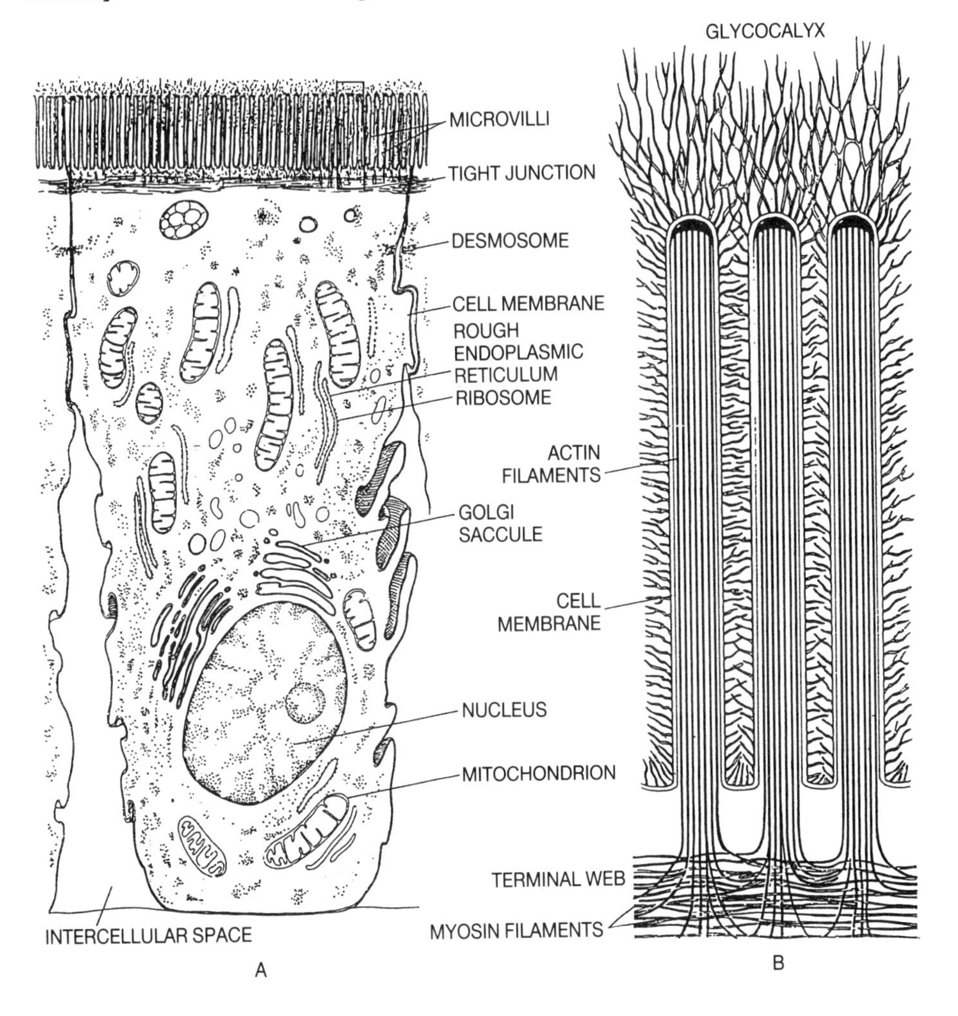

Fig. 6.4. (A) Structure of the absorptive epithelial cell in the small intestine. (B) Structure of the microvilli.

(brush border) at the top of the cell towards the interior of the tract (Fig. 6.4A), almost 1.5 nm long. The structure of the brush border was clarified by electron microscopy in the 1950s. At that time the existence of microvilli ($\approx$200 000/mm^2 in the jejunum) was confirmed. The microvilli multiply by a factor of about 20 the surface area of the small intestine. The interior of microvilli (Fig. 6.4B) consists of fibres, especially the protein fibres actin and myosin, while the exterior is covered by the cell membrane.

The membrane is comprised essentially of a phospholipid bilayer, in which glycoprotein molecules are located. The phospholipids are arranged such that the hydrophilic (polar) end is directed towards the two membrane surfaces, inner and outer, and the hydrophobic (non-polar) groups towards the membrane centre (Fig. 6.5). Currently accepted theory concerning the position of glycoproteins on the membrane holds that the protein part penetrates the membrane to a varying degree whereas the carbohydrate part is located in the outer part of the cell, forming the glycocalyx (Figs 6.4B and 6.5). This can be seen under the electron microscope as a network of thin fibres. Glycoproteins act either as enzymes (in most cases) or as carriers in the permeation of molecules through the membrane and are in that case described as transfer proteins.

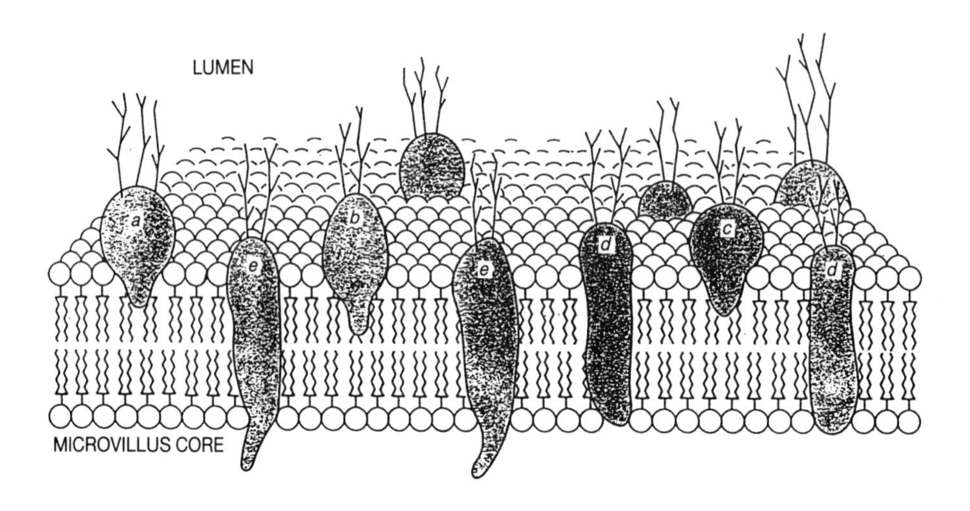

Fig. 6.5. Structure of the microvillus membrane. The protein group of the glycoproteins penetrates the interior of the bimolar phospholipid layer. The carbohydrate chains protrude into the lumen forming the glycocalyx; a, b and c are disaccharidases; d is alkaline phosphatase, which hydrolyses many of the phosphate compounds in food; e are aminopeptidases.

Quite often, membrane enzymes have their active centre directed towards the exterior of the cell, and they possess a thin chain anchor which continues on to the other end of the lipid bilayer. Principal enzymes residing in the microvillus membrane are disaccharidases, alkaline phosphatase and aminopeptidases which catabolize disaccharides, phosphate compounds and peptides, respectively. The functions of the transfer proteins (whose molecular weight is about 50 000) are less well understood and it is believed that their function is based on conformational changes in their structure (Fig. 6.6). Transfer proteins are thought to form microscopic channels which allow small-sized cations or anions to pass selectively. Those passages are called *aqueous pores* (see section 6.1.2.2 on the permeation mechanisms of epithelial cells), because they are filled with water and offer continuity between the interior and the exterior of the cell (Fig. 6.6). However, due to the high degree of specificity of most transport proteins, the membrane of GI epithelial cells may be considered primarily as a continuous lipid barrier to the uptake of drugs.

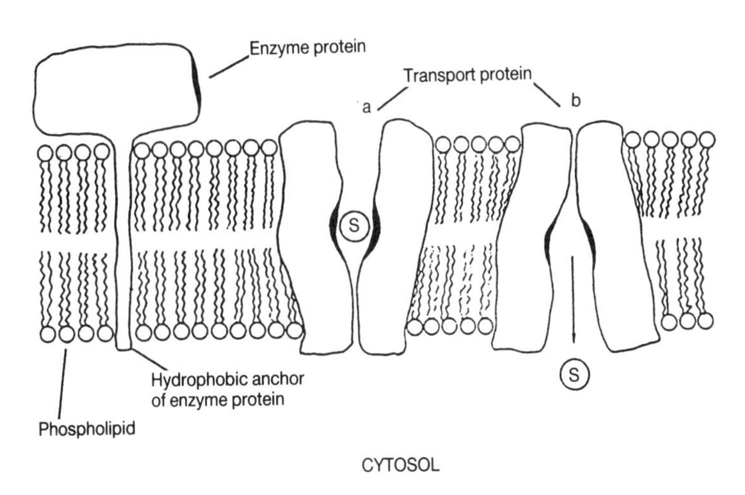

Fig. 6.6. Relationship between the phospholipid layer, the enzyme proteins and the transfer proteins in conjunction with the transfer process of a small water-soluble molecule (S) to the interior of the cell through the aqueous pores. The active centre of the enzyme protein and the micromolecule-transfer protein binding site are shaded. (From *J. Small Animal Pract.* **21**: 555–569 (1980) with permission.)

To complete the description of the microvillus cell membrane, it is worth mentioning that across the GI epithelia the electric potential (described by the Nernst equation†) is negligible (0–4 mV) compared to the value displayed in other epithelial cells (20–90 mV). Consequently, the permeation of the mucosa of the GI tract is not significantly affected by the charge of the penetrant compound, except in so far as it affects drug lipophilicity.

Other common cell types found in the small intestine include M and goblet cells. The lymphoid follicles (Peyer's patches) found in the jejunum and ileum afford protection against pathogenic substances. Primary contact between the lumen and the Peyer's patches is mediated via the M cells. Glands in the small intestine are found mainly in the duodenum (Brunner's glands) and secrete mucus and bicarbonate ions. The goblet cells are found either on the surface epithelium or in the depressions between the villi (called crypts) and secrete mostly mucus.

The mucosa of the large intestine

In the human intestine, no villi are found beyond the ileo-caecal sphincter. The walls of the ascending colon are usually sacculated into permanent haustra. Secretory cells are found on the surface or in crypts, and produce a fluid having very low enzyme content and consisting almost exclusively of mucus. The main absorptive function of the large intestine is based on the active uptake of Na^+ ions and consequently water (as water absorption depends on the absorption of osmotically significant Na^+ ions). Although

† In general, the outside of the membrane wall is positively charged in relation to the inside and therefore cations (e.g. weak bases) are accumulated in the interior of the cell.

drugs are usually absorbed to a lesser extent than in the small intestine, some of them are satisfactorily absorbed by the colon (Table 5.5).

6.1.2.2 Mechanisms of permeation of gastrointestinal epithelium

In general, permeation of the epithelial cells by xenobiotics and physiological substances depends primarily on the permeability of the microvilli cell membrane (transcellular transport). Paracellular transport, or movement through the tight junctions between absorptive cells, represents an alternative route of uptake.

Transcellular transport

The transcellular route is considered to be the most common pathway for drug transport from the GI fluids to the blood and lymphatic vessels. Transport through the epithelial cells encompasses permeation of the cell epithelial membrane, movement across the intracellular space, and permeation of the lateral or basolateral membranes.

However, the major obstacle for the permeation process appears to be the cell membrane. Physical barriers to movement across the cytosol are not well defined, and the role of the basolateral and lateral membranes appears to be of secondary importance. Although its structure is complex (Figs 6.5 and 6.6), the epithelial cell membrane appears to behave as a lipid barrier to the permeation of many drugs. In contrast to the permeation of the stagnant aqueous layer, transcellular transport requires partitioning of the drug into the membrane lipid fraction. More lipophilic (less polar) compounds are mainly transported into the cell by a partitioning/passive-diffusion process, while hydrophilic (polar) compounds must either be transported by a specialized mechanism (such as the mediation of a carrier or (rarely) pinocytosis) or by the paracellular route.

Permeation of the cell membrane by passive diffusion: The pH-partition hypothesis. The principle of passive diffusion, as well as of certain specific cases of non-reversible passive transport, have been discussed in chapter 2. This process is now discussed in more detail from the standpoint of intestinal uptake of drugs.

Considering the lipid nature of the cell membrane, one would logically expect that the permeation of the drugs through the membrane of the small intestine depends to a large degree on their lipophilicity. Extensive research on the permeation of cell membranes has shown that there is a strong correlation between permeation and the partition coefficient of the drug between an aqueous and an organic phase. The partition coefficient, usually expressed in its logarithmic form, log P, constitutes a measure of lipophilicity. The higher the partition coefficient (i.e. the more lipophilic the drug), the more easily the drug appears to be able to partition into the lipid membrane, facilitating the diffusion of the particular drug across the cell (Table 6.1). The permeation process, being passive in nature, is mainly controlled by the concentration of drug remaining to be transported from one to the other side of the membrane. These principles are followed by the majority of drugs with the exception of highly branched compounds, which are less permeable than one would expect on a theoretical basis. The reason for this inconsistency is that the permeation of branched molecules into the lipid layer is hindered by their stereochemistry, since entrance of branched molecules results in greater disturbance in the arrangement of the lipid layers. Ionization of the drug in the GI fluids relative to the

Table 6.1. Structural influences on drug lipophilicity

Lipophilicity increases by:	Lipophilicity decreases by:
Replacement of oxygen by sulfur Replacement of hydrogen by halogen Increase of the length of an alkyl or hydrocarbon chain	Addition of groups which ionize or permit the formation of hydrogen bonds (e.g. OH, COOH, NH_2, NR_3^+, SO_2H, SO_2NH_2)

pH (see section 2.3.1.2) also affects passive uptake. It is important to know what percentage of drug is non-ionized, as this form, having a higher partition coefficient than the ionized, is able to permeate cell membrane more easily. These observations led to the *pH-partition hypothesis*, which claims that *only* the non-ionized form of the drug permeates the membrane. The ability of the drug to permeate the lipid barrier is therefore related to the pK_a of the drug, the pH on the luminal side of the membrane and the partition coefficient of the non-ionized form of the drug.

Data in Tables 6.2 and 6.3 are in general agreement with these considerations. Table 6.2 shows the effect of the pK_a value on the uptake of several substances by the small intestine of rats. Table 6.3 relates the uptake of four barbiturates to the partition coefficient. However, based on these tables, there are cases where the uptake of weak acids and bases is not in agreement with the pK_a values. A typical example is the uptake of

Table 6.2. Uptake of drugs by the small intestine of rats in relation to their pK_as[a]

Acids	pK_a	Uptake (%)[b]	Bases	pK_a	Uptake (%)[b]
5-Sulfosalicylic	Strong	<2	Acetanilide	0.3	42
o-Nitrobenzoic	2.2	5	Theophylline	0.7	29
5-Nitrosalicylic	2.3	9	*p*-Nitroaniline	1.0	68
Salicylic	3.0	60	Antipyrine	1.4	32
m-Nitrobenzoic	3.4	53	*m*-Nitroaniline	2.5	77
Acetylsalicylic	3.5	20	Aniline	4.6	54
Benzoic	4.2	51	Aminopyrine	5.0	33
Phenylbutazone	4.4	65	*p*-Toluidine	5.3	59
Acetic	4.7	42	Quinine	8.4	15
Thiopental	7.6	55	Ephedrine	9.6	7
Barbitone	7.8	30	Tolazoline	10.3	6
p-Hydroxy-propiophenone	7.8	61	Mecamylamine	11.2	3
Phenol	9.9	51			

[a] Data published in the *Journal of Pharmacology and Experimental Therapeutics* **123**: 81–88 (1958).
[b] Expressed as percentage reduction of concentration of the drug in normal saline, perfused for 7 min with a flow of 1.5 ml/min along the whole small intestine. The perfusion technique is described in section 6.4.2.2.

Table 6.3. Permeability of barbiturates through the small intestine of rats in relation to the partition coefficient calculated in a chloroform/water system[a]

Barbiturate	Partition coefficient	% Uptake
Barbitone	0.7	12
Phenobarbitone	4.8	20
Butethal	11.7	24
Pentobarbitone	28.0	30

[a] Data published in *The Absorption and Distribution of Drugs*, Saunders L., p. 81, Baillière Tindal, London (1974).

salicylates by the small intestine of rats, which is greater than would be predicted from pH-partition considerations. This behaviour is also observed in humans, where the median pH of the jejunum is about 6.5 and, since more than 99.9% of the salicylic acid molecules are ionized at this pH, uptake should be extremely low. However, it is known that when salicylic acid is administered per os as an enteric coated dosage form, its uptake is satisfactory. It has been proposed that the existence of a lower pH in the microclimate of the mucosal surface can account for this discrepancy. In a similar manner, the pK_a of quinine or of its optical isomer, quinidine, is 8.4. Based on the pH-partition hypothesis, at a pH of 6.6 approximately 1.6% of these drugs are non-ionized and therefore available for uptake. In this case, the maintenance of the pH in the mucosa microclimate of the jejunum at values below 8.4 should result in even less of the non-ionized form being present. Nevertheless, experimental observations show that both isomers have a satisfactory uptake from the small intestine. It is possible that uptake of the ionized form occurs through the paracellular route. Yet another explanation is based on the active secretion of organic cations by the blood into the small intestine. It is possible that the carrier mediating this secretion process also facilitates the transport of organic cations in the opposite direction, i.e. from the small intestine to the blood.

Example 6.1: Based on the Henderson–Hasselbach equations (section 2.3.1.2) and the principles of the pH-partition hypothesis, demonstrate the region of the GI tract from which famotidine (weak base, $pK_a = 6.7$) is expected most easily to permeate the cell membrane of the epithelial cells. Ignore any effect of the pH in the microclimate of mucosal surface.

Answer: The Henderson–Hasselbach equation for a weak base can be written as follows:

$$\mathrm{pH} = \mathrm{p}K_a + \log \frac{[\mathrm{B}]}{[\mathrm{BH}^+]} \quad \text{and} \quad \frac{[\mathrm{B}]}{[\mathrm{BH}^+]} = 10^{(\mathrm{pH}-\mathrm{p}K_a)}$$

The last equation, for the case of a weak base with $pK_a = 6.7$ and for various pH values, yields:

pH	Region of the GI tract where similar pH values prevail	$[B]/[BH^+]$
1.0	Stomach in fasted state	2.0×10^{-6}
3.0	Stomach in fed state	2.0×10^{-4}
6.5	Jejunum	6.3×10^{-1}

Based on the calculations above, according to the pH-partition hypothesis it is predicted that famotidine will permeate the membrane of the epithelial cells most easily in the jejunum, where it is mostly in the non-ionized form.

Example 6.2: Calculate the (theoretical) contribution of the non-ionized and the ionized form of ibuprofen (pK_a 4.4) in equilibrium conditions, considering uptake (a) from the stomach (pH 1.2), and (b) from the jejunum (pH 6.5).

Answer: The following diagram describes the distribution of ibuprofen:

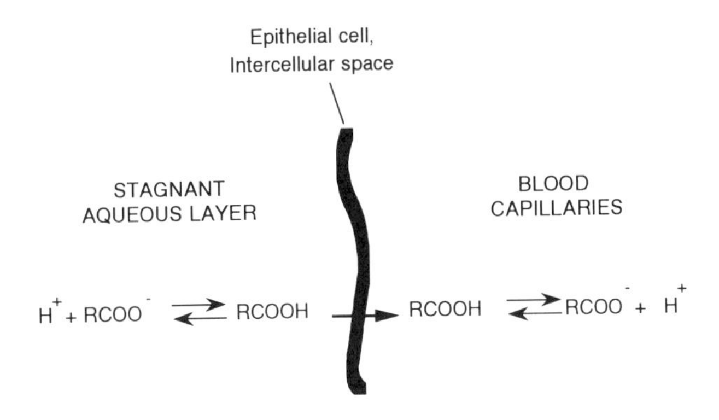

Assuming that at equilibrium the concentration of the non-ionized form is 1 on both sides of the membrane, the concentrations of the ionized forms on both sides of the membrane can be calculated using the Henderson–Hasselbach equation:

$$pH = pK_a + \log \frac{[A^-]}{(HA)} \quad \text{and} \quad [A^-] = [HA]\, 10^{(pH - pK_a)}$$

Therefore

In the plasma: $[RCOO^-] = 1 \times 10^{7.4-4.4} = 1 \times 10^3$

In the stomach: $[RCOO^-] = 1 \times 10^{1.2-4.4} = 6 \times 10^{-4}$

In the jejunum: $[RCOO^-] = 1 \times 10^{6.5-4.4} = 1 \times 10^2$

Based on the above calculations, one would predict that ibuprofen is taken up quantitatively from the stomach, as the total concentration in the blood is a thousand times higher than the total concentration in the stomach. In contrast, in the region of the jejunum the uptake of ibuprofen appears to be less satisfactory, as the concentration in the plasma is only ten times higher than the concentration in the jejunum.

It should be remembered, however, that although the above argument is correct from a physicochemical point of view, it is based on the assumption of equilibrium between the ionized and the non-ionized form in both areas. However, drug concentrations in the GI tract and the blood are unlikely to reach equilibrium because of kinetic considerations (supply, distribution and elimination). Moreover, the huge differences in the surface area between the stomach and the small intestine establish the region of the small intestine as the most important region of drug uptake.

Mathematical consideration of the drug uptake based on the pH-partition hypothesis. The basic consideration of the passive diffusion process on the basis of the pH-partition hypothesis is expressed as follows. The mucosa constitutes a complex barrier in the transport of drug molecules from a region of high concentration (GI fluids) to a region of low concentration (capillaries), the total resistance of which equals the sum of the individual resistances of the stagnant layer, the cell membrane (which depends mainly on the lipophilicity of the permeating molecule) and the membrane–water interface located in the interior of the epithelial cell. It is assumed that from the interior of the epithelial cell to the capillaries and/or the lymph vessels there are no significant resistances (Fig. 6.1). Assuming that the drug does not accumulate in any region between the GI fluids and the capillaries, Fick's law for diffusion (section 2.3.1), which describes the total process of drug uptake, is represented by the equation

$$J_u = P_{app} C_g \tag{6.2}$$

where J_u is the flux of the drug uptake, and P_{app} is the *apparent permeability coefficient*, given by equation (6.3)[†]

$$P_{app} = \frac{1}{\dfrac{1}{P_{aq}} + \dfrac{1}{P_{mem}} + \dfrac{1}{P_{int}}} \tag{6.3}$$

where P_{aq} is the permeability coefficient of the drug in the stagnant aqueous layer, equal to D_{aq}/h_{aq} (equation (6.1)); P_{mem} is the permeability coefficient of the non-ionized molecules in the lipid membrane, equal to $(PD_{mem}f_{s,aq})/h_{mem}$ (where P is the partition coefficient, D_{mem} is the diffusion coefficient through the membrane, $f_{s,aq}$ is the fraction of the non-ionized form and h_{mem} is the thickness of the membrane); and P_{int} is the permeability coefficient during the transport of the drug from the epithelial cytosol to the vessels. P_{int} is equal to $(f_{s,aq}P_{aq})/f_{s,int}$. Since $f_{s,int}$ is the fraction of the non-ionized form in the mucosa,[‡] P_{int} depends on the pH of the cell interior.

† Equation (6.3) is based on the fact that the apparent resistance to uptake, R_{app}, is equal to the inverse of permeation, i.e. $R_{app} = 1/P_{app} = R_{aq} + R_{mem} + R_{int}$.

‡ $f_s = 1/(1 + 10^{pH_s - pK_a})$ for weak acids and $f_s = 1/(1 + 10^{pK_a - pH_s})$ for weak bases.

From the above relationships it follows that in cases where:

(a) the drug is a weak acid and the pH in the mucosa is much higher than the pK_a; or
(b) the drug is a weak base and the pH in the mucosa and the pH is much lower than the pK_a; or
(c) sink conditions prevail during uptake of the drug, i.e. the concentration in the cytosol is less than 20% of the concentration of the drug in the GI fluids[§]

then $f_{s,int}$ becomes negligible and equation (6.3) takes the form

$$P_{app} = \frac{1}{\frac{1}{P_{aq}} + \frac{1}{P_{mem}}} \tag{6.4}$$

Under conditions in which equation (6.4) is operative, one can make the following comments:

(a) When the membrane permeability is very low (due to poor partitioning, i.e. $P_{mem} \ll P_{aq}$), then the process of uptake is membrane controlled and independent from the hydrodynamic conditions prevailing in the lumen.
(b) When membrane permeability is very high (because of a high partition coefficient, i.e. $P_{mem} \gg P_{aq}$), then uptake is controlled by the diffusion through the stagnant layer (diffusion controlled) and it depends on factors which control the transport through the stagnant layer.

In summary, as the lipophilicity of the drug increases, uptake also increases (because P_{mem} increases) until P_{mem} reaches values higher than P_{aq}. After that point, further increase of lipophilicity does not accelerate the uptake any more, and diffusion through the aqueous layer (Fig. 6.7) becomes the rate-limiting step.

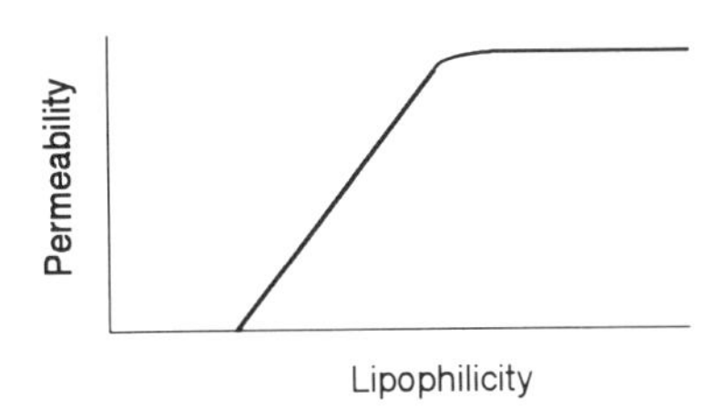

Fig. 6.7. Relationship between the permeability of the epithelial cell membrane of the GI tract and drug lipophilicity, on the basis of the pH-partition theory.

Recent developments related to drug uptake by passive diffusion. On the basis of the pH-partition hypothesis, the permeability of the GI tract (mainly of the small intestine) increases according to lipophilicity (Fig. 6.7). Although this is often correct, in several cases (two examples were mentioned above concerning salicylates and quinine) it is necessary to modify the original expression to allow for the ability of the ionized form to

§ Sink conditions can be assumed in the overwhelming majority of cases because of the continuous drainage of the drug into the capillary bed.

permeate the epithelial membrane. Fig. 6.8 displays experimental data concerning the relationship between permeability (expressed as uptake rate constant) and lipophilicity. Although the form of the plot resembles Fig. 6.7, there is a major scattering of the points, and the plot is sigmoid. As the solvent provides only an approximate estimate of the ability of the drug to permeate the membrane, some scatter is inevitable. The tailing effect at low partition coefficient values, however, is believed to be due to the uptake of these hydrophilic compounds via the paracellular route. Greater attention has recently been given to the study of uptake through aqueous pores, a route that was previously considered to be of minor importance.

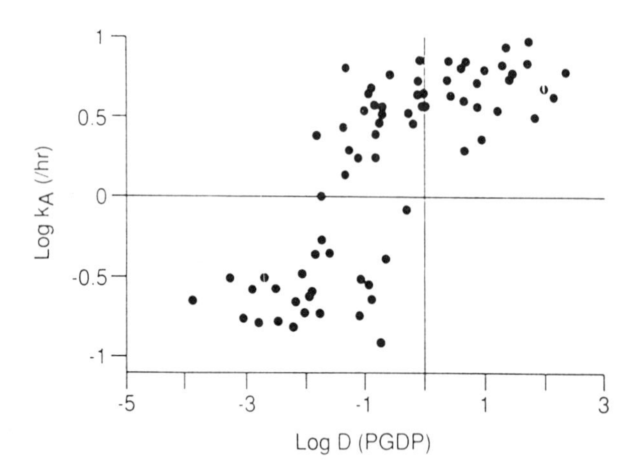

Fig. 6.8. Plot of the logarithm of the first order constant of uptake rate versus the logarithm of the partition coefficient (in a system of propylene glycol dipelargonate (PGDP)/water) for compounds of various structure. (The use of PGDP has been proved to provide better correlations than octanol.) (From *Drug Delivery to the Gastrointestinal Tract*, Hardy JG, Davis SS and Wilson CG (eds), Ellis Horwood (1989), p. 136, with permission.)

Permeation of the cell membrane via carrier mediation. In section 2.3.2 the characteristics of the two types of carrier-mediated transport, i.e. active transport and facilitated diffusion, were described.

Many nutrients and electrolytes are taken up by carrier mediation (which is usually an active process). Until the 1970s no specific permeation processes for drugs had been reported. However, the observation that organic acids and organic bases are secreted actively by the blood into the small intestine led to the assumption that these carriers may also be involved in intestinal uptake. Facile uptake of drugs with basic properties (not predicted on the basis of the pH-partition hypothesis) could be explained in this way. During the 1980s it was demonstrated that the uptake of certain semi-synthetic derivatives of penicillin, the most common cephalosporins, L-dopa, L-methyldopa, aminoglycosides, certain anticancer drugs (such as 5-bromouracil and 5-fluorouracil) and certain lithium salts is carrier mediated. There is also some evidence that cardiac glycosides are absorbed, at least to a certain extent, by a carrier-mediated process.

Mathematical consideration of drug uptake by carrier mediation. As in the case of uptake based on the pH-partition hypothesis, here the total process depends on transport through both the aqueous layer and the membrane. However, here the concentration gradient is the driving force only for the transport through the unstirred water layer. Considering the uptake as a two-step process, i.e. from the GI fluids to the membrane and from the membrane to the interior of the epithelial cell, the flux through the stagnant aqueous layer is described by equation (6.1). The equation which describes the flux of a molecule through the cell membrane by carrier mediation is analogous to the Michaelis–Menten equation (section 2.3.2.1):

$$J_m = \frac{J_{max} C_{br}}{K_M + C_{br}} \tag{6.5}$$

where C_{br} is the concentration of the drug at the interface between the aqueous layer and the cell membrane. Equation (6.5) can be rearranged in terms of C_{br}:

$$C_{br} = \frac{J_m K_M}{J_{max} - J_m} \tag{6.6}$$

For continuity of the flux from the aqueous layer to the membrane, the transport rates in these two sections must be equal, $J_l = J_m$. At steady state, J_l or J_m represents the flux of drug uptake, J_u, i.e. $J_l = J_m = J_u$. In equation (6.1), $C_g = C_{g0} - C_{br}$, where C_{g0} is the initial drug concentration in the GI fluids. By combining equations (6.6) and (6.1) one obtains

$$J_u^2 - \left(J_{max} + K_M P_{aq} + P_{aq} C_{g0}\right) J_u + J_{max} P_{aq} C_{g0} = 0 \tag{6.7}$$

The solution of equation (6.7) gives the following equation (where only the negative value of the square root gives a meaningful solution):

$$J_u = \frac{J_{max} + K_M P_{aq} + P_{aq} C_{g0} - \left\{\left(J_{max} + K_M P_{aq} + P_{aq} C_{g0}\right)^2 - 4 J_{max} P_{aq} C_{g0}\right\}^{1/2}}{2} \tag{6.8}$$

Permeation of the cell membrane through the aqueous pores. In cases where permeation of small hydrophilic molecules is not correlated with the pH and the partition coefficient, it is believed that the transport of the drug molecule to the interior of the epithelial cell is accomplished to a considerable degree through the aqueous pores or channels formed by proteins located in the cell membrane (Fig. 6.6). It is worth mentioning that while permeation of the drug through the membrane lipids is possible throughout the length of the GI tract, entrance into the cell through the membrane pores is favoured only in the small intestine. Based on data collected from perfusion studies, the radius of the pores in human small intestine is estimated to be approximately 0.7 nm in the jejunum and 0.3 nm in the ileum. In general, it is considered that drugs which have a potential of uptake through the aqueous pores must have a molecular weight below about 300.

Examples of drugs which have been found to have a high degree of uptake through the membrane pores in relation to their total uptake include cimetidine (MW 252), caffeine (MW 194), hydrochlorothiazide (MW 298) and atenolol (MW 266).

Special cases of intracellular uptake. In some cases, contemplation of more than one mechanism of permeation of the epithelial cell is required. For example, the bile salts appear to be taken up by a combination of passive and active mechanisms, with the dominant mechanism depending on the region of the GI tract (section 5.2).

The mathematical analysis of the simultaneous uptake of the drug by different mechanisms requires a consideration of the individual mechanisms. In this case, the flux through the stagnant aqueous layer is described again by equation (6.1), whereas the equation which describes the flux across the membrane varies according to the mechanisms involved. For example, if sink conditions prevail and the transport is accomplished by passive diffusion of the non-ionized species and by carrier-mediated transport of the ionized species, the equation describing the transport process from mucosa would be the following:

$$J_m = \left(P_{mem} f_{s,aq} + P_p\right) C_{br} + \frac{J_{max} f_{i,aq} C_{br}}{K_M + f_{i,aq} C_{br}} \tag{6.9}$$

where P_p is the permeability coefficient of ionized and non-ionized species through the aqueous pores and equals to $(D_{aq} F_R)/h_{mem}$; F_R is a dimensionless number which expresses the Renkin filtration factor ($0 \leqslant F_R \leqslant 1.0$); and $f_{i,aq}$ is the fraction of the ionized species at the interface between the aqueous layer and the membrane.

Equality of the fluxes ($J_l = J_m = J_u$) in this case does not lead to an algebraic solution for a direct estimation of J_u in relation to C_{br}, as in equation (6.8). Such a calculation is in this case possible only by numerical methods.

Finally, in cases where drug is transported simultaneously by two carriers, or where transport is accompanied by simultaneous biotransformation at the membrane (as occurs with prostaglandins), the mathematical treatment is quite complicated and the reader is referred to the appropriate literature cited at the end of this chapter.

Influence of water exchange during the intracellular uptake of the drugs. Concluding the description of the intracellular permeation mechanisms, it is worth mentioning that regardless of the mechanism the transport of drugs to the interior of the epithelial cell is influenced by the water exchange (secretion or absorption), which takes place during the uptake of the drug (solvent drag effect).

The mean water secretion by an adult into the GI lumen is about 6–7 l/d. If one takes into consideration another 1–2 l/d ingested orally and 100–200 ml/d eliminated in faeces, approximately 9 litres of water are absorbed by the GI tract each day. It has been established that drug uptake is proportional to the transport of water from the GI tract to blood. More specifically, administration of hypertonic solutions of drugs leads to increased secretion in the lumen, an event that delays the absorption not only of water but of coexisting drug molecule(s) as well. By contrast, administration of hypotonic or isotonic solutions accelerates drug uptake because of increased absorption of water.

Sulfisoxazole, metoclopramide and salicylic acid are examples of drugs for which net water secretion/absorption has been shown to influence absorption. This phenomenon appears to be associated with the interaction between water and drug molecules, at the membrane interface as well as in the bulk solution. It also appears that in the case of carrier-mediated uptake the absorption or secretion of water results in an increase or decrease, respectively, in the rate of drug uptake.

Permeation of the cell membrane by pinocytosis. Pinocytosis is characterized by a folding of the membrane and inclusion of the molecule in the vesicle. The drug molecule is then released into the cytoplasm. This mechanism of transport is rare and an important contributor to the overall uptake rate only in the case of macromolecules. With regard to nutrients there is some indication that pinocytosis is involved in the absorption of vitamin B_{12}. In addition, botulism (a severe form of food poisoning) is induced by the absorption of the botulism toxin (MW $\approx$900 000), which is believed to occur by pinocytosis.

Paracellular transport

Permeation of the tight junction of the epithelial cells. From a morphological point of view, the epithelial cells which line the GI tract are in such tight contact that the membrane seems continuous when studied by electron microscopy. However, the sites of contact are functionally permeable by water, electrolytes and other (ionized or not) molecules of small size.† More specifically, the radius of the opening is a little bigger than the size of the aqueous pores and ranges between 0.5 and 5 nm. There is, however, some evidence that compounds such as insulin and cardiac glycosides can be taken up through the paracellular route, which would imply that under certain conditions the pore size can extend up to 1–2 μm. It has been hypothesized that in the presence of compounds which form complexes with calcium ions, an elevation in the local pH, and changes in the water exchange can account for the observed transport.

Persorption. The entrance of particles with a size of up to 150 nm from the top of a villus through the temporary opening formed during the shedding of two neighbouring epithelial cells into the lumen is called persorption. Naturally, the entrance of molecules in the interstitial fluid in this manner is expected to be quite rare and has not been studied extensively.

6.2 TRANSFER OF THE DRUG FROM THE INTERIOR OF THE EPITHELIAL CELL INTO THE BLOOD

From the interior of the epithelial cell the drug enters the intracellular space through the basolateral cell membrane and, after moving across the capillary wall (or under certain conditions the membrane of the lymph vessels), it is transported by the venous blood (or the lymph) into the general circulation.

† Besides the GI epithelium, permeation of the epithelia of the gallbladder, the choroid plexus and of the proximal glomerular tubule is possible through the paracellular route (leaky epithelia). On the contrary, such a process is not possible in the epithelia of the distal glomerular tubule or the bladder.

As transport from the interior of the epithelial cell to the capillaries and lymph vessels is passive, this process does not usually present a limitation. However, profound alterations in the blood flow rate and/or the inability of the drug molecule to penetrate the wall of the lymph vessels may hamper the rate of drug transport to the systemic circulation.

6.2.1 Transfer of the drug into the portal circulation via the capillaries

The GI tract constitutes the region of the body which has the most blood flow per gram of tissue and it receives approximately 30% of the stroke volume. Transport of drug to the systemic circulation through the blood vessels, which collect from mucosa of the GI tract to the portal vein, constitutes the principal way by which orally administered drugs are assimilated. The lymph is usually of lesser importance because of the much lower flow rate and the high degree of lipophilicity required for incorporation into chylomicrons.

6.2.1.1 The network of blood vessels supplying the gastrointestinal tract

The supply network of the GI tract, commonly referred to as the splanchnic circulation, covers all of the layers of the gut wall. However, it is more dense in the mucosal than in the outer layers. For example, during relaxation in the small intestine 75% of the total flow is distributed to the mucosa.

There are three arteries supplying the gastrointestinal system (Fig. 6.9). Supply of blood to the stomach occurs primarily by branches of the celiac artery. Arterial blood

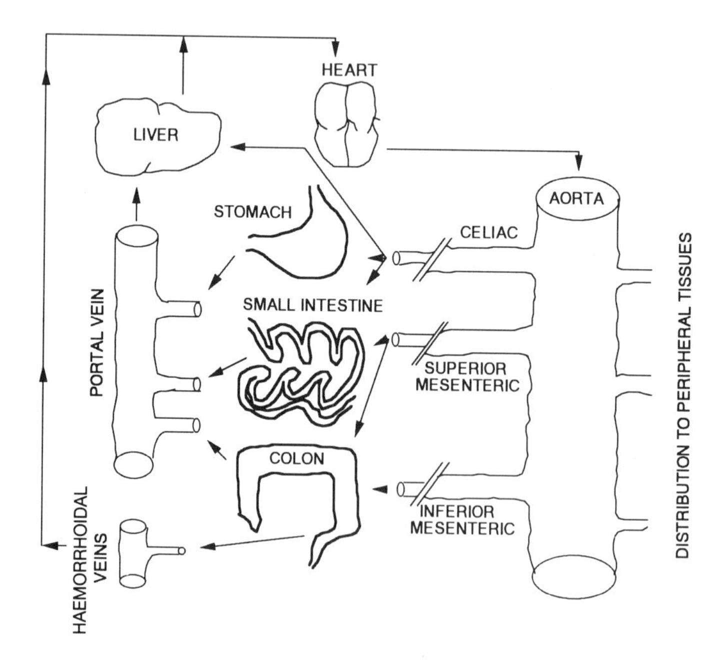

Fig. 6.9. Structure of splanchnic blood flow. In general, the blood flow rate is considered to be approximately 25 ml/min per kilogram.

reaches the duodenum by branches of the superior mesenteric artery, while for the rest of the small intestine blood is supplied primarily by branches of the superior mesenteric artery. Finally, the large intestine is supplied by successive branches of the superior and inferior mesenteric arteries. The arteries enter the organs they supply and divide into smaller formations, called arterioles, which have an inner diameter of less than 25 μm. The arterioles are the principal source of resistance to the flow of blood. Gating of flow is achieved by the opening and closing of pre-capillary sphincters located in the arterioles, and is supported by the exceptionally thick wall of the arterioles. This regulates the rate of capillary perfusion. The pre-capillary sphincters are made mainly of smooth muscle. After passing through the arterioles, blood enters the capillaries. In relaxation (and when food is not consumed) only one-third of the capillaries are open to blood flow. During this period, the flow rate in the mucosa is only about half that of the splanchnic flow, i.e. approximately 13 ml/min per kilogram body weight (or about 1 l/min).[†] In contrast, during digestion the sphincters do not contract and the flow rate through the capillaries is doubled. The capillaries, unlike the arterioles, have an exceptionally thin wall. Because of the simple construction of the wall (see also section 8.1) and their large surface (relative to their volume), capillaries constitute the main area where exchange of liquids, electrolytes, metabolites, nutrients and drugs is accomplished.

The wall of the capillaries of the GI tract comprises a simple layer of endothelial cells, between which there are large pores. The size of the pores is such that molecules with a molecular weight smaller than 1000 pass freely. Thus the permeation of the capillary wall by drugs is mainly achieved by diffusion through the pores. For lipophilic drugs transmural movement may also be possible. In contrast, drugs of high molecular weight (such as proteins) cannot enter the capillary and accumulate in the interstitial fluid, pass to the lymph and enter the systemic circulation very slowly through the thoracic duct. Apart from the size of the molecules, permeation of the capillary wall depends on the osmolality between the interstitial fluid and the capillaries. The osmolality of the interstitial fluid is influenced by the active uptake of many ions (such as Na^+), taking place regardless of the concentration gradient of the ions between the aqueous layer and the stagnant interstitial fluid.

From the capillaries, the blood (containing any absorbed drug) is collected into the venules, and then into the veins. Venous blood drained from the stomach, the small intestine and most of the large intestine is united in the portal vein and after passing through the liver reaches the systemic circulation via the inferior vena cava. By contrast, veins from the lower rectum are collected in the haemorrhoidal veins which drain into the inferior vena cava, providing direct access to the systemic circulation. This differentiation is of great importance in cases where the drug is biotransformed extensively in the liver. Oral administration and uptake from the small intestine may result in the biotransformation of a portion of the drug during the first pass through the liver, before its arrival in the general circulation (section 9.4). In contrast, administration from the rectum results in circumvention of the first-pass effect.

† In the large intestine, supply is considerably more dense and in an anaesthetized patient during surgical operation it has been determined to be 18 ml/min per 100 g of tissue.

Under some circumstances arrival of the drug in the systemic circulation will be influenced significantly by the blood flow rate in the GI system. The blood flow rate depends on many factors, which include haemodynamic factors (splanchnic flow rate is proportional to the stroke volume, the arterial pressure and the total blood volume), the autonomous nervous system (mainly the parasympathetic system, stimulation of which causes vasodilation and increase of flow), various neurohumoral substances (vasopressin, catecholamines and angiotensin decrease, while glucagon, chelocystokinin and gastrin increase the flow), local metabolic activity (during absorption or secretion of nutrients the flow increases), certain autoregulating and countercurrent factors, and finally on the presence of enteric ischaemia (observed mainly in patients with congestive heart failure, where the blood tends to 'stagnate'). The importance of the blood flow rate in drug uptake varies according to the drug. The more readily a drug reaches the capillaries, the more dependent on splanchnic blood flow rate is its arrival in the general circulation likely to be.

Hydrophilic drugs, for which the uptake process is limited by permeation of the cell membrane, and very lipophilic drugs for which diffusion across the stagnant layer is limiting, are unlikely to be affected greatly by the blood flow rate.

Drugs which are highly soluble and permeate the mucosa quickly (i.e. have little resistance to uptake) may be more likely to exhibit changes in absorption with changes in flow rate. Table 6.4 presents some substances for which uptake is influenced to a large degree by the blood flow rate.

Table 6.4. The uptake of these substances is influenced by the blood flow rate

Ethanol	Benzoic acid
Aminopyrine	Salicylic acid
Antipyrine	Cimetidine

6.2.2 Transfer of the drug to the systemic circulation via the lymph vessels

Transport of the drug to the systemic circulation via the lymph vessels is generally a path of minor importance, because the lymph vessels are less accessible than the capillaries. In addition, the lymph flow is exceptionally slow.

However, fats, fat-soluble vitamins and other highly lipophilic molecules arrive in the major circulation via the lymph. A major advantage of this pathway compared to the blood vessels is that one can directly access the systemic circulation without passing through the liver. In addition, permeation of the drug through the wall of the lymph vessels does not depend on molecular size (i.e. the molecular weight). In general, compounds of a molecular weight greater than 16 000 may reach the systemic circulation only through the lymph. These considerations suggest three possible advantages of lymphatic transport:

(1) targeted delivery of drugs which act specifically on the lymphatic system (such as interferons and interleukins, which are administered in certain cases of cancer, etc.);
(2) the possibility of administration of drugs with high molecular weight; and
(3) avoidance of the first-pass effect.

6.2.2.1 The network of the lymph vessels which supplies the gastrointestinal tract

The lymph vessels, in contrast to the blood vessels (where arteries and veins form a circuit), begin from blind vessels. In the small intestine, these are the central lacteals of the villi. In the mucosal region of the colon, lymphatic vessels are not readily discernible by light microscopy. However, ultrastructural analysis has indicated that the colonic mucosa does possess lymphatic drainage although not as extensive as that of the small intestinal mucosa. In fact, lymphatic plexuses are found near the muscularis mucosa and within the submucosa of the colon.

In the GI tract, the lymph is drained at a rate of the order of a few millilitres per minute. The lymph plexuses of the entire GI tract are collected into the mesenteric lymph duct at the cisterna chyli (Fig. 6.10). After passing through the thoracic duct, the lymph is brought into the venous section of the major circulation. The total flow rate of the lymph in the thoracic duct is approximately 100–200 ml/h.

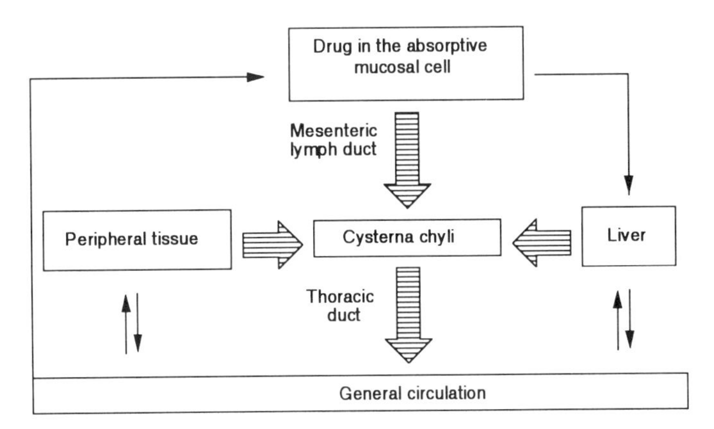

Fig. 6.10. Schematic representation of the transport of drugs to the general circulation via the lymph.

6.2.2.2 Factors that influence drug transport from the epithelial cell to the systemic circulation via the lymph vessels

The arrival of a drug molecule in the lymph is normally associated with feed in and the transport of triglycerides in the lymph vessels.

Fats, although taken up from the GI fluids in the form of fatty acids and monoglycerides, are reconverted to triglycerides in the cytoplasm and enter the lymph vessels in the form of lipoproteins, of which the most important are the chylomicrons (section 7.1). The concentration of chylomicrons in the lymph generally ranges between 1% and 2%. The anabolic process of simple lipids is complicated. Most drugs enter the lymph vessels bound to the triglyceride part of the chylomicrons and of the very low density lipoproteins (VLDL, section 7.1) (Fig. 6.11). After arrival in the systemic circulation the drug is released from the chylomicrons, either due to hydrolysis of the triglycerides (by the lipoproteinic lipases of the blood), or because of diffusion of the drug from the intact chylomicrons to the water of the plasma. For these reasons, the possibility of a drug being transported via the lymph depends on the physicochemical properties of the administered drug, as well as the quantity and the properties of the coadministered lipid carrier which is used to induce the intracellular production of chylomicrons.

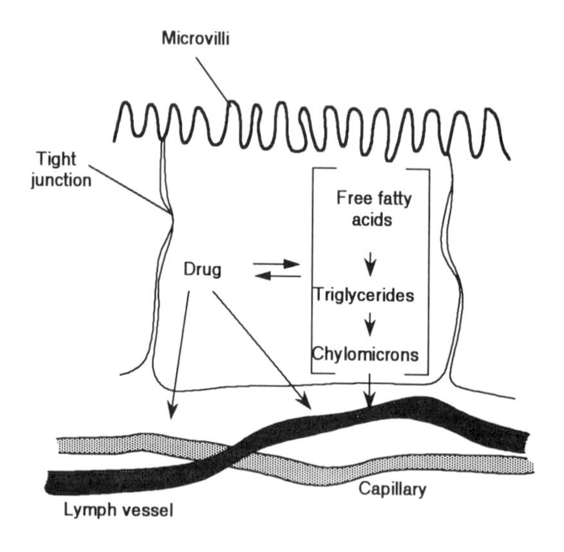

Fig. 6.11. Transport mechanism of a drug from the small intestinal mucosa to the lymph.

The physicochemical properties of the drug

In general, it is difficult to derive rules related to the properties required of a molecule for lymphatic transport. The main requirement appears to be a very high degree of lipophilicity. Lipophilicity in this instance implies very high fat solubility as well as a highly favourable oil/water partition coefficient. In general, in order for 50% of the quantity of a drug molecule to be transported to the lymph, the partition coefficient of the drug between water and chylomicrons (note: the partition coefficient between water and 1-octanol may not accurately predict partitioning into chylomicrons) must be at least 1 : 50000 (i.e. the log P of the molecule must be at least 4.7), and of course the saturation solubility of the molecule in the lipid phase must not be a restriction.

The coadministered lipid carrier

The relative lymph flow rate in the draining lymph vessels, situated in the small intestine, to the venous flow rate, concentrating in the portal vein, is 1 : 500. However, in contrast to the capillaries, the limiting factor for the entrance of the lipophilic molecules in the lymph vessels is usually not lymph flow rate, but the flux of the chylomicrons to the lymph, which in turn depends on the coadministration of lipids.

In order to increase transport of drugs to the lymph vessels, lipid carriers are usually coadministered with the drugs. These carriers are hydrolysed in the lumen, taken up (mainly in the form of fatty acids) and anabolized, during their stay in the cytoplasm, to lipoproteins. The triglyceride part of these lipoproteins binds the lipophilic drug and the complex enters the lymph. It is believed that fatty acids with a chain of at least 12 carbon atoms are the most competent lipid carriers. The administration of diglycerides or triglycerides is less appropriate, because the time required for luminal hydrolysis prior to uptake delays the intracellular re-formation and binding to the transported drug.

6.3 METHODS OF ENHANCING THE PERMEATION OF DRUGS THROUGH THE GASTROINTESTINAL MUCOSA

Strategies to improve the percentage uptake of the drug by the GI mucosa can be pursued, once the rate-limiting step to the uptake process is known (Fig. 6.1). Many times, the rate-limiting step is the transport through the epithelial cells. Increasing the proportion of the drug that permeates the mucosa can be accomplished by using prodrugs that are taken up more easily than the parent compound or, in the case of compounds metabolized during uptake, inhibitors of the enzymes of the epithelial cell membrane.

6.3.1 Penetration enhancers

The most usual way of increasing the extent of uptake is the coadministration of compounds which facilitate the transport of the drug across the membrane. These compounds are called *penetration enhancers* or *penetration promoters*. This method is used mainly in cases of hydrophilic drugs which are expected to have difficulty permeating the lipid structure of the membrane. However, it is worth mentioning that in contrast to the great effect of penetration enhancers on rectal or transdermal administration, their ability to improve uptake by the small intestine appears to be modest. The reduction in efficacy is thought to be mainly due to dilution of the penetration enhancer by the GI fluids (the intensity of the influence is proportional to the concentration of the enhancer).

The mechanism of action of the penetration enhancers varies. Usually it is related to the interaction of the lipid part of the enhancer with the polar component of membrane phospholipids (Fig. 6.12).

Substances which increase the extent of uptake can be divided into three categories:

(1) Substances that act very quickly, have a strong effect and cause injury to the membrane (which is rapidly reversible). Examples are certain fatty acids with 10–20 carbon atoms (such as oleic, linoleic and arachidonic) and their monoglycerides, and esters of fatty acids with glucose.

(2) Substances that again act very quickly, cause temporary histological destruction, but have average activity. Such compounds include the salicylates and certain bile salts.

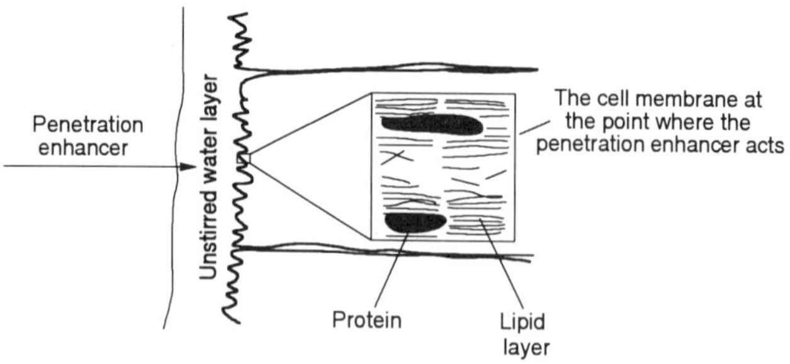

Fig. 6.12. Linear representation of perturbation of the lipid layer, caused by penetration enhancers during their permeation through the epithelial cells.

(3) Substances that have average to strong activity and cause sustained histological changes. Typical examples are certain surfactants, such as sodium lauryl sulfate, ethylenediaminetetraacetic acid (EDTA) and citric acid.

The use of penetration enhancers in the small intestine is restricted owing to the non-specific action of these compounds and the existence of significant side effects. The fatty acids (which were believed at first to act exclusively by increasing the proportion of drug that reaches the lymph) are among the most promising substances. However, in order to secure their action, apart from specificity and biocompatibility, their simultaneous presence with the drug in satisfactory concentrations at the uptake sites is required.

Certain ions can also act as penetration enhancers in specific cases. It has been shown that the transport rate of drugs with acidic or basic properties can be increased by conjugation with counter ions, presumably because of the charge reduction and subsequent transport in the form of ion-pairs. Candidate drugs for conjugation with counter ions have low bioavailability and are completely ionized at GI pH (as, for example, bretylium bromide and atenolol). On the other hand, the counter ions should have or result in high lipophilicity and saturation solubility of the ion-pair, be biocompatible and not present stability problems (for example, negatively charged alkylated salicylates).

6.3.2 Prodrugs with advantageous membrane permeability and inhibitors of the enzymes of the cell membrane

A typical example of a drug for which prodrugs with better membrane permeability can be made is methyl-dopa. This drug has a structure similar to an amino acid and is taken up to a limited degree from the small intestine by means of an amino acid carrier. In contrast, the dipeptides L-α-methyl-dopa-L-phenylalanine and L-α-methyl-dopa-L-proline, which are taken up by the small peptide transporter, have permeation coefficients 5–20 times larger. These dipeptides are hydrolysed in the cytoplasm to the parent compounds.

If the drug is extensively biotransformed during permeation of the epithelial cell membrane (first-pass effect, section 9.4), the use of compounds which inhibit the activity of certain enzymes of the cell membrane leads to an increase of the proportion of the drug that reaches the capillaries. This method is mainly used in cases where the drug is a peptide or a protein, and, therefore, inhibition of peptidase activity in the gut is sought.

6.4 METHODS OF STUDYING UPTAKE

Assessment of drug uptake can be accomplished with experiments which:

— evaluate the participation of the stagnant layer in the uptake process;
— investigate the transport process through the mucosa; and
— determine the region of the GI tract in which the drug permeates the mucosa most easily.

In each case a variety of experimental methods are available, which are generally classified as *in vitro* and *in situ*. Whole animal methods, despite the possibility that they can be extrapolated more easily to humans, provide information only for the overall process of absorption.

6.4.1 Estimation of the thickness of the stagnant aqueous layer

The measurement of the thickness of the stagnant aqueous layer is based on measuring the electric potential between the interface of the epithelium with the aqueous layer and the serosal layer *in situ* or using *in vitro* preparations. When there are no important differences between the interface and the serosal layer in the constitution of the components, the potential difference is zero. In cases where osmotically active compounds or electrolytes are and/or the active transport of ions (Na^+, Cl^-, Ca^{2+}) through the mucosa is disturbed, a potential difference between the interface and the serosal layer is observed.

The experiment consists of measuring the potential difference as a function of time while the concentration at the membrane is continuously increasing owing to diffusion through the unstirred water layer (*Diamond method*). Because of the unstirred water layer, a solute added to the bulk solution does not appear at the membrane instantaneously. Rather, its concentration at the membrane builds up gradually from zero to the final value with a half-time inversely proportional to its diffusion coefficient and directly proportional to the square of the thickness of the unstirred water layer.

6.4.2 Study of transport through the mucosa

6.4.2.1 In vitro experiments

In vitro experiments are used to study the transport of the drug through different types of membranes or biological materials, aiming to establish contributions to transport such as the ability of the drug to diffuse in aqueous media, diffusion and partitioning behaviour in lipid media, binding to various types of membranes, etc. Such experiments may utilize:†

† These *in vitro* techniques are used in studies of drug transport through cell barriers in general and are not used exclusively for the study of permeation of drugs through GI epithelial cell membrane.

— devices of set geometry, usually called diffusion cells;
— segments of the GI tract of laboratory animals (or, very rarely, of humans). Two well-established techniques are the everted sac technique and the everted ring technique;
— cell cultures of laboratory animal or human gut epithelia.

Diffusion cells
Diffusion cells are used in combination with synthetic membranes or segments of membranes from the GI tract of small laboratory animals (Fig. 6.13). These cells usually consist of two compartments and have one of the forms displayed in Fig. 6.13. A solution of the drug is placed in the donor compartment and the rate of its arrival in the receptor compartment (which usually contains a drug-free buffer solution) is measured.

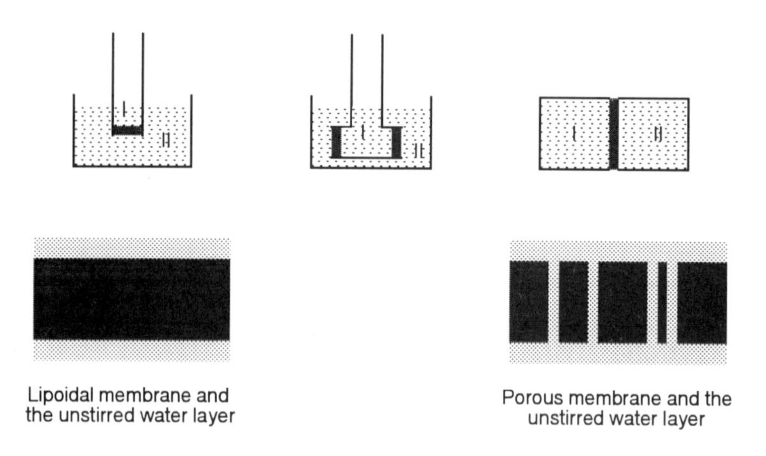

Fig. 6.13. *In vitro* techniques of estimating the transport of drug through synthetic membranes. Characteristic types of membranes and cells.

Synthetic membranes include polymer compounds of silicone to simulate a lipoidal membrane, or cellulose membranes to simulate a porous membrane. The permeation of a drug through a lipophilic membrane requires partitioning and diffusion through the membrane material. As a result, the lipid membranes are considered to reproduce the behaviour of the biological membrane more closely than the porous membranes. The usefulness of the porous membranes lies in the ability to discern contributions to the transport of the drug by the diffusion through the membrane pores, regardless of its lipophilicity (or degree of ionization). The mathematical description of the permeation process through lipoidal membranes is similar to the one described earlier in this chapter for passive diffusion through the GI epithelial cell membrane. For porous membranes, the apparent permeability coefficient under the prerequisite of similar stirring in both compartments, is given by the following equation:

$$P_{\mathrm{app}} = \frac{1}{\dfrac{2}{P_{\mathrm{aq}}} + \dfrac{1}{P_{\mathrm{p}}}} \tag{6.10}$$

where P_p is the permeability coefficient of the total (ionized and non-ionized) drug through the aqueous pores and is equal to

$$\left[(1-\alpha)K_r D_{aq} F_R\right]/h_{mem}$$

where α is the fraction of the actual (without the pores) volume of the membrane, K_r is the actual surface area of the membrane and F_R is the Renkin filtration factor ($0 < F_R < 1$). The Renkin factor depends on the molecular radius of the molecule which permeates the membrane compared with the radius of the membrane pores.

The everted sac technique

This technique was originally developed in the mid-1950s by Wilson and Wiseman and offers the capability of studying the transport of drugs through the entire intestinal wall. It is based on the initial eversion of a segment (about 2.5–3 cm) of the intestine of small laboratory animals, usually of rats or rabbits. The segment is then converted to a sac, filled with buffer solution and tied at both ends by a thin thread. The sac is immersed in a pre-oxygenated (95% O_2 to 5% CO_2) solution of the drug of a specific concentration, exposing the mucosa directly to the oxygenated liquid (Fig. 6.14). The whole preparation is placed in a container (usually, an Erlenmeyer flask) and is shaken mildly in a water-bath at 37°C. It is possible to make several such sacs and place them in flasks in the incubation water-bath. At predetermined time intervals, the sac is removed and the concentration of the drug in the internal (serosal) liquid is determined. One of the major disadvantages of the method is the difficulty of taking more than one sample per sac, but this can be overcome by modifying the method appropriately. Another disadvantage is the small volume of the serosal liquid (about 1 ml). This usually precludes quantitative determination of depletion of the drug from the exterior solution. On the other hand, even

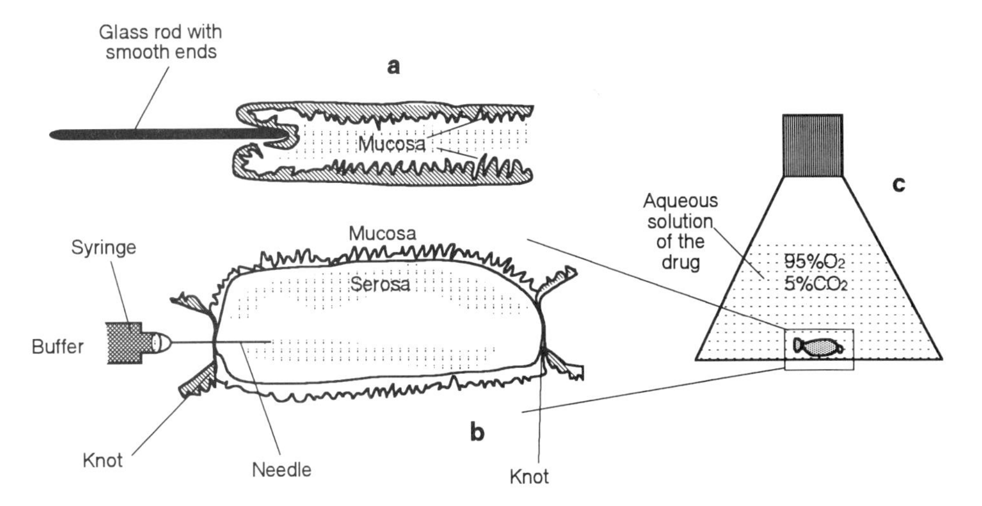

Fig. 6.14. *In vitro* estimation of drug transport through the GI wall. The everted sac technique, as developed originally by Wilson and Wiseman. (a) Inversion of the sac, (b) placing of buffer solution in the interior of the sac, and (c) placing of the sac in the drug solution.

when only a small portion of the drug passes through the gut wall there will be a significant change in its concentration in the serosal liquid.

Example 6.3: In an *in vitro* study of drug uptake using the everted sac technique, the following rates of permeation were observed, after incubating the sacs for 15 min in three different solutions of the drug:

Initial concentration of the drug (mg/l):	29.2, 60.4, 82.1
(Initial) rate of permeation (10^{-3} μg/mg tissue per 15 min):	41, 80, 119

The volume of each sac was 1.10 ml and the volume of drug solution was 20.0 ml. Determine whether the kinetics of permeation of the studied drug follows the principles of passive diffusion.

Answer: Transport to the interior of the sacs is a reversible process and the following equation describes the initial rate of transport (section 2.3.1):

$$\frac{dm_0}{dt} = AP_{app}(C_0 - C_{AE}) \tag{6.11}$$

where C_{AE} here is the concentration after reaching equilibrium. At equilibrium, the sum of the quantities of the drug inside and outside of the sac will be equal to the initial quantity placed in the external solution, and the concentrations on both sides will be equal. Therefore for the first sac it follows that

$$X_{AE,1} + X_{BE,1} = 29.2 \text{ (mg/l)} \times 0.0200 \text{ (l)} = 0.584 \text{ mg}$$

In addition

$$C_{AE,1} = C_{BE,1}$$

i.e.

$$X_{AE,1}/20.0 = X_{BE,1}/1.10 \quad \text{or} \quad X_{BE,1} = X_{AE,1}/18.2$$

where the subscripts AE,1 and BE,1 denote the equilibrium state inside and outside of the first sac, respectively. From the above equation it follows:

$$X_{AE,1} + X_{AE,1}/18.2 = 0.584 \text{ mg}$$

and

$$X_{AE,1} = 0.554 \text{ mg}$$

Therefore

$$C_{AE,1} = 27.7 \text{ mg/l}$$

In a similar manner it is found that

$$C_{AE,2} = 57.2 \text{ mg/l} \quad \text{and} \quad C_{AE,3} = 77.8 \text{ mg/l}$$

Therefore

	dm_0/dt (10^{-3} μg/mg tissue/15 min)	$C_0 - C_{AE}$ (mg/l)
Sac 1:	41	29.2 – 27.7 = 1.5
Sac 2:	80	60.4 – 57.2 = 3.2
Sac 3:	119	82.1 – 77.8 = 4.3

According to equation (6.11), a plot of dm_0/dt versus $(C_0 - C_{AE})$ should give a straight line if uptake is passive. Based on Fig. 6.15 and as regression analysis verifies the linear relationship between the two variables ($R = 0.992$), it appears that the kinetics of permeation are consistent with passive diffusion.

It is worth mentioning that it is necessary to report the transport rate in relation to the weight of tissue, because the thickness of the membrane often varies with the preparation. Thus, experimental data should be normalized according to the weight of each sac.

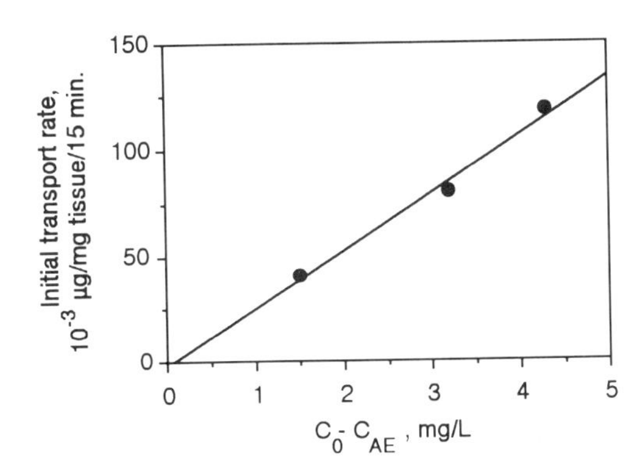

Fig. 6.15. Plot of dm_0/dt versus $(C_0 - C_{AE})$ for the data of Example 6.3.

The everted ring technique

This technique was originally developed in the mid-1950s. The idea of the accumulation of the drug against an apparent concentration gradient within the tissue was first introduced by Agar, Hird and Sidhu (1954) using strips of intestine and was further developed by Crane and Mandelstam (1960).

The rate of uptake of a compound is studied using rings, which are prepared by dissecting an inverted segment from the intestine of a small laboratory animal (usually a rat). The appropriate section of intestine is isolated, inverted and dissected in slices of a thickness usually between 1 and 3 mm. The slices are then placed in an oxygenated isotonic drug solution at 37°C and incubated for a predetermined period under gentle shaking. The incubation time is calculated from preliminary experiments (timed uptake study), in which the period over which uptake is linear is determined. After incubation, the rings are washed, dried and placed in pre-weighed scintillation vials. Each vial is reweighed to determine the wet tissue weight, then the sample is analysed for drug.

The method of everted rings is simple and reproducible and, in combination with other models, it can be used to investigate pre-systemic metabolism by the intestinal mucosa.

This method has been utilized for determination of the intestinal uptake characteristic of sugars, amino acids, peptides and pyrimidine compounds. The main disadvantage of this method lies in the process of dissection. It is possible for the tissue to be injured by the dissection at the section point and so a region very permeable by the drug may be formed, resulting in overestimation of the uptake.

Cell culture techniques

The development of single layers of differentiated cells on porous materials is a very recent technique, developed after 1985 for the investigation of drug transport. It is obvious that although in this chapter only the contribution of this technique in the study of GI drug uptake will be discussed, it can also be used for the study of drug transport through several other epithelia (e.g. buccal, renal, skin) and endothelia (e.g. the blood–brain barrier).

The main disadvantage of this novel method is that the cultivation of intestinal epithelial cells up to now has not been completely successful. The most popular method is to cultivate malignant cells from the large intestine (Caco-2 cells, HT-29 cells, etc.). Differentiated cells of the intestine, originating from Caco-2 cells placed in synthetic polycarbonate membranes, have been used in studying the permeation of bile salts, peptides, vitamins, antibiotics, etc.

The development of a method of cell cultivation which simulates the mucosa epithelium requires not only the series of appropriate cells, but also a porous membrane which (usually after treatment with an appropriate material, such as collagen) makes the reproduction of cells possible while not retarding permeation of the drug. In Fig. 6.16 the principle of constructing such a system of cell culture is presented.

Both uptake mechanism and pre-systemic metabolism can be identified using this technique.

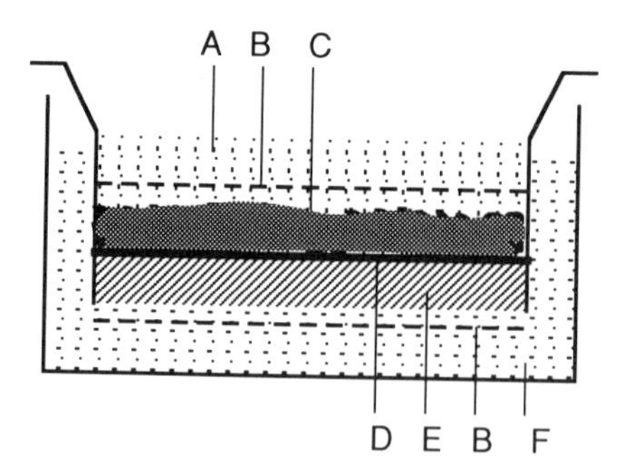

Fig. 6.16. The barriers for drug permeation in a system of cell cultures, which has been developed on a porous membrane. (A) Region in which the drug is initially placed (apical side), (B) the stagnant aqueous layer, (C) layer of cultivated cells, (D) supportive material (not mandatory), (E) porous membrane, (F) region where the drug reaches (basolateral side).

6.4.2.2 In situ *experiments*

In situ experiments for studying intestinal drug uptake were first introduced in the late 1960s and are based on the perfusion of a segment of the GI tract by a solution of the drug and subsequent calculation of the amount of drug which is taken up from the perfusate.

This type of experiment simulates the *in vivo* conditions better than the *in vitro* set-ups, since circulation of the blood is maintained and the drug is taken up by vessels situated in the mucosa. The main disadvantage is that measurement of the rate of decrease of drug concentration in the perfusate does not always represent the rate of arrival of the drug to the vessels (for example, whenever pre-systemic metabolism in the intestinal mucosa occurs). Therefore, in some cases this technique is applied in combination with measurements of the concentration of the drug in the portal vein.

The perfusion technique is used mainly in small laboratory animals, but it can also be applied to larger laboratory animals or humans.

The perfusion technique in small laboratory animals

This can be done using the following methods.

Doluisio method: The animal, after fasting for 12–24 h (the duration varies with the region of intestine to be perfused), is anaesthetized by intraperitoneal injection of urethane. After dissection in the abdominal region, the upper and lower parts of the section of the intestine† under study are connected with small L-shaped tubing, the free end of which is connected to a syringe with a capacity of about 10–30 ml (Fig. 6.17). After washing the segment with normal saline, the syringe, positioned at the upper part of the perfused segment, is filled with a solution containing the drug (usually radiolabelled), and a non-absorbable marker which is used as an indicator of the water flux during perfusion. Part of the content of the syringe is delivered to the interior of the intestine and, depending on the type of study, this solution is collected in the same or a second syringe and analysed for drug.

Single-pass perfusion: in this case the drug solution passes only once through the study region (Fig. 6.18). This technique is superior to the Doluisio method because it offers the possibility of precise adjustment of the hydrodynamic conditions (the type of flow in relation to the volume of the solution), which can influence not only the normal circulation of the blood but also the strain on the intestinal wall. In addition, adjustment of the hydrodynamic conditions results in more accurate simulation of the *in vivo* situation, thus assisting in scale-up of the data collected from laboratory animals to humans. Moreover, the Doluisio method takes longer, because the ratio of surface area of the intestine to the volume of the solution is much smaller (up to 10 times). Finally, it is worth mentioning that in both these perfusion methods it is assumed that transport through the membrane is similar over the whole segment.

† This technique (like single-pass perfusion, see below) is applied mainly to studies in the intestine, but its application to the study of uptake by the stomach has also been described.

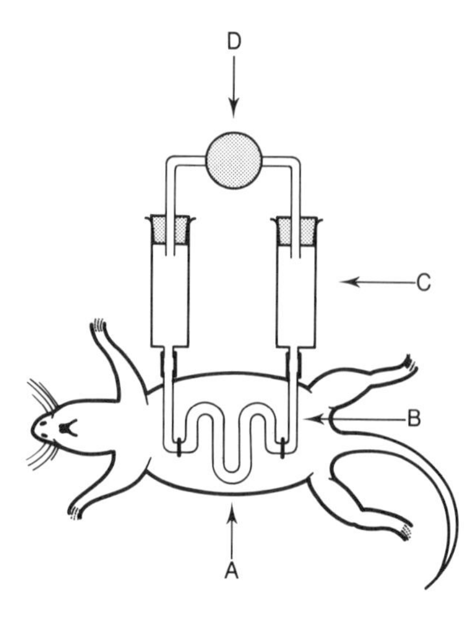

Fig. 6.17. Principle of the experimental device used for the *in situ* determination of the rate of uptake of drugs by the intestine of rats using the Doluisio method. (A) Segment of intestine at which uptake is studied, (B) tube connecting the intestine to the syringe, (C) syringe, (D) peristaltic pump.

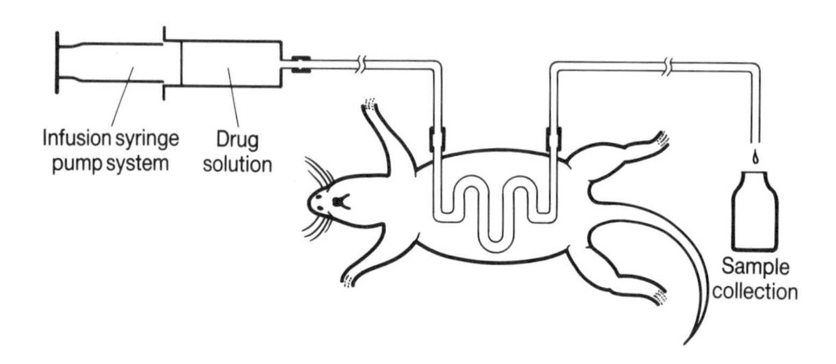

Fig. 6.18. Device for *in situ* study of drug uptake by the technique of single-pass perfusion.

The technique of perfusion in humans

In humans the perfusion technique is performed by intubation. Intubation is achieved by the method discussed in section 5.3.6, where it was presented as a method of studying transit through the GI tract. The application of this method to uptake studies presents certain problems. The main problem is the possible reflux of the administered solution. This problem can be overcome using a triple-lumen tube. Drug is administered via the shortest and aspirate sampled from the middle and longest tubes. The segment from the middle to the longest tube constitutes the study segment.

FURTHER READING

Amidon GL, Leesman GD and Elliott RL. Improving Intestinal Absorption of Water-Insoluble Compounds: A Membrane Metabolism Strategy. *J. Pharm. Sci.* **69**: 1363–1368 (1980).

Bronk JR and Hastewell JG. The Transport of Pyrimidines into Tissue Rings Cut from Rat Small Intestine. *J. Physiol.* (London) **382**: 475–488 (1987).

Diamond J. A Rapid Method for Determining Voltage–Concentration Relations Across Membranes. *J. Physiol.* (London) **183**: 83–100 (1966).

Fleisher D, Lippert CL, Sheth N, Reppas C and Wlodyga J. Nutrient Effects on Intestinal Drug Absorption. *J. Controlled Rel.* **11**: 41–49 (1990).

Ho NFH, Park JY, Amidon G, Ni PF and Higuchi W. Methods for Interrelating in Vitro Animal and Human Absorption Studies. In: *Gastrointestinal Absorption of Drugs.* Aguiar AJ (ed.), American Pharmaceutical Association, Academy of Pharmaceutical Sciences, Washington DC (1979).

Kvietys PR, Wilborn WH and Cranger DN. Effects of Net Transmucosal Volume Flux on Lymph Flow in the Canine Colon. Structural–Functional Relationship. *Gastroenterology* **81**: 1080–1090 (1981).

Muranishi S. Absorption Barriers and Absorption Promoters in the Intestine. In: *Topics in Pharmaceutical Sciences*, Breimer DD and Speiser P (eds), Elsevier Science Publications, Amsterdam (1987).

Neubert R. Ion Pair Transport Across membranes. *Pharm. Res.* **6**: 743–747 (1989).

Prescott LF and Nimmo WS (eds). *Novel Drug Delivery and its Therapeutic Application*, Chs 4–7, 10, Wiley, Chichester (1989).

Sernka TJ, Jacobson ED and Chowdhury TK. *Gastrointestinal Physiology: The Essentials.* Williams & Wilkins, Baltimore.

Strocchi A and Levitt MD. A Reappraisal of the Magnitude and Implications of the Intestinal Unstirred Layer. *Gastroenterology* **101**: 843–847 (1991).

Whalen GE, Harris JA, Green JE and Soergel K. Sodium and Water Absorption from the Human Small Intestine. The Accuracy of the Perfusion Method. *Gastroenterology* **51**: 975–984 (1966).

Wilson CG and Washington N. *Physiological Pharmaceutics: Biological Barriers to Drug Absorption*, Chs 1, 4, 5. Ellis Horwood, Chichester (1989).

Wilson G. Cell Culture Techniques for the Study of Drug Transport. *Eur. J. Drug Metab. Pharmacokinet.* **15**: 159–163 (1990).

Winne D. Unstirred Layer, Source of Biased Michaelis Constant in Membrane Transport. *Biochem. Biopharm. Acta* **298**: 27–31 (1973).

Winne D. Shift of pH-Absorption Curves. *J. Pharmacokinet. Biopharm.* **5**: 53–94 (1977).

Winne D. Influence of Blood Flow on Intestinal Absorption of Xenobiotics. *Pharmacology* **21**: 1–15 (1980).

PART III

7

Protein binding

Objectives

After completing this chapter the reader will be able to identify:

— The characteristics of drug–protein binding
— The mathematical relationships that describe drug–protein binding
— Calculation of binding parameters
— The importance of protein binding to drug distribution in the body
— The methods used for the study of protein binding

By the term 'protein binding' we mean the interaction of micromolecules (here drugs) with proteins. Protein binding may be divided to intra- and extracellular. In the former case the drug is bound to a cell protein which may be the drug receptor; if so, binding elicits a pharmacological response. These types of receptors are usually called *primary receptors*. Extracellular binding of drug to proteins does not usually elicit a pharmacological response and these types of receptors are called secondary or *silent receptors*.

The most important silent receptors are plasma proteins, in particular albumin. The extent of drug binding with plasma proteins varies significantly for different drugs and depends exclusively on the structure of the drug.

The significance of the drug's binding to plasma proteins with regard to its distribution, elimination and pharmacological action is shown schematically in Fig. 7.1. The bound form of the drug in plasma is in dynamic equilibrium with the free form. Only the free form participates in transport of drug into extravascular sites in the body. Thus, it is reasonable to infer that the higher the extent (percentage) and the strength of binding, the more significant its effect on drug distribution.

Although a great number of blood constituents may be capable of binding drugs, it has been shown that most drugs are primarily bound to albumin. Recently, great interest has also been shown in the binding of basic drugs with α_1-acid glycoprotein as well as the interaction of lipophilic drugs with lipoproteins. Relevant properties of these proteins are listed in Table 7.1.

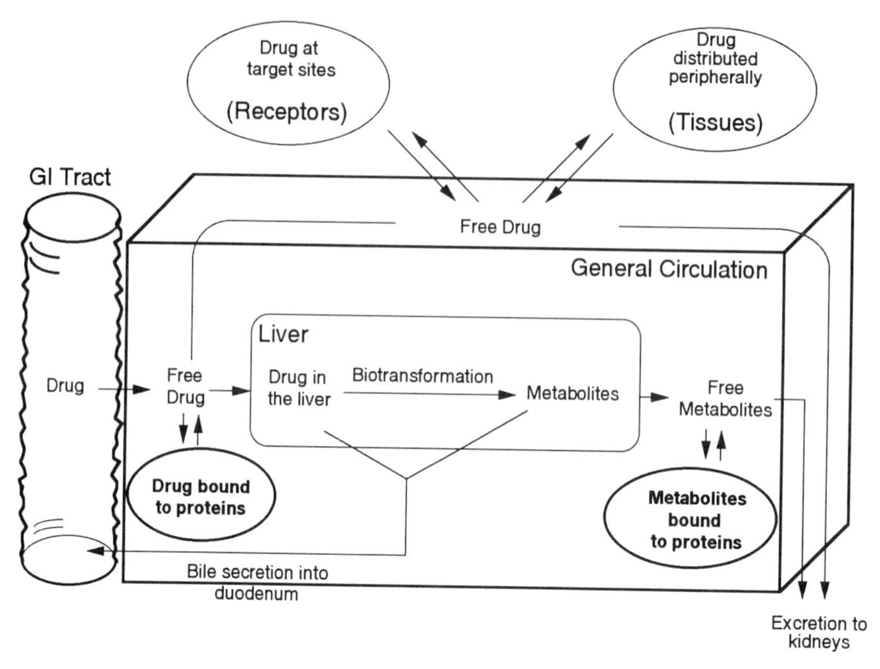

Fig. 7.1. Effect of the drug's binding to plasma proteins on transport in the body.

Table 7.1. Properties of the plasma proteins which most commonly bind drugs

Protein	Molecular weight	Physiological concentration range	
		g/l	Molarity
Albumin	66 500	35–50	$(5.0–7.5) \times 10^{-4}$
α_1-acid glycoprotein	44 000	0.4–1.0	$(0.9–2.2) \times 10^{-5}$
Lipoproteins	200 000–300 000		Variable

7.1 STRUCTURE OF THE MOST IMPORTANT PLASMA PROTEINS

7.1.1 Albumin

The complete sequence of amino acids in the human serum albumin (HSA) molecule was reported in 1975. It was shown that HSA consists of a single polypeptide chain containing 585 amino acids and has a molecular weight of 66 500. The structure of the bovine serum albumin (BSA) molecule was also elucidated in 1975 and it was found that the two albumins have a similar chemical composition. This similarity, in conjunction with the cheaper price of BSA, resulted in the extensive use of BSA as a model for the study of drug–HSA interactions.

A common structural characteristic of the albumins is the disulfide bridge between adjacent cysteine molecules at 17 locations on the polypeptide chain. These bridges stabilize a repeating loop structure, consisting of nine loops (Fig. 7.2), which results in the stability of albumin in acid and basic solutions being higher than other proteins. The detailed three-dimensional conformation of albumin is not known but it is usually represented as a ellipsoid of size 40×140 Å which undergoes a number of changes with pH, as shown in Table 7.2.

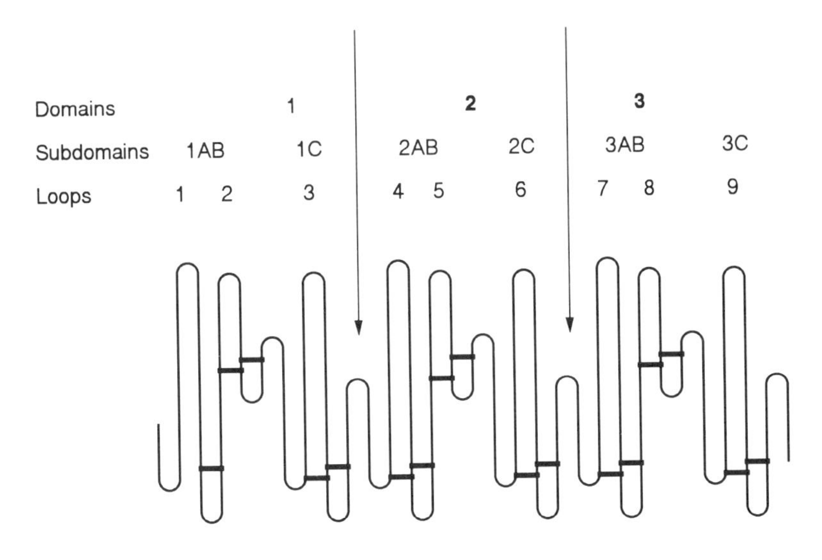

Fig. 7.2. BSA structure, as proposed by Brown (P. Brown Jr, Structure and Evolution of serum albumin. In: *Proceedings of the Federation of European Biochemical Societies*, 11th meeting, Copenhagen 1977, Peters T. and Sjöholm J. (eds), Vol. 50, pp. 1–10, Pergamon Press, Oxford, 1978). The small black lines represent the S–S bonds.

Table 7.2. Albumin conformation at various pH values

pH	Conformation
1–3	E (Expanded): unfolding of the molecule
3–4	F (Faster): moves faster than N in electrophoresis
5–7.5	N (Normal): normal form
7.5–8.5	B (Base): isomeric form gradually transformed to the A form
8.5–11	A (Aged): aged form

The albumin molecule is negatively charged (–17) at physiological pH 7.4. This large charge value makes the albumin molecule hydrophilic and confers high aqueous solubility. The isoelectric pH for albumins is about 5.3, with about 100 positive and 100 negative charged groups present. The concentration of albumin in human plasma ranges between 35 and 50 g/l (3.5–5%), which is equivalent to a molar concentration of about 7.0×10^{-4} M. Under physiological conditions there is negligible fluctuation in plasma albumin concentration for a given individual. The long-chain plasma fatty acids are strongly bound to albumin in a ratio of about 1–2 mol of fatty acids per mole of albumin. Thus, even the commercially available albumin products contain fatty acids. A special treatment with active charcoal is required for the preparation of fatty acid-free albumin.

7.1.1.1 Binding sites on the albumin molecule

Like other macromolecules, albumin has a number of 'classes of binding sites', and there are several 'binding sites' in each of these classes. These concepts are illustrated in Fig. 7.3. On the left-hand side (A), the macromolecule interacts with the micromolecule at two equivalent binding sites. The interaction can thus be characterized as having one 'class of binding sites', with two 'binding sites'. On the right-hand side (B), there are two 'classes of binding sites', classified as spherical and conical, with three and two binding sites each. Each class is characterized by its unique strength of chemical bond between the macromolecule and the micromolecule, which is usually expressed by the association constant, K_{as}. In general, for m existing classes of binding sites, each class is accompanied by a number of binding sites $n_1, n_2, \ldots, n_i$ and the corresponding binding constant $K_{as1}, K_{as2}, \ldots, K_{asi}$ for $i = 1$ to m.

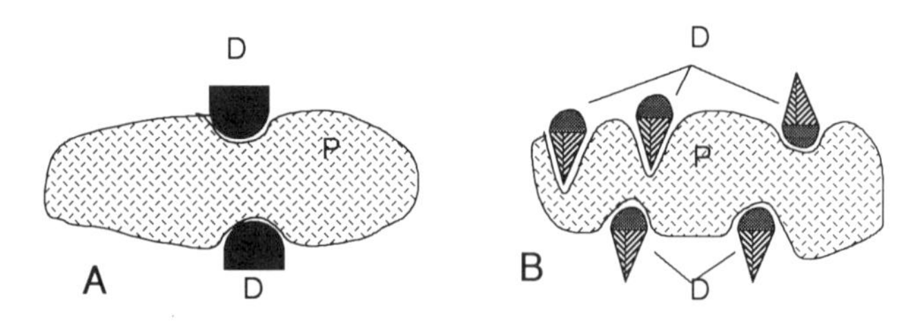

Fig. 7.3. Theoretical scheme for the drug (*D*)–protein (*P*) interaction: (a) one class of binding site with two binding sites; (b) two classes of binding site with two and three binding sites, respectively.

Let us now consider the specific binding sites on the albumin molecule. A simplified model of the structure of albumin is shown in Fig. 7.4. According to this model the hydrophobic surfaces of subdomains AB and C form hydrophobic channels with cavities of polar character at the edges of the channels. The size of each channel is appropriate to accommodate the hydrocarbon chain of a fatty acid. This model predicts a maximum of six binding sites, one for each of the six AB and C subdomains.

7.1.2 α_1-Acid glycoprotein

Although drug binding to human plasma can usually be explained by HSA binding, the binding of some basic drugs to HSA may be much lower than their overall binding to plasma. For these drugs another protein, α_1-acid glycoprotein (α_1-AGP), also contributes to plasma binding. Some selected examples of basic drugs which bind to α_1-AGP are presented in Table 7.3. Binding to α_1-AGP is characterized by only *one* class of binding

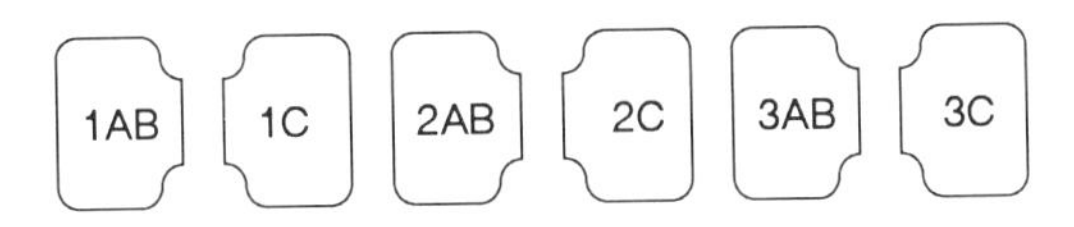

Fig. 7.4. According to its molecular structure, albumin consists of three domains, 1, 2 and 3. Each domain contains two subdomains leading to a total of six binding sites. (Redrawn from *Lipid–Protein Interactions*, Jost PC and Griffith OH (eds), Vol. 1, pp. 25–68, Wiley, New York (1982).)

site with high binding constant values, ranging from 0.5 to 550×10^5 M^{-1}. Recently, drugs with acidic properties have also been found to interact with α_1-AGP.

Table 7.3. Some drugs which are bound to α_1-acid glycoprotein

Amitryptiline	Dipyridamole	Pindolol
Warfarin	Thioridazine	Progesterone
Desipramin	Imipramine	Propranolol
Diazepam	Nortriptyline	Chlorpromazine

7.1.3 Lipoproteins

Lipoproteins are macromolecular compounds with a relatively hydrophilic surface and a hydrophobic core. The hydrophilic surface consists of phospholipids, cholesterol and proteins (named *apolipoproteins*), while the internal part is composed of triglycerides and cholesterol esters. The molecular weight of lipoproteins ranges from 1.8×10^5 to 4×10^8; they are divided into four classes according to their density and size (Table 7.4). The main physiological role of plasma lipoproteins is the circulation of water-insoluble lipids to the tissues through the blood.

Table 7.4. Physical characteristics of lipoproteins

Lipoprotein	Density (g/L)	Size (MW)	Diameter (nm)
Chylomicrons (CM)	0.950	4×10^8	>100
Very-low-density lipoproteins (VLDL)	<1.006	19.6×10^6	30–90
Low-density lipoproteins (LDL)	<1.063	2.3×10^6	18–25
High-density lipoproteins (HDL)	<1.210	$(0.18–0.3) \times 10^6$	8–12

Owing to the heterogeneous character of lipoproteins they bind with both ionized and non-ionized drugs at pH 7.4. Many hydrophobic drugs can also bind lipoproteins, as shown in Table 7.5. Drug–lipoprotein binding is non-specific, i.e. there are no specific classes and binding sites, and binding is not dependent on concentration. Rather, 'binding' reflects partitioning of the drug to the hydrophobic core of the lipoprotein molecule.

Table 7.5. Some drugs which are bound to plasma lipoproteins

Aloperidol	Diltiazem	Cyclosporin A	Reserpine
Amphotericin B	Diclofenac	Nicardipine	Rifambicin
Amitryptiline	Dipyridamole	Nifedipine	Trifluoperazine
Verapamil	Imipramine	Pindolol	Phenytoin
Digitoxin	Quinidine	Propranolol	Chlorpromazine

Binding of drugs to lipoproteins can play an important role in the transport of drugs to the tissues. Fig. 7.5 illustrates an enhanced transport process of the drug–lipoprotein complex by the lipoprotein receptor pathway. Thus, the drug permeates the biological membrane not only by passive diffusion but also through a lipoprotein receptor located on the membrane.

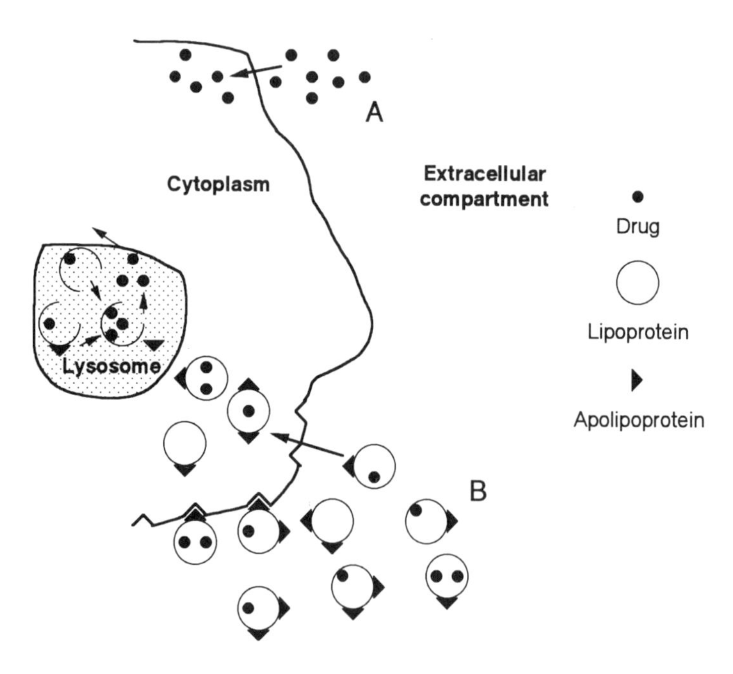

Fig. 7.5. Entry of the free and lipoprotein-bound drug in the cell (A) by passive diffusion, and (B) by the assistance of a lipoprotein receptor located on the cell membrane. (Redrawn from *Protein Binding and Drug Transport*, Symposia Medica Hoechst, Tilement JP and Lindenlaub E (eds), Vol. 20, pp. 73, Schatauer Verlag, Stuttgart, 1986.)

7.2 DRUG–PROTEIN BINDING

7.2.1 Reversibility of the interaction

The reversible character of the drug–protein interaction can be experimentally observed in dialysis experiments (Fig. 7.6). Plasma and a drug known to bind with plasma proteins are initially placed together in a sealed bag made from a semi-permeable membrane. Owing to its pore size, this membrane allows the permeation of only the free drug. The bag is placed in phosphate buffer pH 7.4 of equal volume to that of the bag solution and the system is shaken gently (Fig. 7.6a). By sampling and analysing for the drug in the outer solution it can be observed that, with time, the free drug crosses the membrane and moves from the inner to the outer solution (Fig. 7.6b) until the drug free concentration in both compartments of the system equilibrates (Fig. 7.6c).

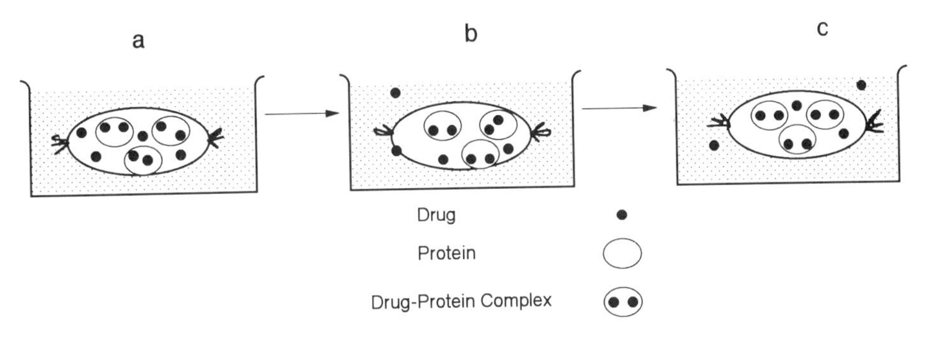

Fig. 7.6. Schematic representation of the approach to equilibrium in a dialysis experiment: (a) initial concentration distribution through (b) to (c) equilibrium concentration distribution.

The drug–protein interaction is usually represented by the following reaction:

$$P + D \rightleftharpoons PD \tag{7.1}$$

where P, D, and PD represent the protein, the drug, and the drug–protein complex respectively. When the bag is placed in the outer solution the initial equilibrium inside the bag is perturbed. According to the Le Chatelier principle, the reaction proceeds until the concentrations of the free drug inside and outside the bag have equilibrated.

7.2.2 The Protein–drug binding interaction

The reversibility of the drug–protein interaction indicates that the bonds formed between the drug and the protein are not covalent. The types of non-covalent bonds involved in the interaction are

— electrostatic bonds;
— van der Waals' forces;
— hydrogen bonds; and
— hydrophobic interactions.

These bonds participate to varying degrees in the formation of the complex. The great majority of drugs are weak acids or bases and are therefore partly ionized at physiological pH. However, some drugs, like non-steroidal anti-inflammatory drugs, penicillins, cephalosporins and the quartenary ammonium salts, are completely ionized at physiological pH. In all these cases electrostatic bonds are initially formed between the ionized part of the drug and the charged groups of the macromolecule, such as the $-COO^-$ group of the glutamic acid, the $-NH_3^+$ of lysine, or the $-NH^+$ group of histidine on the albumin molecule. This initial electrostatic attraction is followed by the development of van der Waals' forces and hydrogen bonds. The potential number of hydrogen bonds formed between the C=O, N—H and O—H groups of the drug and the protein molecules is extremely high, and thus makes an important contribution to binding, as well as determining the exact sites of interaction with the protein molecule. In addition, both the drug and the protein can form hydrogen bonds with surrounding water molecules. The aqueous medium is also of great importance for the formation of hydrophobic bonds. The hydrophobic interactions, which involve the non-polar parts of the drug and the protein, result from entropically driven displacement of water molecules (which are highly ordered at the non-polar interfaces) to the bulk solution (Fig. 7.7).

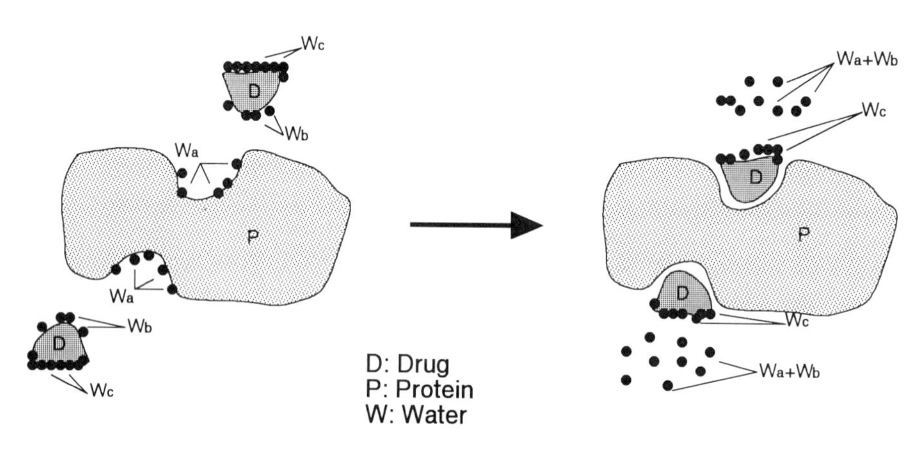

Fig. 7.7. Schematic representation of hydrophobic bond formation, with displacement of the water molecules from sites a and b.

In rare cases, covalent bonds in drug–protein interactions are observed. Such interactions are likely to result in very slow elimination from the body and may result in cumulative toxicity. A classic example of covalent bond formation is the acetylation of the ε-amino groups of lysine on the HSA molecule by aspirin, which is hydrolysed to salicylic acid. In this particular case, however, the interaction does not appear to cause therapeutic problems. A similar interaction is the non-reversible binding of the anticancer drug dichloro-diamino-platin II (cisplatin) to HSA. The covalent bond is most likely formed with the sulfhydryl groups (—SH) of cysteine on the HSA molecule.

7.2.3 Fundamental equations in protein binding

The Scatchard model is widely used to interpret protein binding data. This model is based on the assumption that the binding sites are independent and non-interacting. This means that the micromolecules interact to the greatest extent with the class of binding site for which they have highest chemical affinity. The binding proceeds in an independent manner with micromolecules also binding to the second, third (etc.) classes of binding site. The relative magnitude of association constants determines the extent of occupancy of the various binding sites.

In order to derive the equations based on the Scatchard model, let us consider the reversible general reaction (7.1) for the drug binding to n_1 sites of the first class (highest chemical affinity), where P is the molar concentration of the free protein and, for the purposes of derivation, represents the molar concentration of the free binding sites on the protein; D_f is the molar concentration of the free drug while D_{b1} is the molar concentration of the bound drug to the first class of binding sites. The concentration of free binding sites on the protein is given by the following equation:

$$P = n_1 P_t - D_{b1} \tag{7.3}$$

where P_t is the molar concentration of the total protein. Consequently, the binding constant, K_{as_1}, for the equilibrium (7.1) can be written as follows:

$$K_{as_1} = \frac{D_{b1}}{(n_1 P_t - D_{b1}) D_f} \tag{7.4}$$

Solving equation (7.4) for D_{b1} results in

$$D_{b1} = \frac{n_1 K_{as_1} D_f}{1 + K_{as_1} D_f} P_t \tag{7.5}$$

Equation (7.5) can be generalized for the ith class of the m classes of binding sites:

$$D_{bi} = \frac{n_i K_{as_i} D_f}{1 + K_{as_i} D_f} P_t \tag{7.6}$$

The total concentration of drug bound to the protein, D_b, is given from the sum

$$D_b = D_{b1} + D_{b2} + \ldots + D_{bi} = \sum_{i=1}^{m} D_{bi} \tag{7.7}$$

Combination of the last equation with equation (7.6) gives the generalized equation of the Scatchard model:

$$D_b = \sum_{i=1}^{m} \frac{n_i K_{as_i} D_f}{1 + K_{as_i} D_f} P_t \tag{7.8}$$

Equation (7.8) can also be used in the following form:

$$r = \frac{D_b}{P_t} = \sum_{i=1}^{m} \frac{n_i K_{as_i} D_f}{1 + K_{as_i} D_f} \tag{7.9}$$

where r is the molar concentration ratio of the bound drug to the total protein. Essentially, r represents the number of drug moles bound per mole of total protein.

In protein binding studies, it is possible to calculate the free and bound drug concentration for a given total drug concentration, if the binding parameters n and K_{as} are known. This problem is equivalent to the solution of the Scatchard equation for D_f or D_b. In the simplest case, in which one class of binding site predominates, equation (7.9) becomes

$$r = \frac{D_b}{P_t} = \frac{D_t - D_f}{P_t} = \frac{nK_{as}D_f}{1 + K_{as}D_f} \tag{7.10}$$

Solution of equation (7.10) for D_f results in the quadratic equation

$$K_{as}D_f^2 + (nK_{as}P_t + 1 - D_tK_{as})D_f - D_t = 0 \tag{7.11}$$

with only one acceptable root:

$$D_f = \frac{-(nK_{as}P_t + 1 - D_tK_{as})}{2K_{as}} + \frac{\left[(nK_{as}P_t + 1 - D_tK_{as})^2 + 4K_{as}D_t\right]^{1/2}}{2K_{as}} \tag{7.12}$$

Substituting the values of n, K_{as}, P_t and D_t in (7.12) permits calculation of D_f. Then, the bound drug concentration, D_b, is calculated by the difference:

$$D_b = D_t - D_f$$

A knowledge of the values for D_f, D_b and D_t allows the calculation of the free (f_f) and bound (f_b) fraction of the drug, according to the following equations:

$$f_f = \frac{D_f}{D_f + D_b} = \frac{D_f}{D_t} \tag{7.13}$$

$$f_b = \frac{D_b}{D_f + D_b} = \frac{D_b}{D_t} \tag{7.14}$$

$$f_f + f_b = 1 \tag{7.15}$$

The percentages of the free and bound drug are obtained by multiplying through the right parts of equations (7.13) and (7.14) by 100.

Example 7.1: If the binding constant of a drug is $K_{as} = 1.00 \times 10^5\ M^{-1}$ and the total protein concentration is $P_t = 7.20 \times 10^{-4}$ M, calculate the free drug concentration, D_f, and the free drug fraction, f_f, assuming there is one class of binding site, with one binding site, for total drug concentrations, D_t, of 2.00, 4.00, 8.00, 16.0, 24.0 and 48.0×10^{-4} M. Plot D_f and f_f versus D_t.

Answer: From equation (7.12), for $n = 1$ and the various D_t values, the free drug concentrations are calculated to be

$D_f(\times 10^{-5}$ M):	0.375	1.17	13.1	88.8	168	408
$f_f = D_f/D_t$:	0.019	0.029	0.164	0.555	0.700	0.850

The plot of Fig. 7.8 shows that both the free drug concentration and free drug fraction increase non-linearly with increasing total drug concentration. It is interesting to note that the f_f value asymptotically approaches unity.

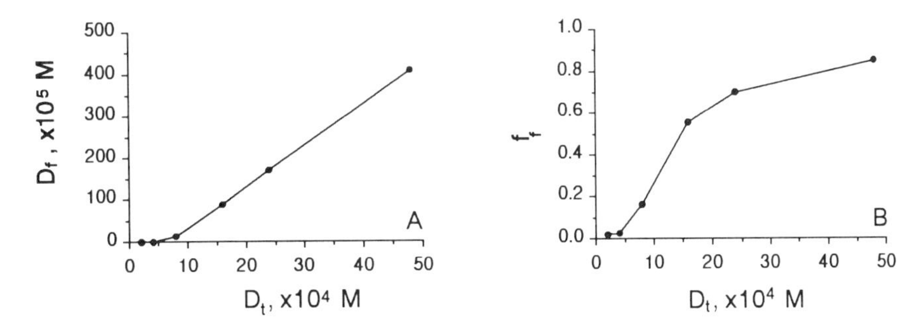

Fig. 7.8. Plot of free drug concentration, D_f (A) and fraction of drug in free form, f_f (B) versus total drug concentration D_t for the data of Example 7.1.

7.2.3.1 Estimation of binding parameters from in vitro *experiments*

The primary objective of every protein binding study is to estimate the fundamental parameters, the binding constants, K_{as_i} and the number of binding sites, n_i, for each class of binding site.

In the case of one binding class, equation (7.10) can be applied. This equation is the basis of several graphical treatments of experimental data, which are designed to estimate the binding parameters n and K_{as}.

Direct plot

A plot of r against the free drug concentration, D_f, in accordance with equation (7.10), is shown in Fig. 7.9A. This type of curve is similar in form to an adsorption isotherm. From equation (7.10) and Fig. 7.9A, it is evident that for a given total protein concentration r approaches the saturation value, n, as free drug concentration increases. Further, for $r = n/2$, equation (7.10) gives $D_f = 1/K_{as}$. However, the extrapolation of asymptotic curves, such as that in Fig. 7.9A, for the calculation of $r_{max} = n$ from experimental data is neither easy nor accurate. Only rough estimates for n and K_{as} can be obtained from these direct plots.

For low D_f values $K_{as}D_f \ll 1$, and so $K_{as}D_f + 1 \approx 1$. In this case equation (7.10) can be simplified to $r = nK_{as}D_f$. This means that the slope of the curve in Fig. 7.9A near the origin is equal to nK_{as}. This tangent can be used to calculate the nK_{as} value, but the calculation is subject to error similar to that of the previous method. For these reasons, the transformation of equation (7.10) into linear forms is more reliable for presentation of data and estimation of the binding parameters. Methods which utilize linear regression analysis for the calculation of the parameters n and K_{as} include the Scatchard, Klotz and Hitchcock plots.

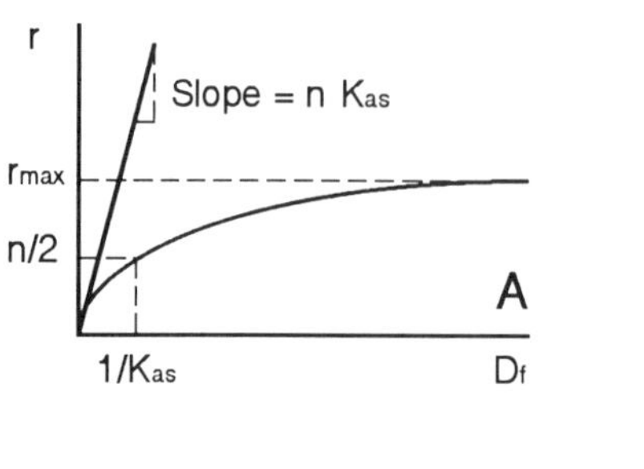

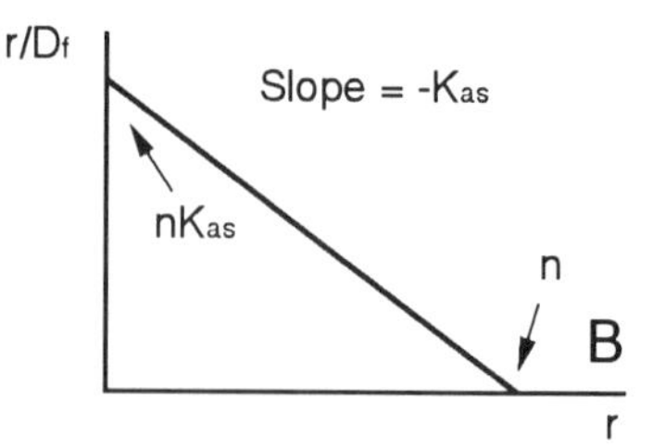

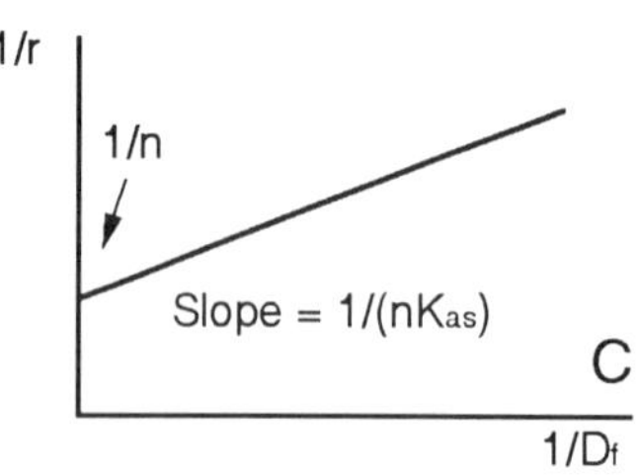

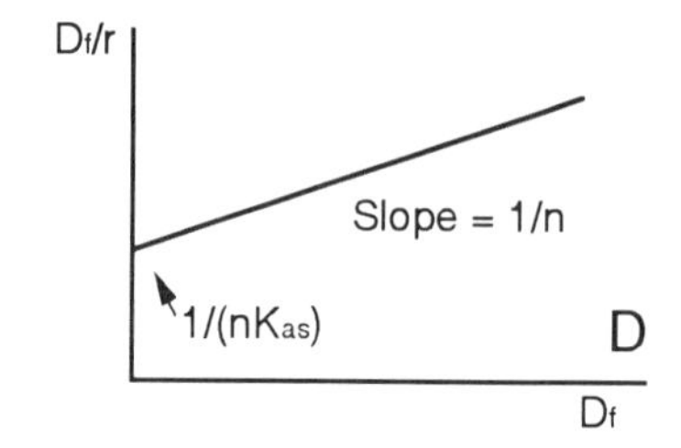

Fig. 7.9. Plots used for the study of drug–protein interactions. (A) Direct plot, (B) Scatchard plot, (C) Klotz plot (double reciprocal plot) and (D) Hitchcock plot.

Scatchard plot

Equation (7.10) can be transformed to a linear version as follows:

$$\frac{r}{D_f} = nK_{as} - K_{as}r \tag{7.16}$$

According to equation (7.16), the plot of r/D_f against r gives a straight line with slope equal to $-K_{as}$ (Fig. 7.9B). The y axis intercept corresponds to nK_{as} while the x axis intercept corresponds to n.

Example 7.2: From an *in vitro* protein binding study, where the total protein concentration used was $P_t = 1.00 \times 10^{-4}$ M, the following data were obtained:

$D_f(10^{-4}$ M):	0.25	0.50	0.66	1.22
$D_b(10^{-4}$ M):	0.40	0.65	1.21	0.90

Calculate K_{as} and n.

Answer: The following values for r and r/D_f are calculated from the data:

$r = D_b/P_t$:	0.40	0.65	0.80	1.10
$r/D_f(10^4\ M^{-1})$:	1.60	1.30	1.21	0.90

Linear regression analysis of r versus r/D_f (Fig. 7.10) results in a slope of $-K_{as} = -0.98 \times 10^4\ M^{-1}$, therefore $K_{as} = 0.98 \times 10^4\ M^{-1}$. The intercept is $nK_{as} = 1.97 \times 10^4\ M^{-1}$, therefore $n = 1.98 \approx 2$. The correlation coefficient is $R = -0.996$ (statistically significant at the 0.05 level).

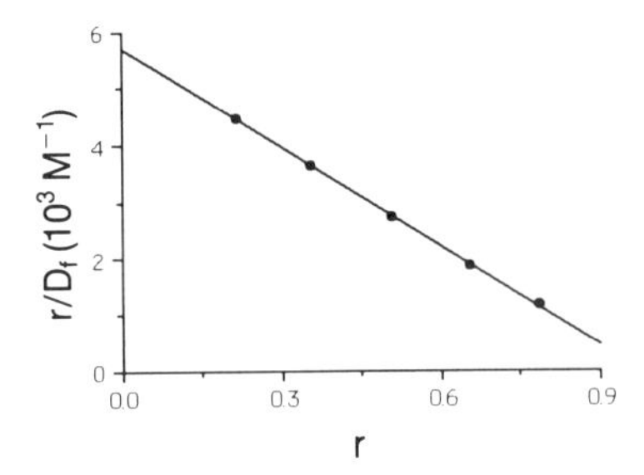

Fig. 7.10. Scatchard plot (using equation (7.16)) for the data of Example 7.2.

Klotz plot
The Klotz plot, which is sometimes called the double reciprocal plot, is also derived from equation (7.10):

$$\frac{1}{r} = \frac{1 + K_{as}D_f}{nK_{as}D_f} = \frac{1}{n} + \frac{1}{nK_{as}}\left(\frac{1}{D_f}\right) \quad (7.17)$$

According to equation (7.17), the plot of $1/r$ against $1/D_f$ is linear, with slope equal to $1/nK_{as}$ (Fig. 7.9C). The intercepts of the straight line after extrapolation to both axes, $1/r$ and $1/D_f$, give the values of $1/n$ and $-K_{as}$, respectively.

Hitchcock plot
Equation (7.10) can be rewritten

$$\frac{nK_{as}D_f}{r} = 1 + K_{as}D_f$$

Dividing both sides by nK_{as} gives

$$\frac{D_f}{r} = \frac{1}{nK_{as}} + \left(\frac{1}{n}\right)D_f \quad (7.18)$$

Equation (7.18) is the Hitchcock equation, according to which the plot of D_f/r versus D_f yields a straight line with slope equal to $1/n$. The intercept of the back-extrapolated line with the y axis is $1/(nK_{as})$ (Fig. 7.9D).

The y and x intercepts as well as the slope of the various linear plots used in protein binding studies are listed in Table 7.6. These linearized methods of data analysis suffer the disadvantage that both the x and y axis variables are subject to experimental error.

Further, the various methods of analysis 'weight' the data points differently according to concentration. According to equation (7.17), the Klotz plot 'overestimates' the data points corresponding to low free drug concentrations. The opposite, i.e. overestimation of the data points corresponding to high D_f values, applies to the Hitchcock plot. The advantage of the Scatchard plot is that it offers a uniform weight to data points corresponding to both low and high D_f values. Moreover, the researcher can use either the y

Table 7.6. Interpretation of the intercept and slope of the regression lines for the various linearized plots

Plot	*y* intercept	*x* intercept	Slope
Scatchard	nK_{as}	n	$-K_{as}$
Klotz	$1/n$	$-K_{as}$	$1/K_{as}$
Hitchcock	$1/(nK_{as})$	$-(1/K_{as})$	$1/n$

intercept or the x intercept in conjunction with the slope for the estimation of n and K_{as}. For these reasons, the Scatchard plot is widely used and it is particularly useful for the interpretation of complex protein binding data.

In cases where more than one class of binding site exists, the Scatchard plot is not linear but takes the form of a hyperbola. Fig. 7.11 shows a Scatchard plot for two independent and non-interacting classes of binding sites, with n_1, n_2 the number of binding sites and K_{as1}, K_{as2} the binding constants, respectively. The equations describing the asymptotes of the hyperbola (Fig. 7.11) are

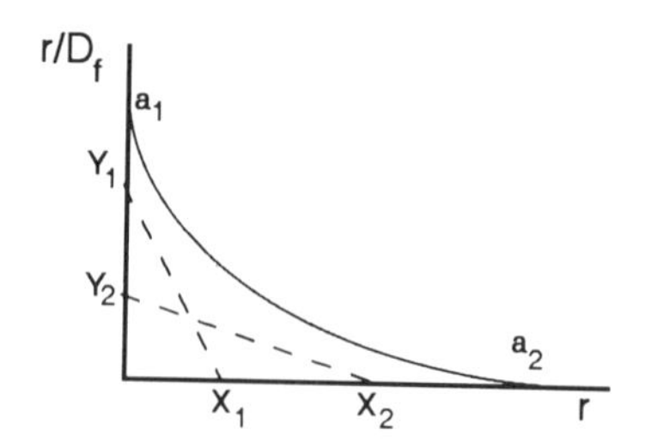

Fig. 7.11. Scatchard plot for two independent and non-interacting classes of binding sites. Y_1X_1 and Y_2X_2 are the asymptotes of the hyperbola.

$$Y_1 = n_1K_{as1} - K_{as1}X_1 \quad \text{and} \quad Y_2 = n_2K_{as2} - K_{as2}X_2 \tag{7.19}$$

From equations (7.19) it can be seen that

(1) the slopes of the asymptotes correspond to the binding constant values for the two classes of binding sites;

(2) the following equations are valid:

$$X_1 = n_1, \quad X_2 = n_2, \quad Y_1 = n_1K_{as1} \quad \text{and} \quad Y_2 = n_2K_{as2} \tag{7.20}$$

The estimation of all binding parameters can therefore be achieved from the slopes of the asymptotes and the use of equations (7.20). When curvature of the central part of the hyperbola is observed, it can be concluded that either two classes of binding site with similar binding constants, or more than two classes of binding sites, are operating. Despite the analytical power of the Scatchard plot when two classes of binding sites are operating, this technique becomes impractical when the experimental error is significant, because identifying the asymptotes becomes problematic. Consequently, the method of choice for analysing complex binding phenomena is the non-linear regression analysis according to the appropriate equation of the generalized Scatchard model (equation (7.9)). For example, the appropriate equation for two classes of binding sites is

$$r = \frac{n_1 K_{as1} D_f}{1 + K_{as1} D_f} + \frac{n_2 K_{as2} D_f}{1 + K_{as2} D_f} \tag{7.21}$$

All the above-mentioned analyses and conclusions are valid when the binding sites are independent and non-interactive. Phenomena related to the interaction of binding sites which are termed as *cooperativity* or *allostery* are outside the scope of this book.

7.2.3.2 Scatchard equation for use in experiments with blood samples

When plasma, serum or whole blood samples are used in protein binding studies, the analysis of the experimental data cannot be performed with the equations described in section 7.2.3.1, since the molar concentration of the binder(s) (protein) is not known. In these cases it is possible to estimate the association constant, K_{as}, and the total *binding capacity*, N, instead of the number of binding sites, n. Rearranging equation (7.16):

$$\frac{D_b}{D_f} = nK_{as}P_t - K_{as}D_b \tag{7.22}$$

and transforming the molar concentrations into weight per volume (W/V) concentrations one obtains

$$\frac{C_b}{C_f} = N K_{as} C_P - \frac{K_{as}}{1000 \text{ MW}} C_b \tag{7.23}$$

where C_b and C_f are the concentrations of bound and free drug, respectively, in μg/ml, N is the binding capacity in mol/g, C_P the total protein concentration of the sample in g/l and MW is the molecular weight of the drug. Linear regression analysis of C_b/C_f against C_b gives a straight line when one class of binding sites is encountered. The slope and the intercept of the regression line are given from the following equations:

$$\text{slope} = -\frac{K_{as}}{1000 \text{ MW}} \tag{7.24}$$

$$\text{intercept} = NK_{as}C_P \tag{7.25}$$

From equations (7.24) and (7.25) the parameters K_{as} and N can be easily estimated, since the value of C_P can be calculated by determining the total protein concentration of the sample. Equation (7.23) reveals that the intercept is a unitless number. This means that the binding capacity, N, is expressed in units reciprocal to those of the product $K_{as}C_P$, i.e. mol/g. Actually, N is the product of the number of binding sites per protein molecule and the total protein concentration, and indicates the number of drug moles bound per gram of protein. The product NK_{as} (l/g) is a general indicator of the protein binding capacity and is used frequently as a reference parameter for comparative drug–protein binding studies in plasma or serum from different animal species.

Example 7.3: In a binding study in human serum containing a total protein concentration of 72.1 g/l, the following data were obtained:

Total drug concentration C_t (μg/ml)	*Free drug concentration* C_f (μg/ml)
266	13.5
201	6.40
179	4.90
110	1.90

Calculate the binding capacity, N, and the binding constant, K_{as}, if the molecular weight of the drug is 316.

Answer: For each pair of data, the concentration of the bound drug and the respective ratio C_b/C_f are

C_b (μg/ml)	C_b/C_f
266 − 13.5 = 252	252/13.5 = 18.7
201 − 6.40 = 195	195/ 6.40 = 30.5
179 − 4.90 = 174	174/ 4.90 = 35.5
110 − 1.90 = 108	108/ 1.90 = 56.8

The linearity of the C_b/C_f versus C_b plot in Fig. 7.12 reveals that there is one class of binding site. The regression line has slope = −0.266 and intercept = 83.8.

According to equations (7.24) and (7.25)

$$K_{as} = 8.40 \times 10^4 \text{ M}^{-1} \qquad \text{and} \qquad N = 1.38 \times 10^{-5} \text{ mol/g}$$

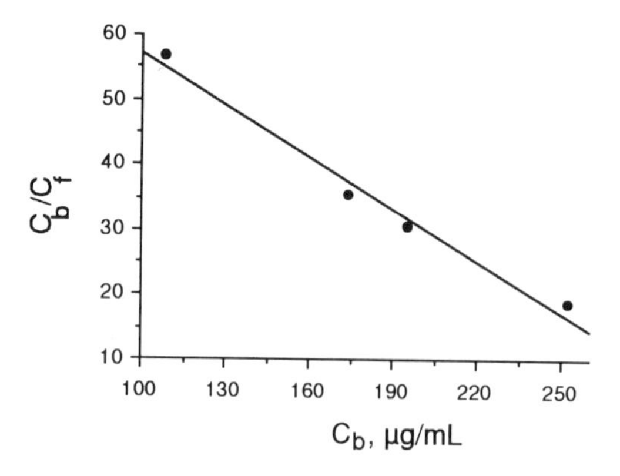

Fig. 7.12. Plot of C_b/C_f versus C_b for the data of Example 7.3.

7.2.3.3 Drug–protein binding under in vivo *conditions*

The knowledge of the fraction or percentage bound drug *in vivo* is of great importance, since only the free fraction of the drug can diffuse through the biological membranes. The equations describing the drug–protein binding in the analysis of *in vitro* data can also be used for the consideration of protein binding under *in vivo* conditions. To simplify the calculations, one usually assumes that one class of binding site prevails. The concentration of bound drug can be calculated from equation (7.10):

$$D_b = \frac{nP_t K_{as} D_f}{1 + K_{as} D_f}$$

Combining equations (7.10) and (7.14), the fraction of the bound drug can be expressed as follows:

$$f_b = \frac{D_b}{D_f + D_b} = \frac{nP_t K_{as}\, D_f/(1 + K_{as} D_f)}{D_f + \left[nP_t K_{as} D_f/(1 + K_{as} D_f)\right]}$$

$$= \frac{nP_t K_{as}}{nP_t K_{as} + 1 + K_{as} D_f}$$

This equation can be simplified by dividing both the numerator and the denominator by the product (nK_{as}):

$$f_b = \frac{1}{1 + \dfrac{1}{nP_t K_{as}} + \dfrac{D_f}{nP_t}} \qquad (7.26)$$

Equation (7.26) contains all the parameters involved in the binding phenomenon, i.e. drug concentration, protein concentration, the binding constant and the number of binding sites. The parameters n, K_{as} and P_t in equation (7.26) can be considered constant for a given drug *in vivo*, since the first two are related to the inherent interaction of the drug under study with the plasma proteins, while the third is constant under physiological conditions for a given individual. Equation (7.26) shows that under these circumstances, the fraction of bound drug depends exclusively on the free drug concentration, D_f. The value of D_f, for known and constant values of n, K_{as} and P_t, changes with the total drug concentration in accordance with equation (7.12). Since the total drug concentration in blood changes during its time course in the body the fraction of the bound drug in plasma is not constant. The change of the bound fraction of drug as a function of the ratio D_f/nP_t is illustrated in Fig. 7.13 (Goldstein plot). The Goldstein plot of Fig. 7.13 has the following features:

(a) the logarithmic scale is used on the abscissa so that changes in f_b over a wide range of D_f values can be represented;

(b) D_f values have been calculated from equation (7.12) for various values of the product ($nP_t K_{as}$), quoted in the legend of Fig. 7.13; and

(c) for each curve the corresponding values of n and P_t have been incorporated in the x axis; thus the plot depicts exclusively the change of f_b as a function of D_f.

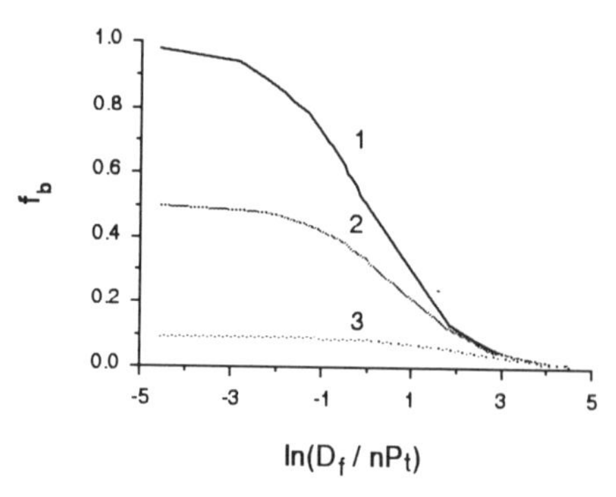

Fig. 7.13. Plot of the bound fraction of drug, f_b, as a function of ln (D_f/nP_t), according to equation (7.26), for various $1/(nP_tK_{as})$ values and for one class of binding site: (1) $1/(nP_tK_{as}) = 0.01$, (2) $1/(nP_tK_{as}) = 1$, (3) $1/(nP_tK_{as}) = 10$.

Fig. 7.13 shows that the fraction of bound drug decreases as the free drug concentration increases. This effect is more pronounced for strongly bound drugs (i.e. a high K_{as} value which corresponds to a small $1/nP_tK_{as}$ value). The shape of the curves also shows that the fraction of bound drug approaches a maximum value which is proportional to the value of the product nP_tK_{as}.

Using the Goldstein plot, it is possible to correlate changes in the bound fraction of drug with changes in the total blood drug concentration over the time course of the drug in the body. Intravenous bolus administration of a dose produces initially high total drug concentration, after which levels gradually decline. The high initial drug concentration in blood after intravenous bolus dosing corresponds to a high initial $\ln(D_f/nP_t)$ value. As levels in the body decline, there is a corresponding increase in the fraction of bound drug (from right to left in Fig. 7.13), with the exact curve depending on the specific value of the product nK_{as} for the drug under consideration. After per os administration the bound drug fraction, f_b, is anticipated to decrease until the peak level is achieved and then start increasing again as the levels in the body decline. However, for many drugs, the levels achieved after clinically relevant doses are within the linear part of the curves in Fig. 7.13. Practically speaking, this means the fraction bound will be approximately constant over most of the dosing interval. The fraction bound (expressed as percentage binding) drugs are listed in Table 7.7 with respect to their therapeutic concentrations. Because of the inherently non-linear character of binding phenomena the total drug concentration should always be specified when the percentage of binding is reported.

From *in vivo* drug–protein binding data, one can calculate the percentage of the total drug which is 'retained' in plasma. Since the total body water is 60% and plasma water is only 4% of the total body weight with volumes of 42 litres and 3 litres, respectively, it is possible to calculate the percentage of drug 'retained' in plasma. Assuming only the free drug diffuses out of the blood, that it distributes homogeneously in the body water, and that there is no drug binding in other tissues, the following expressions can be applied under equilibrium distribution conditions:

Table 7.7. Percentage bound of some drugs in plasma at their therapeutic levels[a]

Drug	% bound	Drug	% bound
Acetazolamide	90	Indomethacin	90
Allopurinol	0	Isoniazid	0
Aminopyrine	18	Kanamycin	10
Aminosalicylic acid	65	Meperidine	40
Amitriptyline	96	Methadone	40
Ampicillin	25	Methicillin	45
Antipyrine	4	Methotrexate	45
Atropine	50	Nitrofurantoin	70
Barbitone	10	Nortriptyline	94
Carbamazepine	72	Novobiocin	96
Cephalexin	22	Oxacillin	94
Chloramphenicol	25	Oxyphenylbutazone	90
Chlorpheniramine	70	Oxytetracycline	28
Chlorpromazine	95	Phenacetin	30
Chlorpropamide	80	Phenylbutazone	95
Chlortetracycline	47	Phenytoin	87
Desipramine	80	Prednisolone	90
Diazepam	96	Probenecid	80
Diazoxide	99	Procainamide	15
Dicoumarol	97	Promethazine	8
Digitoxin	95	Quinidine	70
Doxycycline	8	Rifampicin	85
Erythromycin	18	Streptomycin	34
Ethambutamol	8	Sulfadimethoxine	95
Furesamide	75	Sulfamethizole	90
Glutethimide	54	Sulfathiazole	70
Heparin	0	Theophylline	15
Imipramine	85	Thiopental	75

a Data taken from *Textbook of Biopharmaceutics and Clinical Pharmaceutics*, by S. Niazi, p. 101, Appleton Century Crofts, New York (1979).

$$
\begin{aligned}
\%\text{ drug in plasma} &= \frac{\text{quantity in plasma}}{\text{quantity in the body}} \times 100 \\
&= \frac{3(D_\mathrm{f}+D_\mathrm{b})}{39D_\mathrm{f}+3(D_\mathrm{f}+D_\mathrm{b})} \times 100 = \frac{3D_\mathrm{t}}{42D_\mathrm{f}+3D_\mathrm{b}} \times 100 \\
&= \frac{3}{42(D_\mathrm{f}/D_\mathrm{t})+3(D_\mathrm{b}/D_\mathrm{t})} \times 100 \\
&= \frac{3}{42f_\mathrm{f}+3f_\mathrm{b}} \times 100 = \frac{3}{42-39f_\mathrm{b}} \times 100 \qquad (7.27)
\end{aligned}
$$

From equation (7.27) the percentage drug 'retained' in plasma, as a function of the bound fraction of the drug, f_b, can be calculated. Fig. 7.14 illustrates that only highly bound drugs are 'retained' in plasma. Similar calculations, confirmed experimentally, have shown that the percentage of drug 'retained' in plasma becomes significant only when the binding constant is higher than 10^4 M^{-1}. Under these conditions the fraction of the drug bound in plasma acts as a reservoir for supply of free drug to the general circulation, replenishing drug which is metabolized and/or excreted. Despite the approximation that true equilibrium is achieved, when in fact, plasma protein binding is a dynamic phenomenon, the percentage of drug in plasma is a simple and reliable indicator of drug distribution in the body. Binding of drug to extravascular tissue complicates the picture somewhat, and its contribution, along with the importance of protein binding, is further elaborated in the discussion of the volume of distribution in chapter 8.

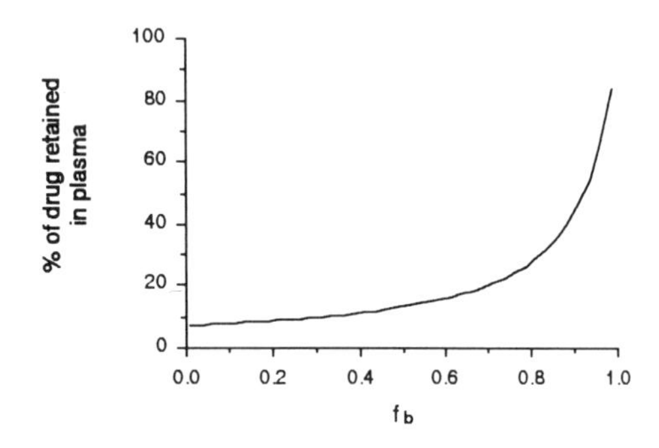

Fig. 7.14. The percentage of drug 'retained' in plasma as a function of the bound fraction of drug, f_b.

7.2.4 Changes in the percentage of protein binding *in vivo*

7.2.4.1 Displacement from binding sites

The linear parts of the curves in Fig. 7.13 are significantly shorter for strongly bound than for weakly bound drugs. For strongly bound drugs, then, significant changes in the bound fraction of drug can result from small changes in drug concentration. This may occur when two drugs are competing for the same binding site(s) on the protein. The net result of competition is the displacement of the weakly bound by the strongly bound drug. The potential magnitude of this effect is illustrated by considering two examples of drugs which are displaced to an extent of 4%. Fig. 7.15 shows the behaviour for two hypothetical drugs which are bound 98% and 60%, respectively, prior to displacement. The displacement phenomenon is greater for the extensively (98%) bound drug, since the relative change of the free drug concentration is very high. Several clinically important displacement interactions have been identified.

For example, when patients stabilized on warfarin are administered phenylbutazone, increased anticoagulation is observed. Phenylbutazone displaces warfarin from binding sites and also reduces the rate of warfarin metabolism. The increased free warfarin levels

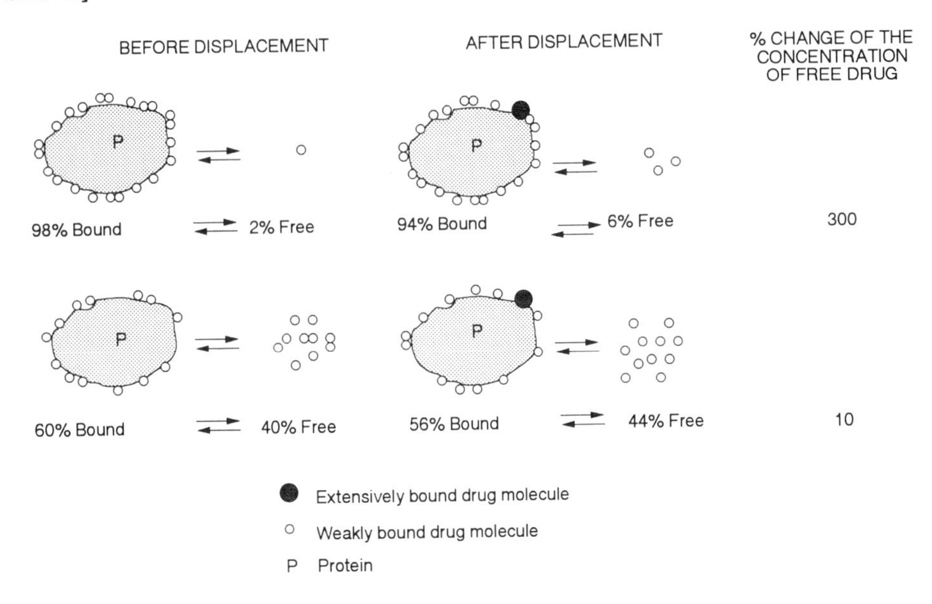

Fig. 7.15. Schematic of the displacement phenomenon.

cause an increase in the prothrombin clotting time. A more detailed description of the warfarin–phenylbutazone interaction is given in chapter 9.

The interaction of bilirubin and sulfonamides was discovered incidentally in a clinical study comparing tetracycline versus a mixture of penicillin–sulfonamide in the management of premature infants. A higher mortality rate and incidence of kernicterus among premature infants with the sulfonamide mixture was observed. The administration of sulfonamides displaces bilirubin from plasma proteins, producing high enough bilirubin levels to result in entry of bilirubin into the brain. A further example is the displacement of diazepam from its binding sites on albumin by fatty foods.

Effects on binding may also be indirect. For example, the use of heparin as an anticoagulant activates lipoprotein lipase, an enzyme which metabolizes triglycerides to free fatty acids. Heparin coadministration with drugs has also been shown to result in decreased protein binding of propranolol, quinidine, diazepam, chlordiazepoxide and oxazepam, possibly via its effects on fatty acid levels.

7.2.4.2 Drug binding to plasma proteins in pathological conditions

For a given drug and a certain concentration range, the percentage of binding to the plasma proteins under physiological conditions can often be considered constant (Table 7.7). However, in several pathological conditions binding is significantly altered. Two important disease states in which protein binding is modified are considered here.

In patients suffering from *uraemia* the binding of acidic drugs with plasma proteins is decreased, while binding of basic drugs remains normal. Various explanations have been proposed for the decreased binding of acidic drugs in uraemia. Certainly, the decreased binding is partly due to the lower albumin concentration associated with this disease state. It also appears that compounds which act as displacers termed 'uraemic metabolites', which accumulate in the plasma of uraemic patients, contribute to the reduction in binding. These compounds are usually organic acids, e.g. *p*-hydroxyphenylacetic acid, *o*-hydroxyhippuric acid, 2-hydroxybenzoylglycine and indole-3-propionic acid, and can thus compete with drugs having acidic properties and displace them from plasma proteins. It is interesting to note that urea and creatinine, which are found in high concentrations in the plasma of uraemic patients, do not affect protein binding. Another hypothesis developed to explain the decreased binding of drugs in uraemia is associated with alterations in the structure of albumin synthesized by uraemic patients. It is postulated that the alterations in the amino acid composition of albumin cause the binding defect in uraemic plasma. Table 7.8 lists selected drugs for which uraemia modifies protein binding.

Table 7.8. Changes in the percentage of drug bound, in uraemic plasma

Drug	Physiological values	Uraemia[a]
Valproic acid	92	77
Benzylpenicillin	66	44
Dicloxacyclin	97	91
Sulfamethoxazole	66	42

[a] Uraemic patients receiving haemodialysis on a long-standing basis.

A great number of studies have documented lower bound fractions for drugs such as tolbutamide, phenylbutazone, azapropazone, phenytoin, diazepam and quinidine in patients suffering from hepatic diseases such as chronic active hepatitis, acute viral hepatitis and cirrhosis. The reduction in binding is more pronounced in chronic liver disease than in acute viral hepatitis, with dramatic reductions observed in cirrhosis. The reasons for the decreased binding are not clear. One hypothesis is that there are structural alterations in the plasma proteins, while another attributes the effects to the displacement of drugs by bilirubin and other compounds, e.g. bile acids, which accumulate in the plasma of patients with hepatic diseases.

7.3 TECHNIQUES USED IN PROTEIN BINDING STUDIES

The analytical techniques used in protein binding studies can be divided in two classes: (a) indirect techniques based on the separation of the bound form from the free micromolecule; and (b) direct methods, not requiring the separation of bound form from the free micromolecule. Indirect techniques are usually applied in biological samples (blood, serum, plasma) for the determination of the percentage of binding, while the direct methods are used for the estimation of the number, and the elucidation of the character, of binding sites in pure aqueous solutions of proteins. The analytical techniques used in protein binding studies are equilibrium dialysis, dynamic dialysis, ultrafiltration, diafiltration, ultracentrifugation, gel filtration (indirect techniques) and ultraviolet (UV) spectroscopy, fluorimetry and ion-selective electrodes (direct methods).

7.3.1 Indirect techniques

7.3.1.1 Equilibrium dialysis

This is the most widely used technique in protein binding studies. According to the classic methodology, a protein solution is placed in a bag made from a semi-permeable membrane. The bag is sealed and immersed in a drug solution of the same volume, thus achieving the initial separation of the drug from the protein. The pore size of the semi-permeable membrane allows the permeation only to the free drug, with the protein and the protein–drug complex remaining in the bag. The whole system is usually shaken gently, to facilitate rapid equilibration. A further reduction in the equilibration time can be achieved by deploying the same total concentration of drug in the bag (internal compartment) as in the external compartment. When equilibrium is achieved, the solution inside the bag contains the free and the bound drug, while the solution outside the bag contains only the free drug; the concentrations of the free drug inside and outside the bag are equal. Consequently, the difference between the total drug concentration inside the bag and the free drug concentration outside the bag gives the bound drug concentration. The time required for a dialysis experiment is of the order of 16–24 h, over which protein denaturation and bacterial growth can occur. Recently, use of cells made from inert materials (teflon, stainless steel), which consists of two compartments of small volume (0.2, 1.0, 2.0 or 5.0 ml) separated by the semi-permeable membrane have been developed, in which the ratio of the membrane surface to the volume of the solution is significantly enlarged, resulting in equilibration times of 4–6 h.

Other potential problems with the dialysis method include binding of the drug to the membrane, protein leakage across the membrane, and volume shifts due to the colloidal osmotic pressure generated by the protein. When the drug is ionized under the experimental conditions used an additional consideration is the effect of the Gibbs–Donnan equilibrium on the results.

Example 7.4: In an equilibrium dialysis experiment, the volume of the solution used inside and outside the bag was 5.00 ml while the protein concentration was kept constant, $P_t = 1.00 \times 10^{-4}$ M. The initial drug concentrations inside each of the four bags used were 11.25, 20.25, 28.00 and 45.50 μg/ml, while the concentrations at equilibrium in the external compartment were 3.25, 6.00, 8.75 and 15.6 μg/ml, respectively. Assuming that drug binding to the membrane is negligible, calculate the binding constant, the number of classes of binding sites and the number of binding sites for each class (the molecular weight of the drug is 250).

Answers: Since the volume of the solution inside the bag is equal to that outside the bag, the initial drug concentration inside the bag represents the total drug concentration, C_t, while the final concentration outside the bag represents the free drug concentration, C_f, at equilibrium. The bound drug concentration, C_b, is calculated by subtracting the free drug concentration, inside and outside the bag, from the total drug concentration. Since at equilibrium the free drug concentration is the same inside and outside the bag, we have

$$C_b = C_t - 2C_f$$

Consequently,

C_f (μg/ml)	C_b (μg/ml)
3.25	$11.25 - 2 \times 3.25 = 4.75$
6.00	$20.25 - 2 \times 6.00 = 8.25$
8.75	$28.00 - 2 \times 8.75 = 10.50$
15.6	$45.50 - 2 \times 15.6 = 14.30$

From these data the following r and r/D_f values are calculated, taking care to express concentrations in mol/l:

$r = D_b/P_t$:	0.190	0.330	0.420	0.572
$r/D_f(10^{-4}\,M^{-1})$:	1.46	1.37	1.20	0.917

Linear fitting of the Scatchard equation (7.16) to these data gives the regression line equation

$$r/D_f = 1.79 \times 10^4 - 1.48 \times 10^4 r$$

The correlation coefficient is $R = -0.97$ and it is statistically significant at a probability level of $P = 0.05$ (see chapter 10); therefore, the assumption that there is only one class of binding site appears to hold. From the regression equation $K_{as} = 1.48 \times 10^4\,M^{-1}$ and $n = (1.79 \times 10^4)/(1.48 \times 10^4) = 1.21$.

7.3.1.2 Diafiltration

In this technique, a volume of protein solution is placed in the diafiltration cell (Fig. 7.16), and a drug solution of known concentration is added at a constant rate from a reservoir of high capacity. The addition results in a continuous exponential increase of the drug concentration in the cell, until it becomes equal to the drug concentration in the reservoir. The free drug concentration is measured in the diafiltrate, usually by continuous spectrophotometric analysis. Since the input rate of the solution from the reservoir is equal to the output rate of the diafiltrate, the volume of the solution in the diafiltration cell is constant and, thus, the protein concentration remains constant. A potential problem with the diafiltration technique arises from the possible binding of the drug with the membrane. For this reason, blank experiments (in absence of protein) are usually performed. In general, though, this technique has significant advantages compared to other equilibrium techniques, in that

— experiments are rapid (~1 h);
— protein concentration remains constant;
— construction of the complete binding curve can be performed with only two experiments (blank and test).

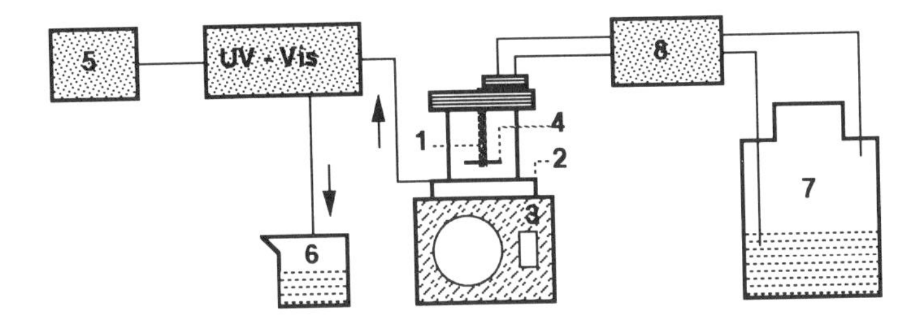

Fig. 7.16. Schematic representation of the diafiltration system: (1) diafiltration cell, (2) membrane, (3) magnetic stirrer, (4) magnet, (5) recorder, (6) ultrafiltrate, (7) reservoir, and (8) switch for pressure channelling to the cell and/or the reservoir.

7.3.1.3 Ultrafiltration

In ultrafiltration the biological sample (plasma or serum) is filtered through a semi-permeable membrane which allows the passage of small molecules (e.g. drugs) but not macromolecules. Laboratory centrifuges are used to provide the pressure needed for ultrafiltration. Usually about 15 μl of filtrate can be produced from 1 ml sample in fifteen minutes. Caution should be exercised with the potential problems of all the indirect binding techniques, i.e. protein leakage through the membrane and the binding of the drug to the membrane.

7.3.2 Direct techniques

These techniques are mainly spectroscopic and only the most frequently used is discussed here.

7.3.2.1 Ultraviolet–visible spectroscopy

Spectral changes, such as a shift of the maximum absorbance wavelength, λ_{max}, or change of absorptivity, may occur due to the interaction of the drug with protein. In such cases, changes in the UV spectrum with parameters such as pH or the concentration of the drug and/or protein may provide an insight as to the type of the bond(s) developed, the group(s) on the drug and the protein molecules that interact, and may also be used to estimate the binding parameters K_{as} and n. The binding of dicoumarol (UV) and azodyes (visible) with albumin are two examples in which spectrophotometric methods have been successfully applied.

FURTHER READING

Behrens PO, Spiekerman AM and Brown JR. Structure of Human Serum Albumin. *Fed. Proc.* **34**: 591 (1975).

Blaschke TF. Protein binding and Kinetics of Drug in Liver Diseases. *Clin. Pharmacokinet.* **2**: 32–44 (1977).

Bowmer CJ and Lindup WE. Decreased Drug Binding in Uraemia: Effect of Indoxyl Sulphate and Other Endogenous Substances in the Binding of Drugs and Dyes to Human Albumin. *Biochem. Pharmacol.* **31**: 319–323 (1982).

Culyassy PF and Depner TA. Impaired Binding of Drugs and Endogenous Ligands in Renal Disease. *Am. J. Kidney Dis.* **2**: 578–601 (1983).

Klotz IM and Hunston DL. Properties of Graphical Representations of Multiple Classes of Binding Sites. *Biochemistry* **10**: 3065–3069 (1971).

Piafsky KM. Disease-Induced Changes in the Plasma Binding of Basic Drugs. *Clin. Pharmacokinet.* **5**: 246–262 (1980).

Scatchard G. The Attractions of Proteins for Small Molecules and Ions. *Ann. NY Acad. Sci.* **51**: 660–672 (1949).

Sudlow GD, Birkett DJ and Wade DN. Further Characterization of Specific Drug Binding Sites on Human Serum Albumin. *Mol. Pharmacol.* **12**: 1052–1062 (1976).

Valner JJ. Binding of Drugs by Albumin and Plasma Protein. *J. Pharm. Sci.* **66**: 447–465 (1977).

8

Distribution of drugs in the body

Objectives

After completing this chapter the reader will be familiar with:

— *The concept of the apparent volume of distribution*
— *The factors which regulate the apparent volume of distribution*
— *The principles of drug transport through the placenta and blood–brain barrier*
— *The characteristics of drug excretion in breast milk and saliva*

8.1 APPARENT VOLUME OF DISTRIBUTION

8.1.1 Definitions

Chapter 7 discussed the binding of drugs to plasma proteins. Protein binding is just one of many interactions which can affect the time course and intensity of drug action. Many drugs act at receptors which are located at extravascular sites and for these drugs the ability to pass from the blood into other fluids and tissues is prerequisite to their pharmacological action. Drugs may diffuse into extravascular body water and/or partition into non-aqueous domains within the body. The extent to which these processes occur is characterized by the apparent volume of distribution.

The body fluids available for the distribution of drug can be classified as shown in Fig. 8.1. Note that the total water content of the body is approximately 42 litres, compared with about 7 litres total blood volume. This classification will serve as a basis for interpreting the phenomena of distribution.

In principle, the drug is made readily available for distribution to the whole body via circulation of the blood. The heart pumps about 5 litres of blood per minute, with the result that almost the entire volume of the blood is circulated through the body every minute. In other words, within 1–2 min of the drug reaching the general circulation it will have been distributed in the total blood volume and have come in contact with all of the major organs. Provided it can penetrate the pores of the capillaries, the drug then diffuses from the general circulation into the interstitial fluid. The interstitial fluid constitutes approximately 20% of tissue volume and is rich in plasma proteins. For example, 60% of the total body albumin is found in the interstitial fluid. The facile exchange of substances

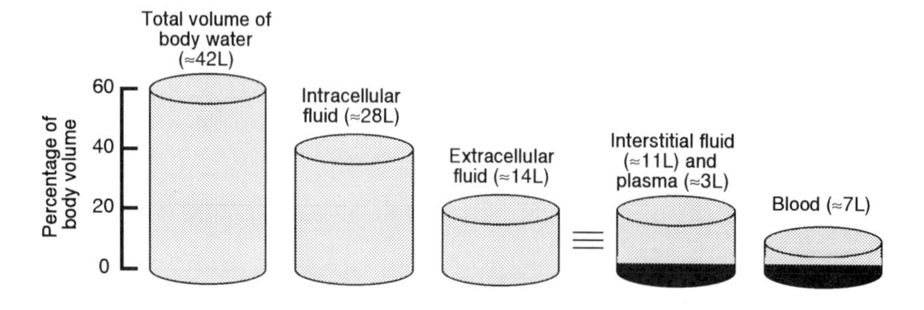

Fig. 8.1. Classification of the body fluids. For comparative purposes the total blood volume is also shown.

between blood and the interstitial fluid is the result of the large surface area of the capillaries, as well as the low flow rate of the blood at the points of exchange.

The capillaries are narrow cylindrical tubes, with walls formed by a thin single layer of cells (Fig. 8.2).† The endothelial cells contain pores (fenestrae), which vary in size from approximately 9 to 15 nm in diameter. It is estimated that there are on the order of 10^9 of these capillaries in the whole body. These pores allow the easy transfer of small hydrophilic substances between the blood and the fluid outside the capillaries. Small lipophilic substances may gain access to interstitial fluid by diffusion through capillary pores or permeation of the lipophilic capillary membrane. Only very large substances such as proteins and drug–protein complexes are confined to blood, as their size does not permit their transport through the pores. Thus, nearly all drug molecules can be transported from blood to the interstitial fluid and vice versa through the pores of the capillaries. The permeation of the capillary wall follows the principles of passive

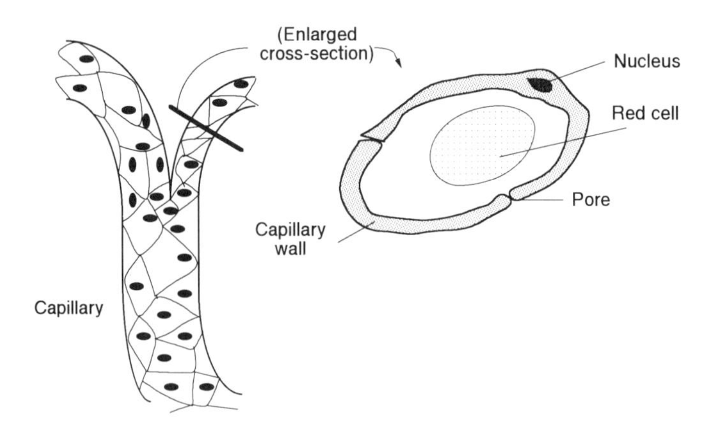

Fig. 8.2. Structure of blood capillaries in cross-section. (Redrawn from *A Primer of Drug Action*, Julien RM (ed.), 2nd edn, p. 12, Freeman, San Francisco (1978).)

† Further information on the structure of the capillaries is given in section 6.2.1.1, in which the transport of the drug from the interior of the gastrointestinal epithelial cell to the blood is discussed.

diffusion (section 3.1), with the result that there is uncomplicated and rapid exchange of the drug between blood tissues.

The next step which may occur in the distribution process is for the drug to enter the tissue cells and be distributed in the intracellular fluid, which comprises approximately 65% of the tissue volume. This process presupposes, as mentioned in chapter 6, either that the drug is lipophilic or that there is a specific uptake mechanism available to the drug. The rate of permeation of the cell membranes is therefore related not only to the blood flow rate, but also to the particular characteristics of the membrane structure of the various tissues. In some cases the drug can exhibit a specific localization, called *tissue binding*, to certain tissues. The nature of this binding is usually non-specific. For example, inside the cells there are large quantities of lipoidal membranes (such as the endoplasmic reticulum and the shell of the subcellular organelles), which may function as sites of accumulation for lipophilic drugs.

In Fig. 8.3, a general schematic for the temporal sequence of the drug distribution processes is shown. Not all drugs follow this sequence at the same rate or to an equal extent, and some do not participate in all of the processes shown. The *apparent volume of distribution*, sometimes referred to as simply the *volume of distribution*, V_d, is a parameter which aims to describe quantitatively the magnitude of participation of a given drug in the distribution processes of Fig. 8.3. The volume of distribution can be calculated from the equation

$$V_d = \frac{\text{amount of drug in the body}}{\text{total concentration of drug in plasma}} = \frac{X_b}{C_t} \tag{8.1}$$

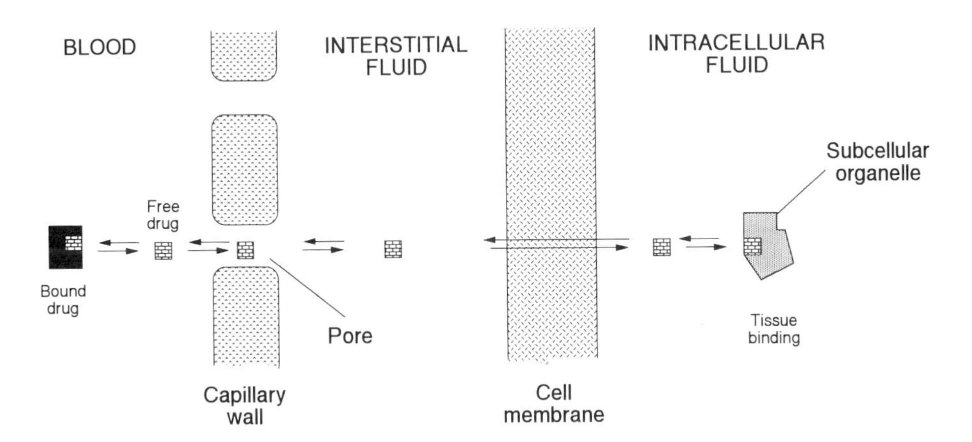

Fig. 8.3. Schematic of the sequence of drug distribution processes in the body.

Equation (8.1) implies that the volume of distribution is the volume of the body fluids in which the drug 'appears' to be distributed. The calculation of V_d requires a knowledge of the amount of drug in the body under steady-state conditions (i.e. when the relative concentrations of drug in various parts of the body have reached a steady value), and experimental determination of drug concentration in blood plasma. The estimated value of the apparent volume of distribution is partly a function of the physicochemical properties of the drug, since these determine the interaction of the drug with the plasma proteins and the tissue components, as well as its ability to diffuse through the biological membranes.

From equation (8.1) it is easily observed that when a drug exhibits extensive distribution, the measured concentration in plasma will be very small. This is also evident from Fig. 8.4, which illustrates the distribution behaviour of four hypothetical drugs administered in equal doses of 100 mg.† Drug 1 is strongly bound to the plasma proteins and is completely retained in plasma. In such cases the volume of distribution is approximately 3 litres. For drugs like drug 1 a direct physiological significance can be attributed to any change in the volume of distribution, in terms of the volume of blood plasma. Drug 2 diffuses into the interstitial fluid, but is not lipophilic enough to penetrate the intracellular fluid. In such cases the volume of distribution has an intermediate value, here on the order of 11 litres. Drug 3 is lipophilic and can pass into the intracellular fluid, resulting in an apparent volume of distribution of the order of 40 litres. For drug 4, which apart from its lipophilic properties is able to interact with tissue components, the volume of distribution has a very large value ($V_d \gg 40$ litres). Very large values for volume of distribution are generally indicative of extensive penetration of extravascular domains and the specific localization of the drug to one or more tissues.

To illustrate the volumes of distribution attributable to the distinct compartments of the body shown in Fig. 8.4, we now consider some specific compound examples. The

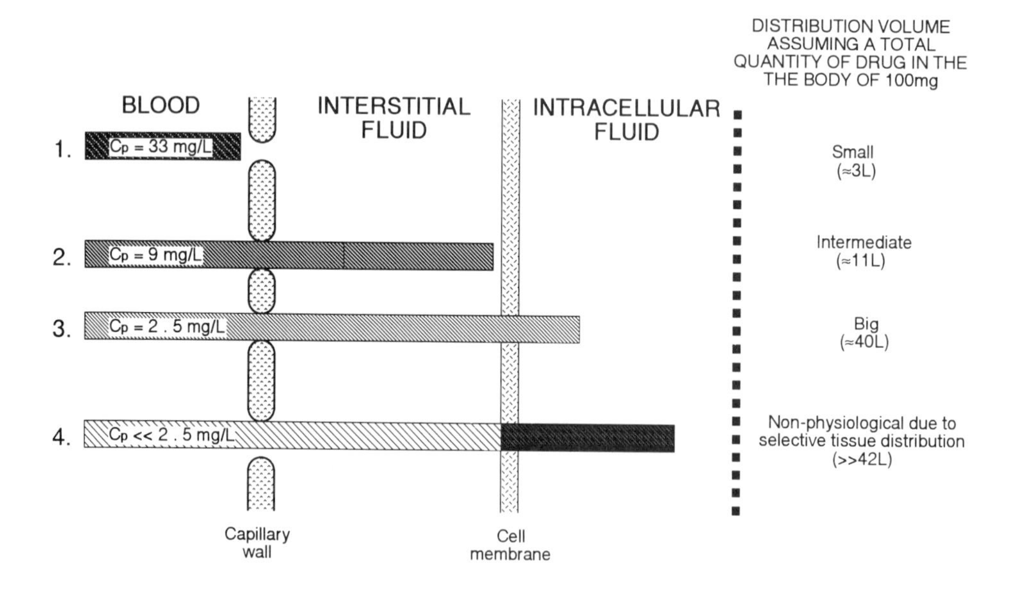

Fig. 8.4. Representation of the concept of apparent volume of distribution. The value of the concentration of the drug, determined in plasma, C_p, is inversely proportional to dilution (i.e. volume of distribution of drug) in the body.

† More precisely, 100 mg of drug are in the body when steady-state conditions are achieved.

macromolecular dye Evans blue is administered at a dosage of 100 μg as a method of estimating plasma water, and consequently the volume of blood, after determining the patient's haematocrit.† Its strong binding to the plasma proteins and size preclude distribution to extravascular sites, leading to a concentration of ≈33 μg/l if the volume of distribution is 3 litres. Other compounds such as inulin, bromide, iodide and inorganic salts of sodium are also used to estimate the volume of the interstitial fluid. However, these compounds, especially the sodium salts, are distributed partly to the intracellular fluid, which results in overestimation of the volume of the interstitial fluid. The total volume of water in the body can be measured after administration of $^{2}H_2O$ or $^{3}H_2O$, both of which distribute in the total water of the body.

Unlike Evans blue and deuterated or tritiated water, which can be used to estimate blood volume and total body water, respectively, no direct physiological interpretation can be placed on the volume of distribution calculated for a given drug. The only exception to this rule occurs when the drug, like Evans blue, is retained completely in the plasma, in which case V_d will be about 3 litres. In cases where the volume of distribution ranges from 3 to 40 litres, it is not possible to distinguish between tissue penetration and tissue binding contributions to the overall distribution volume. When the volume of distribution exceeds the total body water (i.e. $V_d > 40$ litres) it is reasonable to conclude that tissue penetration and binding contribute to the distribution of the drug in the body. However, the sites at which the drug is distributed cannot be specified without additional data (e.g. autoradiography studies). A classic example of extensive distribution is that of the tricyclic antidepressants imipramine and nortriptyline. At therapeutic levels these drugs are bound 90% to the plasma proteins. However, they present volumes of distribution (Table 8.1) on the order of 1000 and 1400 litres, respectively, which indicates that they are extensively distributed to extravascular tissues. Although at first glance this seems contradictory, it can be explained on the basis of Fig. 8.4. At steady state, the greater portion of drug in the body is localized in the tissues, despite the strong binding of these drugs in plasma. In other words, the amount of drug at steady state in the various compartments of Fig. 8.4, is not only a function of the equilibrium constants of the processes of Fig. 8.4, but also of the 'capacity' of the compartments for the drug under study. It is evident that the 'capacity' of a tissue depends on the physicochemical properties of the drug. For example, fat tissues tend to detain large quantities of hydrophobic drugs (e.g. digoxin, cyclopropane, pentothal).

The estimated value of the volume of distribution of a specific drug may depend partly on the weight of the individuals participating in the study. For this reason, values of the volume of distribution are usually expressed as mean values in units of l/kg (Table 8.1). Table 8.1 illustrates the large range in values for the apparent volume of distribution of various drugs.

It must be emphasized that calculation of the volume of distribution requires determination of the drug concentration in plasma after achieving steady state among the

† The haematocrit value is an index of both the number and size of the red cells. Its value (expressed as percentage) corresponds to the volume ratio of packed red cells to total blood volume. The total blood volume can be calculated, if the plasma volume is multiplied by 100/(100-haematocrit). The normal values of haematocrit for men and women are 47% and 42%, respectively.

Table 8.1. Mean values (l/kg) of the apparent volume of distribution of certain drugs and of ethanol[a]

Acyclovir	0.70	Gentamycin	0.23
Allopurinol	0.60	Glibenclamide	0.30
Amikasin	0.20	Glutethimide	2.8
Amiloride	5.0	Griseofulvin	0.70
Aminocaproic acid	0.40	Hydralazine	5.0
Aminopyrine	0.86	Hydrochlorothiazide	0.80
p-Aminosalicylic acid	0.20	Hydrocortisone	0.40
Amiodarone	70	Ibuprofen	0.14
Amitriptyline	8.0	Imipramine	14
Amoxicillin	0.40	Indomethacin	1.0
Amphotericin B	3.0	Isoniazid	0.60
Ampicillin	0.30	Kanamycin	0.25
Atenolol	0.70	Lidocaine[b]	1.0
Atropine	3.0	Lincomycin	0.50
Benzylpenicillin	0.30	Lithium	0.80
Betamethasone	1.8	Melphalan	0.50
Bromazepam	1.0	Methadone	4.0
Bumetanide	0.24	Methotrexate	0.40
Butobarbitone	0.80	Methyl-dopa	0.35
Captopril	0.70	Methylprednisolone	0.70
Carbamazepine	1.2	Metoprolol	4.0
Cefaclor	0.50	Minoxidil	3.0
Cefadroxil	0.40	Morphine	3.0
Cefalexin	0.23	Moxalactam	0.30
Ceftriaxone	0.15	Naproxen	0.10
Cephaloridin	0.20	Neostigmine	0.70
Cephaxoline	0.14	Netilmycin	0.25
Chloramphenicol	0.70	Nifedipine	1.4
Chlordiazepoxide	0.30	Nitrofurantoin	0.80
Chlorpheniramine	2.4	Nitroglycerin	0.35
Chlorpromazine	20	Nortryptiline[b]	20
Chlorpropamide	0.15	Oxazepam	0.65
Chlortetracycline	1.2	Oxytetracycline	1.5
Chlorthiazide	0.20	Paracetamol	1.0
Cimetidine	2.0	Perphenazine	20
Clintamycin	0.60	Pethidine	4.0
Clofibrat	0.08	Phenobarbital	0.80
Cloxacillin	0.35	Phenylbutazone[b]	0.08
Codeine	5.4	Phenylephrine	4.9
Colchicine	2.3	Phenytoin	0.65
Cyclosporin A	3.5	Piroxicam	0.16

Table 8.1 (continued)

Dapsone	1.5	Prednisolone	0.50
Desipramine	22	Procainamide	2.0
Dexamethasone	0.75	Promethazine	13
Diazepam[b]	1.2	Propoxyphene	2.7
Diclofenac	0.15	Propranolol	4.0
Dicloxacillin	0.08	Quinidine	2.8
Dicumarol	0.15	Ranitidine	1.5
Diflunisal	0.11	Rifampicin	1.5
Digitoxin	0.50	Sulfadiazine	0.35
Digoxin	10	Sulfamethizole	0.35
Diltiazem	4.5	Sulfamethoxazole	0.20
Diphenhydramine	3.5	Sulfasalazine	<1.0
Disopyramide	0.80	Spironolactone	0.05
Disulfiram	8.2	Tetracycline	1.5
Doxycycline	1.5	Theophylline	0.50
Ethanol	0.55	Tolbutamide	0.14
Ethosuximide	0.70	Triamcinolone	1.8
Erythromycin	0.70	Trimethoprim	2.0
Fentanyl	3.0	Valproic acid	0.14
5-Fluorouracil	0.40	Verapamil	4.0
Furosemide	1.0	Warfarin[b]	0.10

[a] The data were selected from *Pharmocokinetic Basis of Drug Treatment*, Benet LZ, Massoud N and Gambertoglio JG (eds), p. 10, Raven Press, New York (1984).
[b] For these drugs the calculated values vary widely. For example, the range between the maximum and the minimum value (ratio in parentheses) calculated for three of these drugs are: diazepam 1.3–0.18 (7.2), phenylbutazone 0.15–0.04 (3.8), lidocaine 1.9–0.58 (3.3).

processes of Fig. 8.4, and also a knowledge of the amount of the drug in the body (equation (8.1)) at this time. The time required for the completion of distribution of a drug depends on the extent of its distribution. Consider for example a dose of digoxin administered as an intravenous bolus. Although the initial distribution of drug in the total blood volume is achieved rapidly, its distribution to heart muscle requires 4–5 h. During this distribution phase, the amount of digoxin in the body and its concentration in blood are decreasing as a result of biotransformation and excretion. In cases like digoxin, determination of the distribution volume is problematic, since the quantities X_b and C_t (equation (8.1)) must correspond to the same temporal point. A special treatment of concentration–time data, for calculation of *the time-dependent volume of distribution*, is required. These calculations are described in the references listed at the end of this chapter.

Example 8.1: What percentage of the total amount of a drug remains in plasma, assuming no significant tissue binding and that the drug is distributed to the total body water, when the percentage bound to the plasma proteins is 62%. Recall that plasma is 4.0% of body weight and that total body water is 60% of total body weight.

Answer: Using the symbols V_0 and V_p for the total volumes of the body fluids and plasma, respectively, f_f for the fraction of the free drug in plasma, and C_f and C_t for the concentrations of the free and total drug in plasma, respectively, the 'percentage drug in plasma' can be calculated as follows:

$$\%\text{ drug in plasma} = \frac{\text{amount in plasma}}{\text{amount in body}} \times 100$$

$$= \frac{100 C_t V_p}{C_f (V_0 - V_p) + C_t V_p} = \frac{100}{\dfrac{C_f}{C_t}\left(\dfrac{V_0}{V_p} - 1\right) + 1}$$

$$= \frac{100}{f_f\left[(60/4.0) - 1\right] + 1} = \frac{100}{14 f_f + 1} = \frac{100}{14(1 - 0.62) + 1} = 16 \tag{8.2}$$

The reader should note that despite the relatively high percentage of binding (62%) in plasma and the negligible binding of this drug in tissues, only approximately 16% of the drug in the body is found in the plasma.

8.1.2 Tissue binding

The degree of tissue binding and the locations at which this occurs vary enormously among drugs. Although the value of the apparent volume of distribution gives a general idea of the distribution of a drug in the body, it does not provide information as to which specific organs or tissues the drug is distributed in.

The effect of protein binding to tissues on the apparent volume of distribution, V_d, can be described mathematically by the following equation:

$$V_d = V_p + \frac{f_{fp}}{f_{ft}} V_t \tag{8.3}$$

which is based on the principle that only the free drug can diffuse into the extravascular tissues. In equation (8.3), V_p is the plasma volume, V_t is the tissue volume, and f_{fp} and f_{ft} are the free fractions in plasma and tissues, respectively. According to this equation, extensive tissue binding, corresponding to $f_{ft} \to 0$, is reflected in a dramatic increase of the apparent volume of distribution, V_d. In general, as the factor f_{fp}/f_{ft} increases, i.e. tissue binding increases in relation to that in plasma, a proportional increase of V_d is observed. Solution of equation (8.3) in terms of f_{ft} gives

$$f_{ft} = f_{fp} \frac{V_t}{V_d - V_p} \tag{8.4}$$

An estimate for f_{ft} can be derived from this equation. Note that the value of V_t is dependent on the tissue considered and, therefore, f_{ft} may vary among tissues.

A number of *in vitro* techniques have been developed for the measurement of drug binding to tissues. The main drawback of these techniques is the low degree of correlation between estimates based on organ binding studies and *in vivo* values. The *in vitro* technique which least affects tissue integrity is the perfusion of isolated organs. This technique has been applied to organs like liver, heart and lung, with rabbit and rat being the most commonly used animals. The extent of binding to the organ under study is based on the inlet and outlet perfusate concentration under steady-state conditions. Experimental variables like the composition and the flow rate of the perfusate can substantially affect the binding of drug to the organ's tissues and must be carefully controlled.

Other techniques utilized for the study of tissue binding result in greater disruption of the tissue. The loss of tissue integrity is least when the technique of 'tissue slices' is used. The proper use of the tissue slice technique necessitates the preparation of thin slices so that there is free supply of oxygen to deep layers of cells. Like the organ perfusion techniques, discrimination between binding and active tissue uptake is not possible. Another technique, which is used extensively because of its simplicity, utilizes tissues homogenates. Usually, the tissues are homogenized with an equal volume of isotonic phosphate buffer and the extent of binding is determined by ultrafiltration. Finally, isolated subcellular particles are sometimes used for the study of binding to specific regions of the cell.

8.1.3 Factors affecting the volume of distribution

8.1.3.1 Age

The rapid changes in both weight and body composition that occur as children grow result in corresponding changes in the volume of distribution of the drugs. In general, the volume of distribution, expressed in units of volume per kilogram of weight, is larger in neonates and decreases gradually during childhood, stabilizing in early adulthood. This change is related to the progressive alterations of tissue composition. During the first year of life, a decrease of the total body water in relation to the total body weight is observed. At the same time, the extracellular fluid decreases continuously, with a parallel increase in the intracellular fluid. Consequently, drugs having hydrophilic properties, which are in principle confined to the extracellular fluid (e.g. ampicillin or amikacin) tend to present larger volumes of distribution per unit body weight for children in the first year of life in comparison to adults. It has also been observed that volumes of distribution of lipophilic drugs are larger in neonates than in adults. Although at first glance this seems contradictory, as the fat tissues in neonates are proportionally small, it has been postulated that the higher blood flow rate in neonates promotes distribution to organs rich in fat such as liver and brain.

The relative changes of composition of the body as adults age should also be noted. Fig. 8.5 displays the mean percentages of the basic constituents of the body at the ages of 25 and 75 years old. A decrease in lean body mass is observed, with gradual replacement by fat tissue. The percentage increase in fat tissue varies between 33% and 48% in females and 18% and 36% in males. The result of these changes with ageing is that there is an increase in the volume of distribution for lipophilic drugs and a decrease in the volume of distribution for hydrophilic drugs. Examples of drugs which show increased

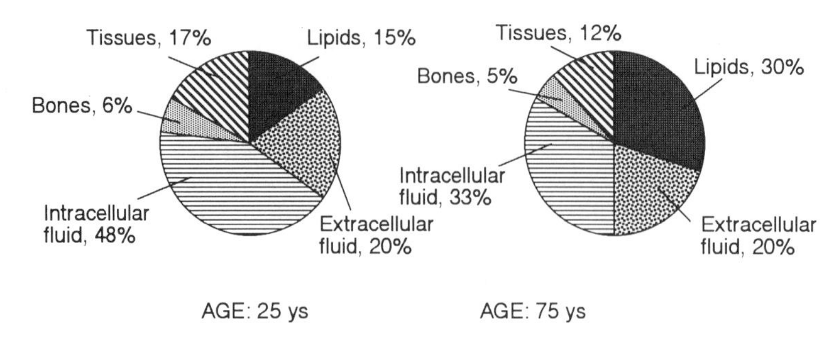

Fig. 8.5. Mean composition of the human body in relation to age.

volume of distribution with age include diazepam and chlordiazepoxide. The structurally similar but less lipophilic drugs, lorazepam and oxazepam, have similar volumes of distribution in young and elderly people. Another observation, related to Fig. 8.5, is that while in the elderly the total water of the body decreases by 10–15%, the extracellular fluid constitutes a greater portion of the total body water than in childhood. These gradual but important changes in the composition of body fluids led scientists to develop equations which allow the calculation of the volume of distribution as a function of age. These equations are based on the magnitude of the volume of distribution at the age of 25 years old (see the references at the end of the chapter for more detailed discussion of these calculations).

8.1.3.2 Pregnancy

The data related to the passage of drugs across the placenta are few and in many cases inconclusive, since administration of drugs to pregnant women is performed only when required by clinical necessity. Experiments in laboratory animals cannot be considered valid, as human physiology is not well modelled by other species in this case. However, it is evident that the physiological and morphological changes associated with pregnancy result in considerable changes in the disposition of drugs in pregnant women. These changes are usually progressive over the course of the pregnancy. For example, upper gastrointestinal transit time is 60% longer in the second or third trimester of pregnancy than the first trimester or the post-partum period.

As far as the distribution of drugs is concerned, the volume of distribution is considerably increased because of increases in plasma volume, the cellular constituents of the blood, fat tissue and body water. Like other physiological changes these increases are progressive from early to late pregnancy and vary according to nutrition and the number of fetuses. The mean changes in blood volume during a normal pregnancy are quoted in Table 8.2. There are attendant increases in the total body water due to an increase in the volume of extracellular fluid and the formation of new tissues. Nevertheless, the increase in total body water varies widely between women because the volume of the accumulated extracellular fluid in the lower limbs varies with the degree of oedema developed (Fig. 8.6).

It is evident that the sizeable increase in the volume of body water will cause a corresponding increase in the volume of distribution of drugs. In addition there is an

Table 8.2. Changes in blood volume (ml) in normal pregnancy[a]

	Non-pregnant	Weeks pregnant		
		20	30	40
Plasma	2600	3150	3700	3850
Erythrocytes	1400	1450	1550	1650
Cellular elements	4000	4600	5250	5500

[a] Reprinted from *Pharmacology and Therapeutics* **10**: 305 (1980) with permission.

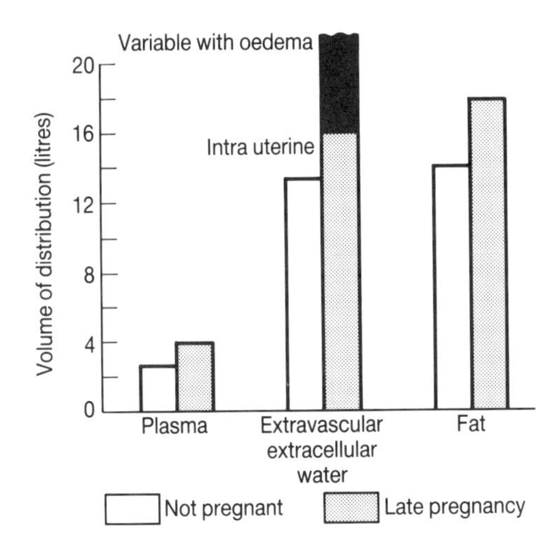

Fig. 8.6. Change in plasma volume, extracellular fluid and fat tissue during pregnancy. (Reprinted from *Pharmacology and Therapeutics* **10**: 301–328 (1980), with permission.)

increase in the mass of fat tissues of approximately 3–4 kg, corresponding to about 30% of the total increase in body weight when there is an overall gain of ≈12 kg (Fig. 8.6). Note that the gain in fat tissue is very dependent on the total weight gain. For example, an increase in total weight of 8 kg is not usually associated with any significant accumulation of fat. By contrast, an increase of 20 kg may be associated with fat accumulations of as much as 50% (10 kg). The increase in fat tissue results in an increase in the volume of distribution of the lipophilic drugs. If the lipophilic pentothal is administered to induce anaesthesia during delivery, for example, its slow release by the fat tissue leads to a delay in recovery from anaesthesia.

The changes observed in the concentration of blood proteins during pregnancy may also result in altered distribution of drugs. The decrease in albumin concentration by mid-pregnancy is about 0.5–1 g/dl, resulting in a mean concentration of 2.5–3 g/dl (Fig. 8.7). As this decrease is offset at least partly by the increase in plasma volume, not all drugs exhibit decreased binding in pregnancy (Table 8.2). Changes in albumin levels are

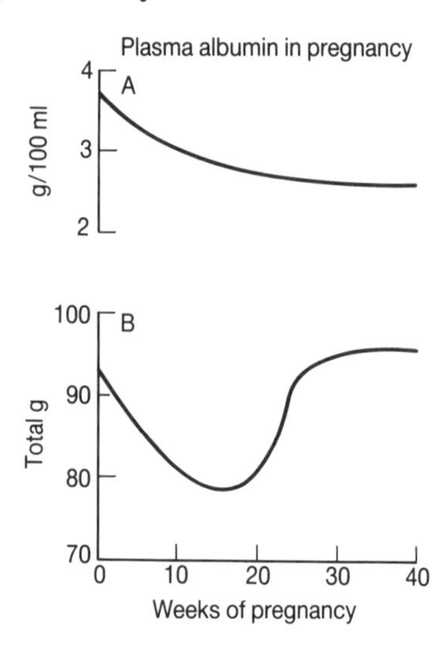

Fig. 8.7. Change (A) in concentration and (B) in total amount of albumin in plasma during pregnancy. (Reprinted from *Pharmacology and Therapeutics* **10**: 301–328 (1980), with permission.)

depicted in Fig. 8.7. Note that in the second half of pregnancy the total amount of albumin regains the same levels as before pregnancy.

8.1.3.3 Pathological conditions

The apparent volume of distribution of drugs is influenced by various pathological conditions, extensive description of which is not within the scope of this book. Here, two examples serve to illustrate the magnitude of disease state effects on volume of distribution.

In renally impaired patients, the volume of distribution may increase, decrease or remain unchanged. Digoxin is a typical example in which renal impairment decreases the volume of distribution. The decrease may be as much as 50% of the values considered normal, ≈400–600 litres or ≈7 l/kg. Clinical observations show that the decrease in volume of distribution of digoxin is correlated to the reduced renal function, as estimated by the clearance of creatinine (section 9.2). Opposite behaviour is exhibited by phenytoin, for which an increase in the volume of distribution is observed in uraemic patients. As mentioned in chapter 7, the binding of phenytoin to the plasma proteins is decreased in uraemic patients, resulting in an increase in the free fraction from 0.12 (the normal value) to 0.25. Consequently, larger amounts of phenytoin are available for distribution. Thus, the estimated volume of distribution of phenytoin is increased from 0.6–0.7 l/kg (normal values) to 1.0–1.8 l/kg (values in uraemic patients).

8.2 TRANSPORT OF DRUGS THROUGH SPECIFIC MEMBRANES

Two cases of the distribution of drugs in tissues of special interest are passage across the placenta and across the blood–brain barrier.

8.2.1 Placental transport of drugs

The membranes separating the maternal arterial supply from the fetal capillary in the intervillous spaces of the placenta have a typical lipid-barrier structure, permitting the transfer of lipophilic drugs across the placenta by the mechanism of passive diffusion. The same is true for drug metabolites, i.e. the lipophilic ones pass across the placenta very readily, while the polar ones penetrate poorly or not at all. The placental transfer of drug and its partition to the maternal–placental–fetal unit is influenced by the degree of ionization of the drug. This influence is especially significant when the value of the pK_a of the drug is close to the pH of the plasma of the mother and the fetus. It should be noted that the pH of the plasma of the fetus is 7.3, resulting in slightly higher concentrations for drugs with properties of weak bases on the side of the fetus. The amniotic fluid is in turn more acidic than the fetal plasma. Its composition is similar to that of the extracellular fluid of the fetus, as these fluids communicate via the permeable epidermis of the fetus. The equilibrium ratio of drug in the fetal plasma is also influenced by the extent of plasma protein binding in the mother's blood. When drug binding to maternal plasma proteins is high, the penetration rate of the drug across the placenta will be slow. It is also worth mentioning that both placental and fetal drug metabolism are possible, as the enzyme systems which exist in the placenta and the tissues of the fetus are capable of initiating all the basic biotransformation processes (section 9.3).

Despite the fact that a large number of drugs, such as antibiotics, barbiturates, sulfonamides and antihistamines, have been found to penetrate the placenta, the fundamental questions regarding the total amount of drug reaching the fetus, the rate at which it crosses the placental membrane, and the duration of its residence in the fetal side remain unanswered. The story of thalidomide provides a grim reminder that drugs which penetrate the placental barrier can have a great impact on the rapidly developing fetus.

8.2.2 Transport across the blood–brain barrier

The term *blood–brain barrier* has its roots in observations in laboratory animals made by German pharmacologists at the beginning of the century. These researchers observed that the intravenous administration of a dye (trypan blue) stained all the tissues of the laboratory animals, except the largest portion of the brain and the spinal cord. These observations led in 1920 to the mistaken conclusion that this barrier is absolute, i.e. the transport of non-physiological substances to the brain is impossible. However, after the development of the electron microscope around 1950, it became possible to study the structure of the endothelial cells comprising the wall of the capillaries in the brain. Today, specific anatomical features associated with the blood–brain barrier, which explain the wide range of penetration rates of substances passing from the bloodstream into the brain and the cerebrospinal fluid (CSF), have been identified.

The blood–brain barrier is generally much less permeable to compounds than other blood/organ interfaces owing to the following structural characteristics of the capillaries in the brain:

(a) in contrast to the porous capillary structure of the peripheral capillaries (Fig. 8.2), the cells of the brain capillaries are tightly joined (section 5.1); and
(b) the basement membrane of the capillary endothelium is surrounded by the end-feet of cells of glial connective tissue, the *astrocytes*. This glial sheath covers 85% of the capillary wall and forms an extra fatty barrier for a drug to reach the cells in the brain.

These unique anatomical features result in reduced permeability of the capillaries in the brain and hence a very slow exchange of substances between blood and brain.

The blood–brain barrier actually consists of two distinct barriers: the barrier between blood and brain and the barrier between blood and the CSF. The CSF's composition is similar to the composition of the extracellular fluid (ECF) of the brain. The lack of tight junctions in the ependymal cells between ECF of the brain and CSF allows a free exchange of substances between these two compartments. The CSF is contained within the ventricles, where it is formed by the choroid plexuses and flows into the subarachnoid space. Thus, drugs may diffuse to CSF either via the choroid plexus or across the subarachnoid membrane (Fig. 8.8).

As far as the blood–CSF barrier is concerned, the junctions between cells in the epithelial layer of the blood capillaries are tight, so the transport of solutes from blood and CSF is restricted. However, certain regions of the central nervous system such as the posterior lobe of the pineal body are known to be much more permeable to drugs. The

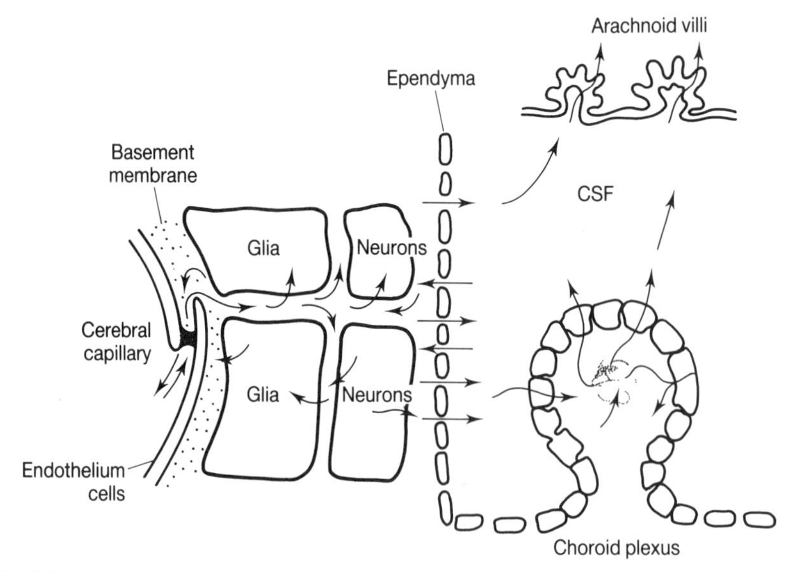

Fig. 8.8. Interrelationship between blood–brain barrier and blood–CSF barrier. Arrows indicate possibilities for solute exchange and transport. (From *Pharmaceutisch Weekbland (Scientific Edition)* **14**: 305–310 (1992) with permission.)

high permeability of these areas may be due either to a highly permeable structure of blood capillaries and/or to a very rich blood supply of these regions. Drug molecules which can penetrate the blood–brain or the blood–CSF barrier and find themselves in the ECF of the brain or the CSF are able to cross the cell membranes of the neurons and other cells and thus gain access to the central nervous system.

Overall, the blood–brain barrier functions as a continuous lipid layer, penetration of which depends mainly on the lipophilicity of the compound. This dependence has been proved experimentally with a large number of drugs. Illustrative examples of passive diffusion through the blood–brain barrier can be found in the lipophilic drugs diazepam and pentothal. The factors controlling the rate of transport of the drugs across the blood–brain barrier are similar to those described in the mechanism of passive diffusion (section 3.1). That is, a high value of the partition coefficient and a low degree of ionization at pH 7.4 are physicochemical properties which favour rapid entry to the brain. The importance of these properties is clearly displayed in the case of pentothal, which is administered intravenously to induce anaesthesia. Pentothal crosses the blood–brain barrier rapidly as a result of its high lipophilicity. Its duration of action is very short, since it passes back out of the brain into blood as soon as its concentration in blood drops, in order to maintain concentration equilibria. In Table 8.3 the physicochemical properties of pentothal are quoted, along with those of the isosteric pentobarbitone. The presence of sulfur in the molecule leads to a very high partition coefficient (see Table 5.1), which imparts unique pharmacokinetic properties of pentothal.

Table 8.3. Physicochemical properties of pentothal and pentobarbitone

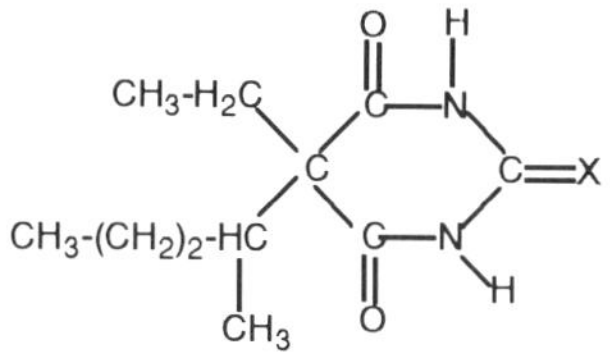	% ionization at pH 7.4[a]	% binding in plasma[b]	Partition coefficient (heptane–water)
X : S, pentothal	39	75	3.30
X : O, pentobarbitone	17	40	0.05

[a] Based on pK_a values 7.6 and 8.1 for pentothal and pentobarbitone, respectively, according to Table 4.4
[b] At therapeutic levels in the blood.

Another factor having an indirect but significant role in the penetration of the blood–brain barrier is the extent of binding to the plasma proteins. The rate of permeation of the blood–brain barrier is proportional to the concentration of the free form of drug in plasma, and equilibration of free drug occurs under sink conditions because the concentration of proteins in the CSF is less than 1% of that in plasma.

The mathematical description of the drug's diffusion through the blood–brain barrier is based on the principles of passive diffusion (chapter 2). Permeation into the CSF thus follows an equation of the form

$$\frac{dC_{CSF}}{dt} = k_1(C_f - C_{CSF}) \tag{8.5}$$

where (dC_{CSF}/dt) is the rate of transport of the free drug from the plasma towards the CSF, C_f is the concentration of the free drug in plasma and C_{CSF} is the concentration of the free drug in the CSF; k_1 is the first order rate constant, and is usually calculated from equation (8.5) using experimental data from laboratory animals (e.g. dogs). In these experiments the plasma drug concentration C_f is maintained at a constant value (usually achieved by continuous infusion of the drug) and the CSF is sampled at various time intervals. Equation (8.5) is then applied in its integrated logarithmic form:

$$\ln\left(\frac{C_f - C_{CSF}}{C_f}\right) = -k_1 t \tag{8.6}$$

k_1 has been shown to be proportional to the lipophilicity of the drug. For example, the rate of entry into the CSF of pentothal (k_{1T}) is greater than that of pentobarbitone (k_{1B}), as shown in Fig. 8.9.

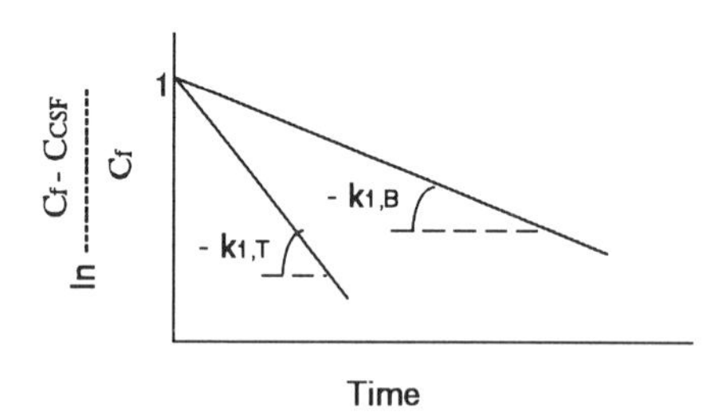

Fig. 8.9. Access of pentothal, T, and phenobarbitone, B, to the CSF.

During the last several years, studies of drug transport through the blood–brain barrier have shown that there are independent carrier-mediated systems for the transport of various drugs at the choroid plexus as well as in the capillaries of the brain. Table 8.4 displays a number of drugs and endogenous substances necessary for the function of the brain which are taken up by carrier-mediated mechanisms. Depending on the substance and the carrier, transport may be either uni- or bidirectional. For example, penicillin G is transported into the brain by the weak carboxylic acid carrier. This carrier has low affinity and capacity (i.e. high K_M and low V_{max}, respectively), so only small amounts of this drug enter the brain. A more powerful transport mechanism for weak acids is situated in the choroid plexus, and this accounts for the transport of larger amounts of penicillin G *from* the CSF fluid *to* the blood. The net result of these processes is that penicillin G achieves low concentrations in the CSF. Ceftriaxone is another anti-biotic which is transported by the weak carboxylic acid transporter into the brain. However, this cephalosporin exhibits low affinity for the exit transport mechanism at the choroid plexus, with the net effect that it achieves high levels in CSF. In other words, the relative affinities of a weak acid for the various carriers of the blood–brain barrier determine the levels it can achieve in the brain. For weak bases, a bidirectional carrier-mediated transport at the capillaries

Table 8.4. Compounds with carrier-mediated transport in the blood–brain barrier

Category		Examples
Ions		Ca^{2+}, Mg^{2+}, K^+, Na^+, HCO_3^-
Physiological substances		Glucose,[a] amino acids, fatty acids
Vitamins		B_1, B_2, B_6, ascorbic acid, biotin
Drugs:	Weak bases	Diphenhydramine, lidocaine, amphetamine
	Weak acids	Penicillins, cephalosporins
	Chemotherapeutics	Vincristine, doxorubicin
	Amino acids (and analogues)	L-Dopa, α-methyl-dopa
	Nucleosides	AZT

[a] Glucose is the first substance for which transport to the brain was studied in detail. The transport process operates bidirectionally. Only D-glucose (and not L-glucose) is transported to the brain.

of the brain is observed. The weak bases listed in Table 8.4 are rapidly transported to the brain, despite the fact that they are almost completely (>99%) ionized at pH 7.4.

Of special interest is the active transport of amino acids to the brain. Amino acids can be classified into one of the following four categories according to their structure; namely, large neutral, small neutral, acidic and basic amino acids. Large neutral amino acids such as phenylalanine, necessary for the synthesis of proteins and neurotransmitters, are transported across the blood–brain barrier in both directions by a specialized mechanism. This carrier is located in the cells of the capillaries. By contrast, the mechanism for the small neutral amino acids, e.g. glycine, function only in the brain-to-blood direction. This is a characteristic example of *non-symmetrical* transport. In the case of glycine, the transport mechanism is located only in the cells of the antiluminal membrane (boundary of brain → capillary wall). Glycine is not accumulated in the cells of the capillaries since it is transferred to the bloodstream by the large amino acid carrier, for which it has some affinity. The directionality of the transport mechanism of glycine suggests that it may be synthesized in the brain cells.

L-Dopa, an amino acid, and α-methyl-dopa, an amino acid analogue, access the blood–brain barrier via the carrier for large amino acids. Both drugs are biotransformed in the brain tissue to their active molecules dopamine and methyldopamine, respectively. Neither of these metabolites can be administered directly because they are inactivated by monoaminoxidase in the cells of the capillaries (Fig. 8.10). The conclusion from these observations is that transport into the brain of L-dopa and α-methyl-dopa is essential to their pharmacological action.

Whenever the transport of the drug through the blood–brain barrier is carrier mediated, the analysis of data is based on the principles of Michaelis–Menten kinetics (section 2.3.2.1). Some methods of studying the quantitative assessment of penetration of the blood–brain barrier are described in the references at the end of this chapter.

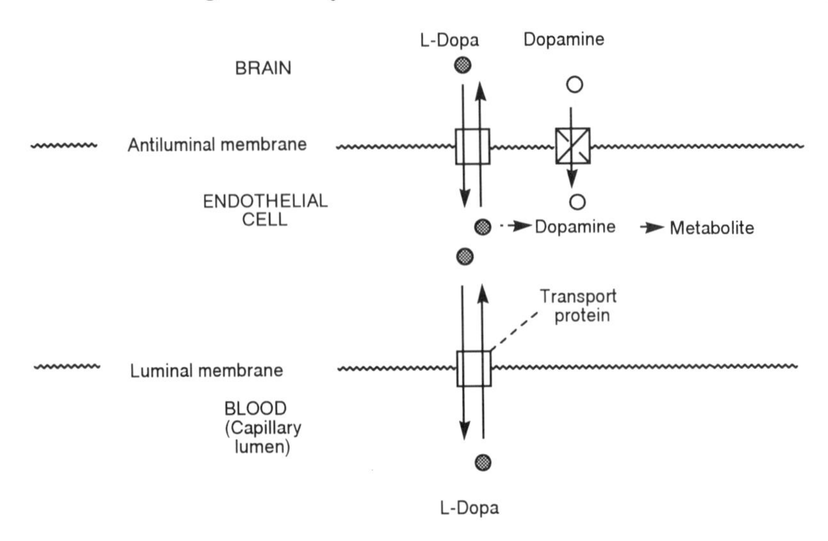

Fig. 8.10. Penetration of the blood–brain barrier by L-dopa.

8.3 EXCRETION OF DRUGS IN BREAST MILK AND SALIVA

8.3.1 Excretion of drugs in breast milk

During pregnancy the breasts become enlarged in response to the high circulating levels of oestrogens, progesterone and prolactin. Oestrogens and prolactin have a synergistic action in the development of the breasts; however, oestrogens antagonize prolactin in the production of milk. After delivery, the concentrations of oestrogens and progesterone fall abruptly. The rise in levels of prolactin combined with the fall in the concentration of oestrogens result in the initiation of milk secretion. Milk is secreted from cells in the mammary epithelium. The secretory cells are positioned in a circle around the alveolar lumen, into which milk is secreted. The milk collects into ducts, then passes to the supply region, where it accumulates between nursing. A large portion of the milk components are synthesized in the secretory cells, while the rest are transported into the cells, and hence the milk, from the blood.

Many drugs are secreted in the milk of nursing mothers, including ethanol, carbamazepine, chlorpromazine, imipramine, metoprolol, metronidazole and pentothal.

The excretion of drugs in milk follows the principles of passive diffusion. Thus, the lipophilicity of the drug is an important factor in determining the fraction of drug which is excreted in the milk. The non-ionized form of the drug diffuses from the blood to the milk and a steady-state ratio of drug concentrations between blood and milk is gradually established. The equilibrium ratio can be calculated from the Henderson–Hasselbach equations (equations (2.35) and (2.36)) using pH 7.4 and 6.8, respectively, for the blood and the milk. The slightly more acidic environment of the milk favours higher ionization of basic drugs in the milk, and therefore greater concentrations of these drugs in milk than in blood. The converse is true for drugs which are weak acids. The partition of the drug is usually defined as the ratio M : P, which expresses the ratio of the drug concentration in milk (M), and plasma (P). The M : P ratio is expressed in terms of the free drug concentrations in both media, since only the free drug participates in the equilibrium. Drug bound to plasma and milk proteins, as well as to lipid components of milk, does not diffuse between the two fluids. Experimentally, the concentrations of the free drug are usually determined in the ultrafiltrate of the two fluids. The overall equilibrium is shown schematically in Fig. 8.11.

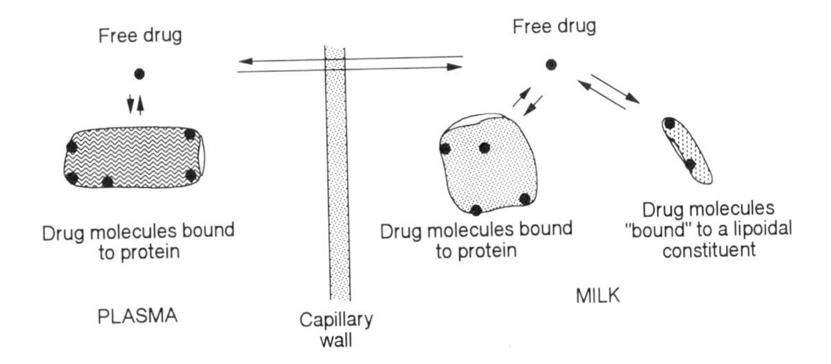

Fig. 8.11. Distribution of drug between blood and milk.

8.3.2 Excretion of drugs in saliva

Over the last two decades, it has been confirmed that for many drugs there is a proportionality between the concentration in saliva and the concentration in plasma. This is of interest since for these drugs it is possible to replace measurement of plasma concentration in pharmacokinetic studies with measurement of concentration in saliva. The use of saliva samples circumvents many of the disadvantages of blood sampling such as pain, stress and possible infection. Before replacing plasma with saliva sampling, one must establish that there is a constant ratio of the drug's concentration in the two media over the total range of the concentrations encountered in clinical practice. Selected examples of saliva to plasma (S : P) ratios found in various studies for different drugs are listed in Table 8.5.

Table 8.5. Ratios of the saliva to plasma concentrations (S : P) of various drugs[a]

Drug	S : P ratio
Antipyrine	0.92
Carbamazepine	0.30
Lithium	3.10
Paracetamol	1.14
Phenobarbitone	0.31
Phenytoin	0.11

[a] Mean values from various sources.

For most drugs that are excreted in saliva it appears that this process follows the principles of passive diffusion. Accordingly, the partition of drug between plasma and saliva depends on the degree of ionization, since only the non-ionized form permeates biological membranes. The partition of the drug in the two fluids, saliva and blood, is described by equation (8.7), which is based on the Henderson–Hasselbalch equation:

$$\frac{S}{P} = \frac{1+10^{\pm(pH_s - pK_a)}}{1+10^{\pm(pH_p - pK_a)}}\left(\frac{f_{fp}}{f_{fs}}\right) \tag{8.7}$$

where pH_s and pH_p represent the pH in the saliva and the blood, respectively. The 'plus or minus' signs are for drugs with acidic or basic properties, respectively. The f_{fp} and f_{fs} are the drug's free fractions in plasma and saliva, respectively, but as the drug binding in the saliva is very low (because of its low protein content), it is usually assumed that $f_{fs} = 1$. From equation (8.7) it is apparent that the measured drug concentration in saliva is proportional to the free concentration of the drug in plasma. This is of particular importance, especially when the normal binding of the drugs in plasma changes (hypoalbuminaemia, uraemia, etc.), and also in the context of the general significance of the free drug concentration from the pharmacological point of view. However, research in this field, with simultaneous measurement of drug in plasma and saliva, has shown that prediction of f_{fp} (i.e. indirect calculation of the percentage of bound drug in plasma) is possible only for a small number of drugs. Two examples are phenytoin and carbamazepine, though the variability in the data is too great to allow application in clinical practice. Also, for drugs with pK_a values similar to the pH of the plasma, the equilibrium of the drug's partition is strongly disturbed by any variation in the saliva pH.

In a few cases, excretion in saliva follows the principles of active transport. A classic example of active transport to the saliva is that of lithium, for which concentrations in the saliva are two- or three-fold greater than the corresponding plasma concentrations, as shown in Table 8.5.

In summary, the following general comments can be applied to the possibility of replacing plasma with saliva sampling. In pharmacokinetic studies involving single oral administration and simultaneous samplings of blood and saliva at appropriate time intervals, it has been found that the saliva and plasma profiles differ considerably during the absorption phase. These results are due to the rapid change of plasma drug concentrations in the absorption phase, which in turn causes instability in the S:P ratio. Thus, measurements in saliva are not appropriate for predicting the concentrations in plasma in oral pharmacokinetic or bioavailability studies, for the large majority of drugs. The only exceptions to this rule are lithium and phenytoin, for which single oral studies have shown that the saliva levels directly mirror the profile of the change of concentration in plasma. However, in prolonged therapies, where a periodic measurement of the drug in plasma is often applied for therapeutic monitoring purposes, measurements in the saliva for certain drugs (such as antiepileptics) may be a reasonable approach. The validity of the saliva method presumes that multiple administration of the drug results in the establishment of steady-state conditions, which are associated with relatively small fluctuations of the concentrations of the drugs in plasma. As yet, however, saliva drug measurements have not been applied in routine clinical practice.

FURTHER READING

Atkinson HC and Begg EJ. Prediction of Drug Distribution into Human Milk from Physicochemical characteristics. *Clin. Pharmacokinet.* **18**: 151–167 (1990).

Benet LZ, Massoud N and Gambertoglio JG (eds). *Pharmacokinetic Basis of Drug Treatment*, Raven Press, New York (1984).

Crooks J, O'Malley K and Stevenson IH. Pharmacokinetics in the Elderly. *Clin. Pharmacokinet.* **1**: 280–296 (1976).

Fenstenmacher JD, Blasgerg RG and Patlak CS. Methods for Quantifying the Transport of Drugs Across the Blood Brain Systems. *Pharmacol. Ther.* **14**: 217–248 (1991).

Jusko WJ and Milsap RL. Pharmacokinetic Principles of Drug Distribution in Saliva. *Ann. N.Y. Acad. Sci.* **694**: 36–47 (1993).

Meisenberg G and Simmons W. Peptides and the Blood Brain Barrier. *Life Sci.* **32**: 2611–2623 (1983).

Mirkin BL and Singh S. Placental Transfer of Pharmacologically Active Molecules. In: *Perinatal Pharmacology and Therapeutics*, pp. 1–69, Academic Press, New York (1976).

Upton RN. Regional Pharmacokinetics. Physiological and Physicochemical Basis. *Biopharm. Drug Dispos.* **11**: 647–662 (1990).

Van Bree JBMM, Baljet AV, Van Geyt A, de Boer AG , Danhof M and Breimer DD. The Unit Impulse Response Procedure for the Pharmacokinetic Evaluation of Drug Entry into the Central Nervous System. *J. Pharmacokinet. Biopharm.* **17**: 441–462 (1989).

Van Bree JBMM, de Boer AG, Danhof M and Breimer DD. Drug Transport Across the Blood Brain Barrier. *Pharm. Weekbl.* **14**: 305–310, 338–348 (1992).

9

Renal and hepatic clearance

Objectives

Upon completing this chapter, the reader will be familiar with:

- *The concepts of extraction coefficient, total body clearance, renal clearance, and hepatic clearance*
- *The physiological and anatomical features of the kidneys which are related to the renal excretion of drugs*
- *The fundamental biotransformation reactions and the principles of drug biotransformation kinetics*
- *The concepts of biliary excretion, enterohepatic circulation, and first-pass effect*

9.1 THE CONCEPT OF CLEARANCE

Clearance is a concept that is especially useful for the quantitative expression of the elimination processes of drugs from the body. It is based on the ability of an organ (e.g. kidneys, liver) to remove drug from the blood which is passing through. Simple mass balance relationship between the rate at which a drug enters the organ and the rate at which it leaves, shown in Fig. 9.1, allow us to quantify clearance.

If Q represents the flow rate (units: [volume]/[time]) of the fluid under consideration (usually blood or plasma) and E is the *extraction coefficient or extraction ratio*, i.e. the

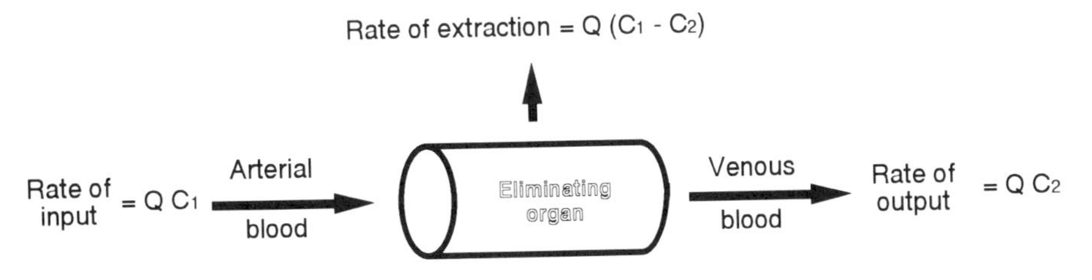

Fig. 9.1. Schematic representation of an eliminating organ (e.g. liver, kidney) with respect to the rates of drug entry, extraction and exit. (Redrawn from *Pharmacology and Therapeutics* **12**: 109–131 (1981).)

fraction of the total drug content in the entering fluid which is extracted (cleared) from the organ as the fluid passes through, then the clearance of the organ, CL_{org}, can be defined as

$$CL_{org} = QE \tag{9.1}$$

The units of clearance are identical to those for the flow rate since the extraction coefficient, E, represents a concentration ratio

$$E = \frac{QC_1 - QC_2}{QC_1} = \frac{C_1 - C_2}{C_1} \tag{9.2}$$

where C_1 is the concentration of drug in the fluid supplying the organ (arterial concentration), and C_2 is the concentration of drug in the fluid leaving the organ (venous concentration).

In conjunction with equations (9.1) and (9.2), the mass balance relationship of Fig. 9.1 allows for the expression of the *extracting ability* of the eliminating organ in two different ways, which give a visual representation of the quantities E and CL_{org}. If all terms of the mass balance relationship of Fig. 9.1 are divided by QC_1, the system is normalized according to the rate of drug entry. This is depicted in Fig. 9.2.

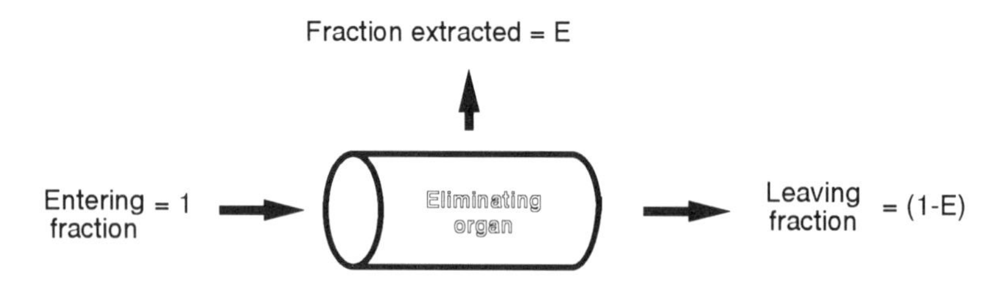

Fig. 9.2. Schematic representation of the extraction coefficient, E, of an eliminating organ.

By dividing all terms of Fig. 9.1 by C_1, the system is normalized according to the arterial drug concentration. This is depicted in Fig. 9.3.

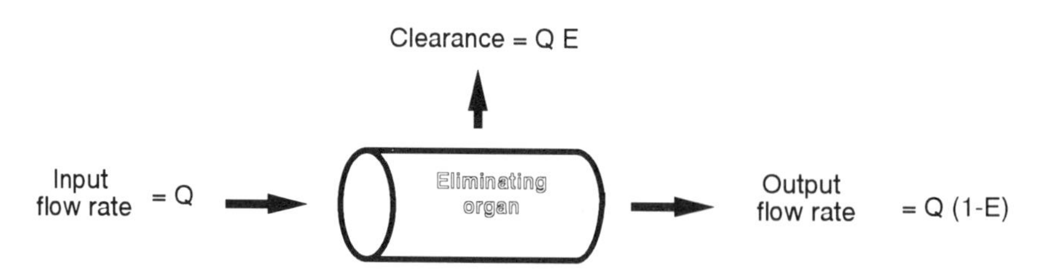

Fig. 9.3. Schematic representation of the clearance from an eliminating organ, $CL_{org} = QE$.

9.1.1 Total body clearance (total clearance)

Combining equations (9.1) and (9.2), one obtains

$$Q(C_1 - C_2) = \mathrm{CL}_{\mathrm{org}} C_1 \tag{9.3}$$

According to Fig. 9.1, the left-hand side of equation (9.3) corresponds to the rate of extraction of the drug from the organ, or, in other words, to the organ's contribution to the elimination rate of the drug from the body. Equation (9.3) may be rewritten in the simplified form

$$(\text{elimination rate})_{\mathrm{org}} = \mathrm{CL}_{\mathrm{org}} \times \text{arterial drug concentration} \tag{9.4}$$

This equation allows the concept of clearance to be generalized since for every eliminating organ of the body a corresponding equation can be written. Furthermore, the term *arterial drug concentration* in equation (9.4) can be specified for every eliminating organ, as the arterial plasma drug concentration. Since the general circulation ensures the rapid movement of drug among the eliminating organs, the concentration of the drug in plasma can be considered to be the same for all eliminating organs at any given time. Consequently, equation (9.4) can be expressed in a generalized form, describing the total elimination rate of the drug from the body:

$$\text{elimination rate} = \mathrm{CL} \times \text{concentration in plasma} \tag{9.5}$$

where CL is the *total (body) clearance* (or, more simply, *clearance*). This definition of clearance as the sum of the clearances of each of the eliminating organs assumes that the various eliminating organs contribute in an additive manner to the total body clearance. Equation (9.5) also reveals that clearance is a proportionality constant, relating the elimination rate of the drug from the body to the corresponding concentration in plasma.

9.1.1.1 Relation of clearance, volume of distribution and elimination rate constant

In most cases, elimination of the drug from the body follows first-order kinetics and the elimination rate is proportional to the quantity of drug in plasma, X_p

$$\text{elimination rate} = -\frac{dX_p}{dt} = k_{1,el} X_p = k_{1,el} C_p V_d \tag{9.6}$$

where $k_{1,el}$ is the first-order rate constant of the elimination, C_p is the plasma drug concentration and V_d is the apparent volume of distribution. Combination of equations (9.5) and (9.6) yields

$$\mathrm{CL} = k_{1,el} V_d \tag{9.7}$$

Equation (9.7) provides a descriptive definition of clearance, according to which 'clearance expresses the fraction of the volume of distribution which is cleared per unit of time'. The rates at which the drug elimination processes (which usually comprise excretion in urine and biotransformation in the liver) occur are mirrored in the magnitude of $k_{1,el}$, which in turn determines to a large degree the magnitude of clearance. Conceptually, total clearance is usually divided into two parts:

(1) renal clearance; and
(2) non-renal clearance, of which biotransformation in the liver is usually the largest component, and which is often characterized as hepatic clearance.

9.2 RENAL CLEARANCE

9.2.1 Structure of the urinary system

The urinary system (Fig. 9.4) consists of a pair of secreting organs, the kidneys, and a number of draining ducts into which the urine is collected and finally eliminated from the body via the urethra. The kidneys are situated on each side of the vertebral column outside the peritoneal cavity in the posterior abdominal wall. The kidneys are approximately 11 cm long, 5 cm wide and 3 cm thick. Two of their major functions are the excretion of the metabolic waste products and the excretion of foreign chemicals (xenobiotics).† Apart from the kidneys, the basic component parts of the urinary system are the renal pelvises, the ureters, the bladder and the urethra (Fig. 9.4).

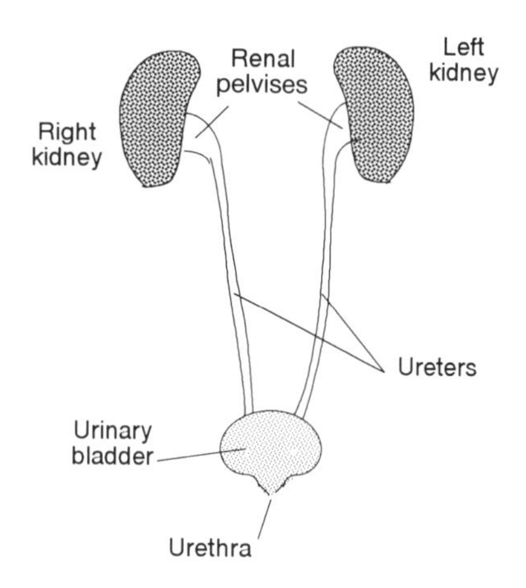

Fig. 9.4. The urinary system. The urine, formed in the kidneys, is collected in the renal pelvis, flows through the ureter into the bladder and is excreted through the urethra.

A cross-section of the kidney shows that the kidney consists of two regions. The outer portion, the *cortex*, has a granular composition, while the inner portion, which does not have a granular appearance, is called the *medulla*. The basic functional unit of the kidney is the *nephron* (Fig. 9.5). The number of nephrons in each human kidney ranges between 1.2 and 1.3 million. Each nephron contains two distinct sections: the glomerulus and the tubule.

9.2.1.1 The glomerulus

Blood reaches the kidneys through the renal artery, which branches extensively to form the afferent arterioles. Each afferent arteriole is divided into multiple capillaries which form a tuft of vessels in the glomerulus. The glomerulus is the filtering component of the nephron. It is composed of a complex system of interconnected capillaries, called

† From the Greek words ξένοσ (foreign), βίοσ (life).

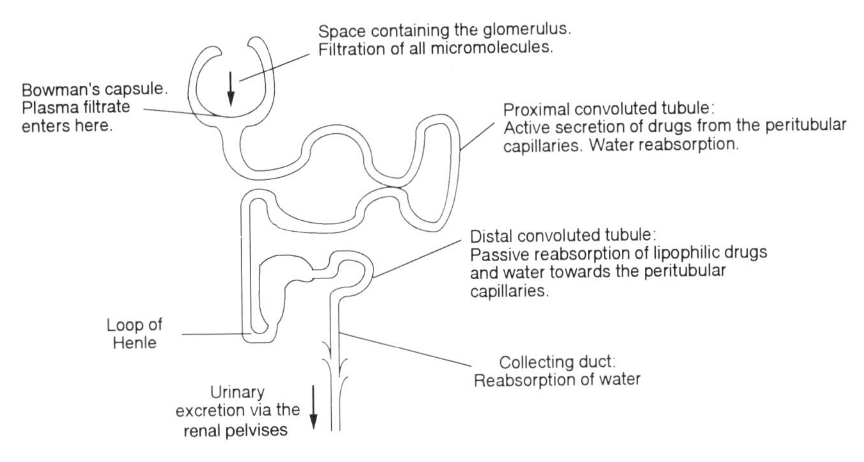

Fig. 9.5. Simplified illustration of the functional components of the nephron. The relative sizes of the components are not to scale.

glomerular capillaries, and a space which looks like a balloon-shaped capsule, called Bowman's capsule. The portion of the blood which undergoes ultrafiltration‡ in the glomerular capillaries flows into the space of Bowman's capsule. About 18% of the plasma entering the glomerulus undergoes ultrafiltration, while the remaining blood leaves the glomerulus through the efferent arterioles, which are formed by recombination of glomerular capillaries. The efferent arterioles subdivide into a second set of capillaries, called peritubular capillaries. These supply the tubules before they rejoin again to form venous channels. The bulk exchange of water and solutes between the tubular lumen and the capillaries is accomplished through the network of the peritubular capillaries.

The glomerular membranes where ultrafiltration takes place are shown in Fig. 9.6. They consist of three layers, with the following spatial arrangement proceeding from the lumen of the capillary to the urinary Bowman's space:

(a) the capillary endothelium with the endothelial cells perforated by many large fenestrae;

(b) a basement membrane (basal lamina) which is composed of a relatively homogeneous network of glycoproteins and mucopolysaccharides; and

(c) a single continuous layer of capsular epithelial cells embedded in the basement membrane, with slit-like pores between them. These epithelial cells are called *podocytes*, and have an octopus-like structure. The pores between the podocytes comprise, in essence, the path through which the ultrafiltrate enters the Bowman's capsule following its permeation through the endothelial cells and the basal lamina. Additional filtration barriers which should also be considered are the thin diaphragms which bridge the slits between the podocytes near the basement membrane and the relatively thick layer of glucosialoproteins on the surfaces of podocytes.

‡ The term *ultrafiltration* is preferred over the term *filtration* in order to emphasize that in this particular process plasma proteins are not filtered.

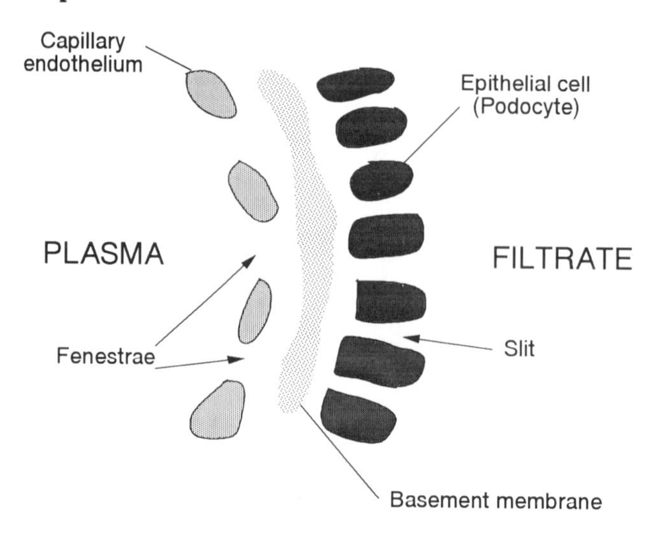

Fig. 9.6. Anatomy of the glomerular capillary wall.

Overall, this anatomical structure results in the permeability of glomerular capillaries being about 50 times higher than the capillaries found in other tissues.

9.2.1.2 The tubule

The initial portion of the tubule is connected to the Bowman's capsule just opposite to the glomerulus. The filtered fluid flows into the tubule and passes through the successive tubular segments. A single layer of epithelial cells, linked together by tight junctions, is found along the entire length of the tubule. However, the structure of the epithelial cells varies widely along the tubule, and for this reason it is subdivided into several segments (Fig. 9.5). The segment nearest to the cavity of the Bowman's capsule is known, because of its shape, as the *proximal convoluted tubule*. The following segment is called *Henle's loop* and consists successively of a thin descending limb, a thin ascending limb and a thick ascending limb. The last segment of the tubule, like the proximal convoluted tubule, has a coiled structure and is called the *distal convoluted tubule*. Following the distal convoluted tubule is the *initial collecting tubule*. This is actually the first portion of the so-called 'collecting duct'. It is worth mentioning that, despite their large number (approximately 10^6), there are no interconnections among the individual tubules. The distal ends of the initial collecting tubules combine to form collecting ducts. These, in turn, are joined together at various levels, culminating in the formation of the renal calyx of the renal pelvis. In short, the fluid which is filtered in the glomerulus follows the route: Bowman's capsule → proximal convoluted tubule → Henle's loop → distal convoluted tubule → collecting duct → renal pelvis → ureter → bladder → urethra. The composition and volume of the original glomerular filtrate change continuously until its entry into the calyx of the renal pelvis. Thereafter, the composition of the urine remains unaltered.

As far as the anatomical arrangement of the various sections of the kidney is concerned, it is interesting to note that the glomerulus and Bowman's capsule, the proximal convoluted tubule and the distal convoluted tubule are located in the periphery of the kidney (the cortex), while the loop of Henle and the renal calyces are situated in the inner part of the kidney (the medulla).

9.2.2 The three processes comprising renal excretion

Renal excretion is a balance of three distinct processes (Figs 9.5 and 9.7): glomerular filtration, tubular secretion and tubular reabsorption.

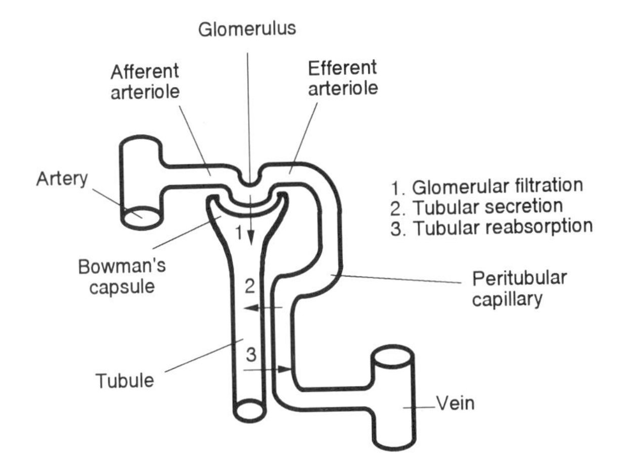

Fig. 9.7. Simplified representation of the regions where the three processes comprising renal excretion take place.

The formation of urine begins with ultrafiltration of the plasma in the glomerulus. The composition of the glomerular filtrate entering Bowman's capsule changes continuously during its transport through the nephron until it reaches the composition of the final urine. Tubular secretion and tubular reabsorption, which take place at various sites along the renal tubules, are the processes which result in the change in composition from that of the ultrafiltrate to that of the urine.

9.2.2.1 Glomerular filtration

Apart from the plasma proteins, the composition of the filtrate is similar to that of plasma. The glomerulus retains macromolecules larger than 8 nm in diameter, while compounds with diameters less than 4 nm penetrate the glomerulus freely. Drugs which are bound to plasma proteins do not permeate the glomerulus; only the free form of the drug is found in the filtrate. As a result, the concentration of drug in the filtrate is almost equal to the concentration of free drug in the plasma. Although the main limiting factor to filtration is molecular size, charge is also a factor since the negative charge of glycosialoproteines in the walls of the capillaries repels macromolecules bearing a net negative charge. Charge repulsion is particularly important in the size range which is borderline for filtration, i.e. 4–8 nm. Thus, albumin with an approximate size of 7 nm and a −17 net negative charge at physiological pH exhibits almost zero permeability of the glomerular capillaries. As a result, the glomerular concentration of albumin is 2000 times less than its concentration in plasma.

Glomerular filtration is driven by the total pressure in the glomerular capillaries which is a balance between the hydrostatic pressure in the glomerular capillaries (~47 mmHg), and the two opposing pressures: (1) the hydrostatic pressure in Bowman's capsule (~10 mmHG); and (2) the difference between the osmotic pressures of the plasma in the glomerular capillaries and the osmotic pressure of the filtrate in the tubule (a net difference of ~25 mmHg), which arises because proteins are present in the blood but not in the filtrate. The net filtration pressure is therefore ~12 mmHg. The pressure gradient decreases along the glomerular capillaries from 12 to 0 mmHg because of a gradual increase in the opposing osmotic pressure. This means that filtration does not take place in the region of the efferent arteriole (nor at more distal locations such as the peritubular capillaries). The combination of the modest pressure gradient and the large number of nephrons results in a large glomerular filtration rate (GFR) of 7.5 l/h (i.e. 125 ml/min or 180 l/d). This value implies that the total plasma volume, ~ 3 litres, is filtered 60 times per day!

The rate at which a drug is eliminated, dX_{ur}/dt, is proportional to the GFR value and the free concentration of the drug in plasma, C_f, i.e.

$$\text{filtration rate} = \frac{dX_{ur}}{dt} = (\text{GFR})\, C_f \tag{9.8}$$

This equation shows the particular importance of the value of GFR for the renal excretion of drugs. In patients with impaired kidney function the value of GFR decreases. Methods for accurately estimating the GFR have been developed, and these are used to adjust the dosage of patients with impaired renal function so that drug toxicity is avoided.

9.2.2.2 Tubular secretion

Tubular secretion (Fig. 9.7) may also contribute to the transport of a compound from the plasma to the urine. This process takes place by an initial transfer of the substance from the peritubular capillaries to the interstitial fluids. The substance then diffuses through the cells of the walls of the tubules, arriving in the lumen of the tubule. Tubular secretion is essentially a process of transport through membranes, which has been discussed in the context of general transport processes of drugs in the human body (chapter 2), and the permeation of the gastrointestinal epithelial cells (section 6.1.2).

Tubular secretion can involve passive transport and/or carrier-mediated transport. However, special emphasis should be focused on the active transport systems at the level of the proximal convoluted tubule. Two separate systems of active tubular secretion of drugs and other organic molecules operate in this region. Neither system is highly specific. One of them mediates the transport of anions and therefore is very important for acidic drugs, while the other system mediates the transport of cations and therefore is important for basic drugs and quaternary ammonium salts. The low specificity of the carrier for acids is demonstrated in the classical example of the competition for active tubular secretion between benzylpenicillin and probenecid, which have little structural similarity apart from both being acids. It is also of interest that metabolites of drugs formed by conjugation with glucuronic acid (glucuronides) and the sulfate esters (sulfates) are actively secreted by the system mediating the transport of anions.

9.2.2.3 Tubular reabsorption

Since all the micromolecular plasma constituents are filtered freely by the glomerulus, the tubular reabsorption processes are vital to the conservation of water and important electrolytes, as shown in Fig. 9.7. Thus, under normal conditions the reabsorption of water is 99%, glucose 100%, and Na^+ 99.5%. For most physiological compounds, the reabsorption process is carrier mediated and is characterized by a *transport maximum*, T_{max}, (equations (2.39) and (2.40)). The value of the T_{max} corresponds to the maximal rate at which the carrier can transport a solute. For example, the value of T_{max} for glucose is about 375 mg/min, so under normal conditions its reabsorption transporter is not saturated and all filtered glucose is completely reabsorbed. In patients with diabetes mellitus, high plasma levels result in very large amounts of glucose being filtered in the glomerulus, resulting in saturation of the active reabsorption process and the appearance of glucose in the urine.

The reabsorption of drugs follows the principles of passive diffusion. This means that lipophilic drugs are reabsorbed much more readily than the hydrophilic ones. Due to the fact that 80–90% of the total reabsorption of water takes place in the region of the proximal convoluted tubule, the concentration gradient of the drug between the tubules and the peritubular tubules is continuously increasing as it moves through the nephron. Hence, if the lipophilicity and the ionization characteristics of the drug favour reabsorption, the whole load of filtered drug can be reabsorbed.

Although tubular secretion and tubular reabsorption are considered separately in the foregoing discussion, bidirectional transport of the solutes is observed in the majority of cases. This means that it is not uncommon for a drug to be actively secreted in the region of the proximal convoluted tubule, and reabsorbed in the distal convoluted tubule. In all cases, the 'net' result of renal excretion will depend on the relative magnitude of these two processes.

The importance of pH in drug reabsorption

Glomerular filtration is the result of the pressure gradient in the glomerulus and therefore is not dependent on the pH of the plasma or urine. Neither is tubular secretion dependent on the variation in urine pH, regardless of whether it is passive or carrier mediated. However, since the major tubular reabsorptive mechanism of drugs is simple passive diffusion, this process can be greatly influenced by the fluctuations in the urinary pH.

It is known that the pH of the urine varies not only during the day, but it is also dependent on diet and certain drugs. The mean value of the urine pH is 6.3; however, it may rise to 8 or fall to 4.5 after administration of sodium bicarbonate† and ammonium chloride,† respectively. These pH fluctuations cause changes in the ionization of drugs, which in turn influences their reabsorption. The degree of ionization can be calculated, using the Henderson–Hasselbach equations (2.35) and (2.36) as shown in section 6.1.2 for oral drug absorption. Use of these equations assumes that only the non-ionized fraction of drug can penetrate the membranes between the lumen of the tubule and the peritubular capillaries. Analysis of the partitioning behaviour of drugs between urine with a pH varying between 4.5 and 8 and plasma with pH 7.4 separated by a membrane results in the following general conclusions for the acidic and basic drugs.

(a) *Drugs with acidic properties*: Strong acids with $pK_a \leqslant 3$ are always ionized to an extent close to 100%, irrespective of the urine pH (4.5–8) and therefore they cannot move across the luminal membrane. On the other hand, very weak acids with $pK_a \geqslant 9$ exist as non-ionized species irrespective of the urine pH and their reabsorption is likewise not dependent on the urine pH. The extent of their reabsorption will be determined from the lipophilic properties of the non-ionized form. It is the weak acids with an intermediate pK_a, i.e. $3 < pK_a < 9$, which are most sensitive to variations in urine pH variations. For these acids, elevation of urinary pH causes greater ionization, resulting in lower reabsorption and therefore greater excretion.

(b) *Drugs with basic properties*: Strong bases with $pK_a \geqslant 10$ are always ionized, irrespective of the urine pH, and therefore are not reabsorbed. Basic drugs with $pK_a < 5$ are present in the urine as the non-ionized species at usual values of urine pH. Their reabsorption is determined mostly from the lipophilicity of the non-ionized form, though in strongly acidic urine (pH 4.5) their reabsorption can be decreased. The basic drugs which are most sensitive to the pH of the urine are those with $5 < pK_a < 10$. For these bases elevation of the urinary pH causes lower ionization, resulting in higher reabsorption and consequently less efficient excretion.

Example 9.1: What is the ratio of the total concentration of amphetamine, a weak base with $pK_a = 9.9$, in region I (tubule) to the concentration in region II (plasma) in equilibrium, assuming that the pH of the urine is (a) 4.5, and (b) 7.0? Recall that the pH of the plasma is 7.4.

Answer: Application of the Henderson–Hasselbach equation for a weak base (section 2.3.1.2) leads to the following equation for the ratio of the concentrations in the urine, C_{ur}, and in the plasma, C_p:

$$\frac{C_{ur}}{C_p} = \frac{1+10^{-(pH_{ur}-pK_a)}}{1+10^{-(pH_p-pK_a)}}$$

For a urinary pH of 4.5, this equation yields

† These compounds are used either in the study of the effect of pH on the excretion of drugs or for the enhancement of the elimination of drugs from the body for toxicological reasons.

$$\frac{1+10^{9.9-4.5}}{1+10^{9.9-7.4}} = 792 \quad \text{for} \quad \text{pH } 4.5$$

and

$$\frac{1+10^{9.9-7.0}}{1+10^{9.9-7.4}} = 2.5 \quad \text{for} \quad \text{pH } 7.0$$

The calculations show that ionization facilitates the excretion of amphetamine when the pH of the urine is acidic. It is worth mentioning that the calculations are based on the assumption of equilibrium between the ionized and the non-ionized form in both compartments. However, drug concentrations in the urine and in blood are unlikely to reach equilibrium because of kinetic considerations.

9.2.3 Use of glomerular filtration rate to investigate the excretion processes of drugs

The calculation of the glomerular filtration rate (GFR) is particularly useful in pathological conditions. Theoretically, an estimate of GFR can be obtained from excretion data for a substance which possesses the following characteristics:

(a) freely filtered in the glomerulus;
(b) not secreted;
(c) not reabsorbed; and
(d) not synthesized or biotransformed in the tubules.

Moreover, it must be possible to maintain a constant concentration of the substance in the plasma. Of the various substances which have been used for the calculation of GFR, creatinine, even though it does not meet all the criteria,† has been extensively used. Plasma concentrations of creatinine remain constant during the day, as it is formed in the muscles from creatine. It thus has the advantage of not requiring exogenous administration to establish a constant plasma concentration. Measurement of GFR using creatinine requires

(a) collection of urine for a fixed period of time, usually 12 h;
(b) measurement of the total volume, V_{ur}, of the collected urine and of the concentration of creatinine, $C_{ur,cr}$, in the pooled urine; and
(c) determination of the concentration of creatinine in the plasma, $C_{p,cr}$.

The equation for the calculation of GFR is based on the following relationship:

$$\text{mass of filtered creatinine} = \text{mass of excreted creatinine} = C_{ur,cr}V_{ur} \tag{9.9}$$

Dividing equation (9.9) by the time period of the collection of urine, Δt, yields

$$\frac{\text{mass of filtrated creatinine}}{\Delta t} = \frac{C_{ur,cr}V_{ur}}{\Delta t} \tag{9.10}$$

† Creatinine is secreted to a small degree in the tubules; thus, the calculated GFR overestimates the real magnitude of GFR. However, the overestimation is not clinically significant.

According to equation (9.8), the left-hand part of this equation is equal to the product ($GFR \times C_{p,cr}$), therefore

$$GFR = \frac{(C_{ur,cr} V_{ur})/\Delta t}{C_{p,cr}} \tag{9.11}$$

Example 9.2: What is the GFR in a patient with a plasma creatinine concentration 10.0 μg/ml, if a urine volume of 0.60 litres was collected over 6 h, and in which the creatinine concentration was 0.75 mg/ml?

Answer: Substituting the values in equation (9.11):

$$GFR = \frac{(0.75 \times 0.60)/6}{10} \frac{(\text{mg/ml})\ (\text{l/h})}{(\mu\text{g/ml})}$$

$$= \frac{(750 \times 0.60)/6}{10} \frac{1}{\text{h}} = 7.5\ \text{l/h} = 180\ \text{l/d}$$

The GFR can be used to help elucidate the processes involved in the excretion of drugs. The three basic processes that contribute to the net rate at which a drug is excreted by the kidneys can be represented as an algebraic sum:

$$\begin{matrix}\text{rate of} \\ \text{excretion}\end{matrix} = \begin{matrix}\text{rate of} \\ \text{filtration}\end{matrix} + \begin{matrix}\text{rate of} \\ \text{secretion}\end{matrix} - \begin{matrix}\text{rate of} \\ \text{reabsorption}\end{matrix} \tag{9.12}$$

While filtration always takes place, the contribution of the other two processes to the overall excretion is highly dependent on the physicochemical properties of the drug. In order to ascertain the contributions of secretion and reabsorption, urine is collected for a certain period of time and its volume and the concentration of drug in it are determined. The maintenance of a constant plasma concentration of the drug, C_p, is also required; this is usually accomplished by continuous intravenous infusion of the drug. Denoting the total volume of urine collected, V_{ur}, over a time period Δt and the drug concentration in it, C_{ur},

$$\text{amount of excreted drug} = C_{ur} V_{ur} \tag{9.13}$$

Applying equations (9.10) and (9.11) for the drug under consideration we obtain

$$\text{amount of filtered drug} = \text{GFR}\ C_p \Delta t \tag{9.14}$$

Comparing the values of equations (9.13) and (9.14) (taking care to express both relationships in identical mass units, e.g. mg) it is easily derived that if

$$C_{ur} V_{ur} < \text{GFR} C_p \Delta t$$

then a portion of the drug has been reabsorbed in the tubules. If

$$U_{ur} V_{ur} > \text{GFR} C_p \Delta t$$

then the drug has been secreted, and if

$$U_{ur} V_{ur} = \text{GFR} C_p \Delta t$$

then renal excretion is either exclusively due to glomerular filtration, or the rates of tubular reabsorption and secretion are equal. The above analysis thus provides a clear indication of the relative contributions of the three processes.

Example 9.3: The renal clearance of a penicillin in healthy volunteers is 300 ml/min. What conclusion can be derived about the processes of excretion?

Answer: The magnitude 300 ml/min is larger than the normal value of GFR expressed in the same units, i.e.

$$\mathrm{GFR} = 180\ \mathrm{l/d} = 125\ \mathrm{ml/min}$$

Therefore, this penicillin is subject to tubular secretion.

Example 9.4: A drug was administered to a healthy volunteer by intravenous infusion at a constant rate, and a steady-state plasma concentration of 11.0 μg/ml was achieved. While the concentration remained constant, urine of a total volume of 0.75 litres was collected, and the concentration of the drug in it was found to be 0.500 mg/ml. What is your conclusion about the processes of excretion?

Answer: According to equation (9.13) the amount of drug excreted is $C_{ur}V_{ur} = 0.500 \times 750\ (\mathrm{mg/ml})\mathrm{ml} = 375\ \mathrm{mg}$. According to equation (9.14) the mass of the drug filtered is

$$\mathrm{GFR}\ C_p \Delta t = 60(\mathrm{l}/8\ \mathrm{h}) \times 11.0\ (\mathrm{mg/ml}) \times 8\ \mathrm{h} = 660\ \mathrm{mg}$$

Since the mass of the drug excreted is smaller than the mass filtered, the drug was reabsorbed.

Example 9.5: Inulin is a compound which meets all the criteria for a compound to be used for the estimation of GFR. It is usually infused at a constant rate to obtain a steady-state plasma concentration over the time period in which urine is collected. Is it possible to ascertain whether a drug is secreted or reabsorbed by comparing the clearance of the drug, CL_D, to the clearance of inulin, CL_{IN} in the same individual?

Answer: The clearance of inulin is identical to the magnitude of the GFR. Consequently, if $CL_D = CL_{IN}$, either the drug is excreted only by glomerular filtration, or the processes of secretion and reabsorption are equivalent. If $CL_D > CL_{IN}$ the drug is secreted, while if $CL_D < CL_{IN}$ the drug is reabsorbed.

Example 9.6: Based on the following data† regarding glucose excretion rate in the urine of a healthy volunteer in various plasma concentration values

Excretion rate (mg/min):	5.00	66.0	151	256	400	520	631
Plasma concentration (mg/dl):	200	301	398	503	605	708	799

derive a rough estimate for the Michaelis–Menten constant of the reabsorption of glucose from the renal tubules.

† These data were taken from *Clinical Pharmacokinetics*, Rowland M and Tozer T (eds), Lea & Febiger p. 399 (1989), with permission.

Answer: Based on the glucose plasma concentration and the GFR value for the healthy volunteer, i.e. 125 ml/min, the drug filtration rates for the various concentrations can be calculated from equation (9.8). For example, when the glucose plasma concentration is 200 mg/dl, the filtration rate is

$$125\ (\text{ml/min}) \times 200\ (\text{mg}/100\ \text{ml}) = 250\ \text{mg/min}$$

In an analogous manner, the following filtration rates can be obtained for each of the resting glucose plasma concentrations:

Filtration rate (mg/min): 376 498 629 756 885 999

By subtracting the excretion rate from the corresponding filtration rate, the reabsorption rate is calculated:

Reabsorption rate (mg/min): 245 310 347 373 356 365 368

Due to the fact that glucose is easily filtered in the Bowman's capsule, its concentration in the filtrate,† C_{fil}, equals its plasma concentration. The graph in Fig. 9.8 shows the change in glucose reabsorption rate, $(\mathrm{d}C/\mathrm{d}t)_{\text{reabs}}$, as a function of the glucose concentration in the filtrate. The shape of the curve in Fig. 9.8 is typical of the Michaelis–Menten kinetics (see section 2.3.2), which, in this case, is given by the equation

$$(\mathrm{d}C/\mathrm{d}t)_{\text{reabs}} = \frac{T_{\max}}{K_{\text{M}} + C_{\text{fil}}} C_{\text{fil}}$$

where $T_{\max}$, the maximum tubular reabsorption rate (transportation maximum) is 370 mg/min, as read from the plateau of the graph in Fig. 9.8. When 50% of the reabsorption is completed, $(\mathrm{d}C/\mathrm{d}t)_{\text{reabs}} = T_{\max}/2$, and application of the above equation under these conditions gives

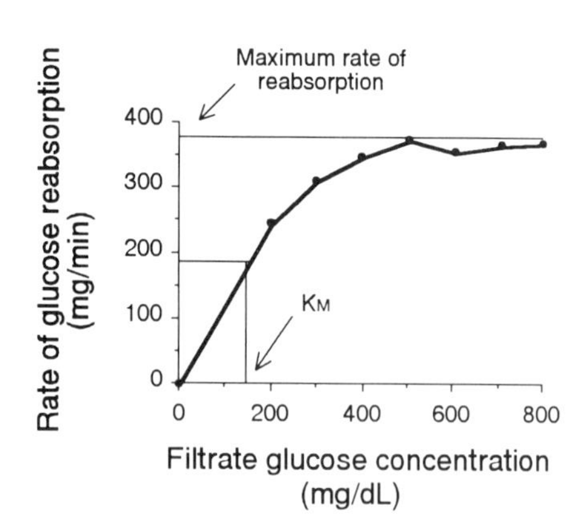

Fig. 9.8. Plot of the glucose reabsorption rate as a function of glucose concentration in the filtrate for the data of Example 9.8.

† The term 'filtrate concentration' is preferred to the term 'concentration in the renal tubules'. The concentration in the tubules is not constant owing to the continuous reabsorption of water and glucose along the tubule.

$$K_M = C_{fil}$$

This means that the value of the Michaelis–Menten constant corresponds to the glucose concentration in the filtrate at which the reabsorption rate is equal to half of the maximum rate of reabsorption. Based on Fig. 9.8, the K_M value is ~170 mg/dl.

9.3 HEPATIC CLEARANCE

As drug molecules pass through the liver (either right after the absorption of drug from the gastrointestinal tract or from the general blood circulation), they can be taken up by the hepatic cells. Drug molecules which enter the hepatocytes meet one of the following three fates:

— returned intact in blood;
— excreted in the bile; and/or
— biotransformed, after which the metabolites enter the blood and/or are excreted in the bile.

9.3.1 Brief description of hepatic tissue structure

The tissues associated with hepatic clearance consist of the liver, the bile ducts and the gall bladder. The liver is the largest composite gland of the body and weighs about 15–20 g/kg body weight. Externally, it is surrounded almost entirely by peritoneum. The liver consists mainly of blood vessels, parenchymal and endothelial cells and bile canaliculi, as shown in Fig. 9.9. The blood supply to the liver is delivered via the portal vein and the hepatic artery.

The total hepatic blood flow in liver is 1.2–1.5 l/min; about three-quarters of the total blood supply of the liver comes from the portal vein, while the remainder is delivered by the hepatic artery. Drugs absorbed from the stomach and the upper part of the intestine are delivered to the liver via the portal vein. The hepatic artery is mainly responsible for the oxygenation of hepatic cells. Exchange of substances and metabolites occurs in special capillaries, called *sinusoids*. The sinusoids, vessels which are extremely rich in blood, are interspersed among the hepatocytes and since their endothelia have wide openings, plasma and hepatocytes are in close contact. The wall of the sinusoids is more permeable than the capillary membranes of the other tissues of the body. A large number of tissue macrophage cells (Kupffer cells) are attached to the endothelium of sinusoids. Venous blood leaves the sinusoids through the hepatic veins, which drain into the inferior vena cava.

Each hepatocyte is surrounded by several bile canaliculi which contain bile. It is interesting to note that while blood flows centripetally in the sinusoids, the bile flows centrifugally in the bile canaliculi, as shown in Figs 9.9 and 9.10. The bile canaliculi join, through Hering's canal, to form bile ducts which subsequently combine to form the common hepatic duct (see Fig. 9.25). The hepatic duct joins the cystic duct (which drains the gall bladder) to form the common bile duct, which in turn empties into the duodenum at the duodenal papilla.

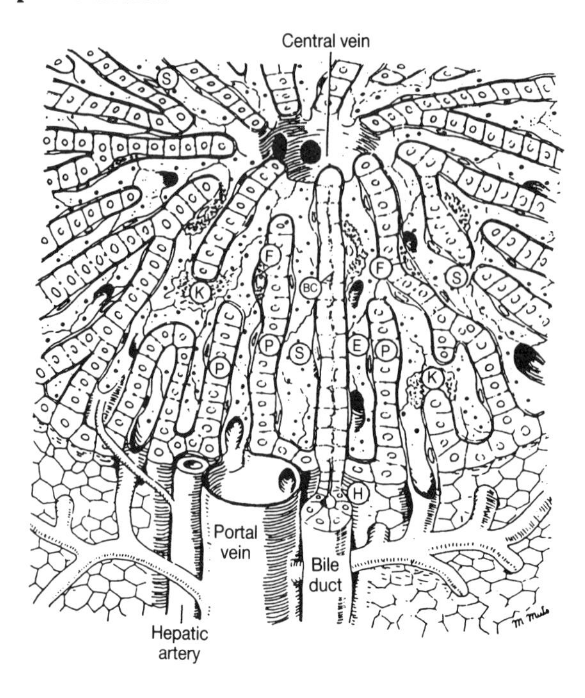

Fig. 9.9. Liver structure. BC, bile canaliculus; H, Hering canal; E, endothelial cell; F, fat-storing cell; P, parenchymal cell; K, Kupffer cell; S, fenestrated sinusoids. (Reproduced from *Journal of Pharmakokinetics and Biopharmaceutics* **18**: 35–71 (1990), with permission.)

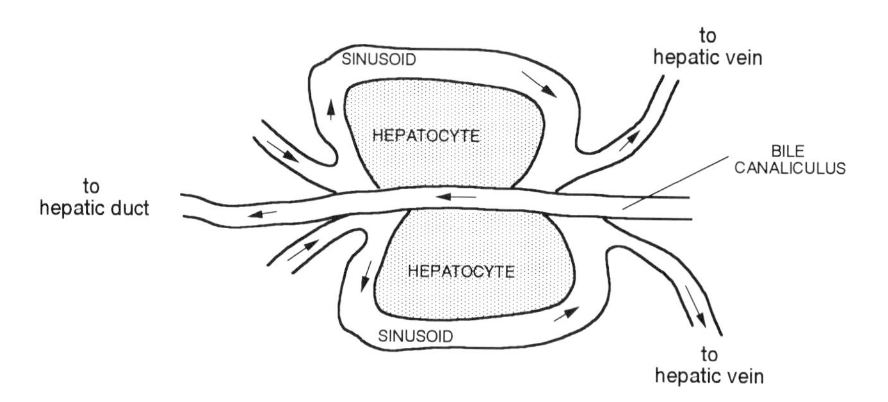

Fig. 9.10. Arrangement of parenchymal cells and bile canaliculi in the liver.

9.3.2 Mechanisms of drug uptake from hepatic cells

According to the classic concept, the rate of hepatic removal of a drug bound to plasma proteins is primarily dependent on the free concentration of drug in plasma. Uptake of drugs which bind to plasma proteins by the hepatocytes presupposes the spontaneous dissociation of drug from its binding protein. These two assumptions appear to be reasonable for compounds that bind weakly and not extensively with plasma proteins. However, there are serious doubts as to the validity of these assumptions for compounds like bilirubin and long-chain fatty acids, which are bound extensively to albumin.

Even compounds which have very low percentages of free drug in plasma can be taken up by hepatocytes, as shown in Fig. 9.11. For water-soluble compounds like glucose, which is not bound to plasma proteins (free fraction = 1), the uptake mechanism consists of simple diffusion of the free drug into the hepatocyte. At the other end of Fig. 9.11 there are, however, non-polar compounds with poor water solubility, e.g. cholesterol esters, which are totally bound to plasma lipoproteins, i.e. their free fraction is essentially zero. For this type of compound, the uptake mechanism of drug from the hepatocytes must involve the bound form of drug. It has been postulated that the lipoproteins, which act as carriers for the cholesterol esters in blood, interact with receptors on the surface of the hepatocyte followed by incorporation of the drug into the hepatocyte. Drugs whose free fractions in blood lie between the two extremes of Fig. 9.11 are probably taken up from the hepatocytes by one or both mechanisms described. Two models for the explanation of uptake which exceeds that expected from free drug concentrations have been proposed.

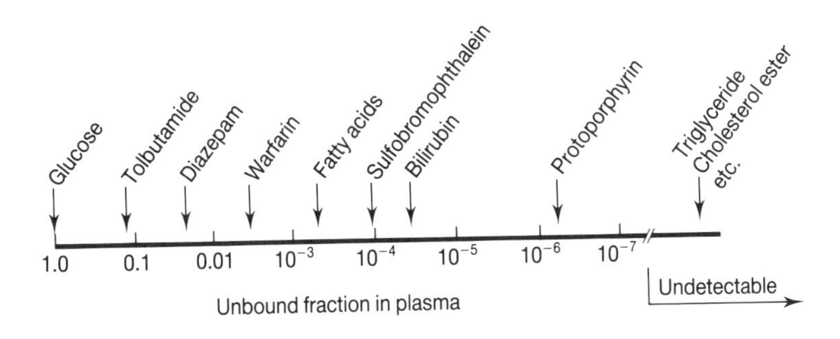

Fig. 9.11. Uptake of drugs by the hepatocytes occurs over a vast range of drug-free fractions in plasma. (Redrawn from *Protein Binding and Drug Transport, Symposia Medica Hoechst*, Tillement JP and Lindenlaub E (eds), Vol. 20, p. 296, Schattauer, Stuttgart (1986).)

The first one is termed the *albumin-receptor model* and is depicted in Fig. 9.12. According to this model the free and bound forms of drug are both taken up by the hepatocyte. The unbound form diffuses into the hepatocyte. In the case of bound drug albumin interacts directly, but temporarily, with a limited number of receptor sites on the membrane of the hepatocyte, facilitating internalization of drug. Compounds with high affinity to plasma proteins are considered to be taken up by the hepatocytes mainly via the bound form, as shown in Fig. 9.12.

The second model is called the *dissociation-limited model.* According to this model, the uptake of the free drug molecule from the hepatocyte is faster than the process of dissociation of the drug from its complex with albumin. In other words, the dissociation rate of the drug becomes the determinant of the uptake rate of the drug from the hepatocytes. This can be diagrammatically represented as follows:

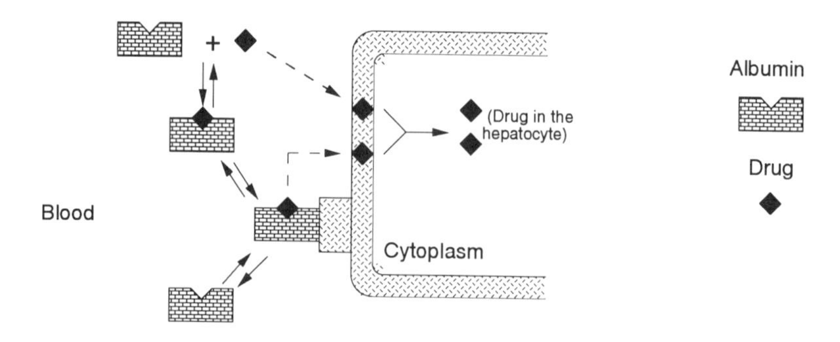

Fig. 9.12. The albumin receptor model of hepatocyte uptake.

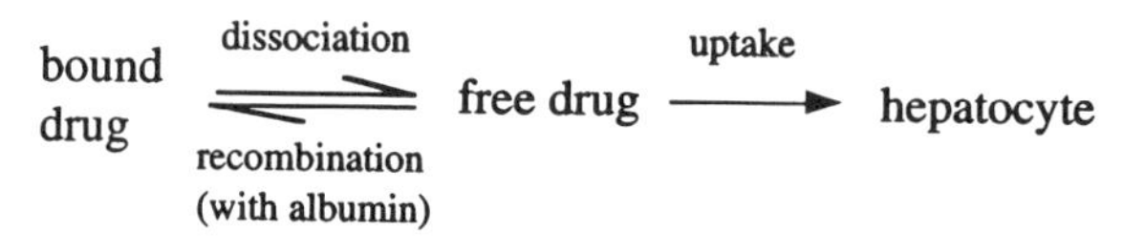

Drug uptake by hepatocytes can be studied with several techniques which resemble those described for drug uptake from gastrointestinal mucosa (section 6.4). Preparations of liver tissue from various animal species can be utilized and in some techniques human material can be also used. The most commonly used techniques are as follows.

Perfusion of the isolated liver

The extent of uptake of the drug under study by the liver is determined from the steady-state concentrations in tissue and free concentrations in the perfusate. The composition of the perfusate and the rate of perfusion are important experimental determinants of the rate of uptake of drug by the liver.

Uptake to liver slices

The use of intact tissue and the possibility of the use of human liver slices are the advantages of the technique. However, caution must be exercised to avoid damage of the liver tissue. The use of buffer rather than plasma as the incubation medium represents another limitation to this technique.

Liver homogenates

During preparation of the homogenate the destruction of the liver tissue is unavoidable. Dilution of the homogenate can also seriously affect the results of the liver uptake capacity. However, the technique is simple and the extent of drug uptake can be measured with the conventional binding techniques, i.e. equilibrium dialysis and ultrafiltration.

Liver subcellular particles

The aim of these studies is to investigate the drug's binding to discrete subcellular particles of the liver cell. This technique requires the isolation of the subcellular component of interest; it has been applied to different components of the cell such as nuclei, membranes and microsomes of various tissues.

More information about the methods of study of drug uptake by the hepatocytes is given in the references at the end of this chapter.

9.3.3 The two processes which comprise hepatic clearance

The hepatic clearance of drugs consists of two processes: biotransformation and biliary excretion. Of these two, biotransformation is usually the main hepatic removal process.

9.3.3.1 Biotransformation

The term biotransformation refers to all biochemical and chemical transformations which occur during the time course of the drug in the body.

Biotransformation occurs mainly in the liver. However, biotransformation can also take place in other tissues or organs, such as the gastrointestinal mucosa, lung, kidney and brain. Such biotransformations are usually characterized as 'extrahepatic'. The product(s) of the biotransformation reaction is(are) called metabolite(s). Drug biotransformation reactions in the liver are enzymatic reactions, and the metabolites formed are, in general, either inactive or less active pharmacologically than the parent compound. This observation was originally explained on the basis of an inherent detoxicating mechanism of the body. Nowadays, the validity of this explanation is not acceptable since there is a plethora of biotransformation reactions which produce active metabolites. For example

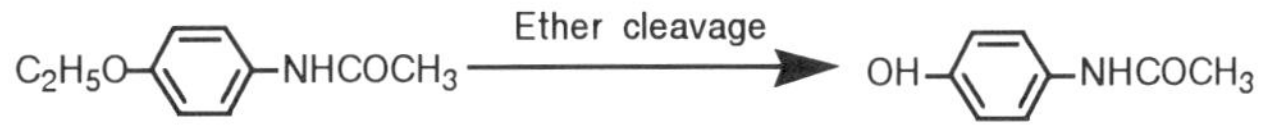

C_2H_5O–C₆H₄–$NHCOCH_3$ —Ether cleavage→ OH–C₆H₄–$NHCOCH_3$

Phenacetin (Active) → Paracetamol (Active)

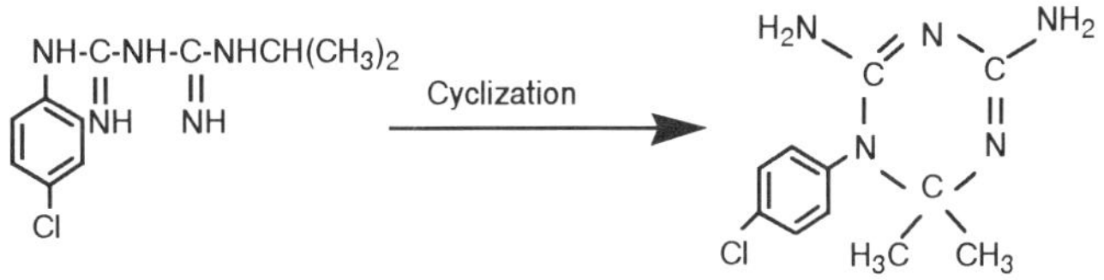

$NH\text{-}C(=NH)\text{-}NH\text{-}C(=NH)\text{-}NHCH(CH_3)_2$ (on chlorophenyl ring, Cl) —Cyclization→ cyclic triazine with H_2N, NH_2, N, C, H_3C, CH_3 (on chlorophenyl ring, Cl)

Chlorguanide (Inert) → Active metabolite

Nevertheless, the metabolites are almost always more polar than the parent drug. This means that the metabolites exhibit higher renal clearance than the parent drug, owing to the decrease in their reabsorption (section 9.2).

Hepatic extraction coefficient

Hepatic clearance is illustrated in Fig. 9.13. The mathematical expression of hepatic clearance can easily be derived by analogy with the general definition of clearance given in section 9.1:

$$\text{hepatic clearance} = \mathrm{CL_h} = Q_\mathrm{h}\frac{C_1 - C_2}{C_1} = Q_\mathrm{h} E_\mathrm{h} \qquad (9.15)$$

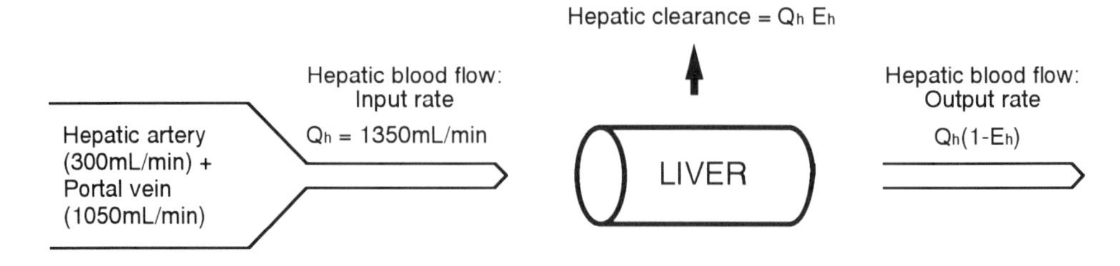

Fig. 9.13. Schematic representation of hepatic clearance.

where Q_h is the blood flow rate in liver and E_h is the hepatic extraction coefficient. Drugs can be classified into three categories according to their E_h values; those with

(a) low hepatic extraction ($E_h < 0.3$);
(b) medium hepatic extraction ($0.3 < E_h < 0.7$); and
(c) high hepatic extraction ($E_h > 0.7$).

Some important drugs in each of these three categories are presented in Table 9.1. Fig. 9.14 gives a mechanistic view of the difference in uptake from the hepatocytes between two hypothetical drugs with high and low hepatic extraction coefficients.

Table 9.1. Classification of certain drugs on the basis of their hepatic extraction coefficient values

Low ($E_h < 0.3$)	Medium ($0.3 < E_h < 0.7$)	High ($E_h > 0.7$)
Amobarbitone	Aspirin	Alprenolol
Diazepam	Codeine	Desipramine
Isoniazid	Quinidine	Isoproterenol
Phenobarbitone	Nortriptyline	Lidocaine
Phenylbutazone		Meperidine
Phenytoin		Morphine
Procainamide		Nitroglycerine
Salicylic acid		Pentazokine
Theophylline		Propoxyphene
Tolbutamide		Propranolol
Warfarin		Salicylamide

The following rates should be fast in order for the drug to have a high hepatic extraction coefficient:

— dissociation from blood proteins;
— uptake from hepatocytes; and
— biotransformation or biliary excretion.

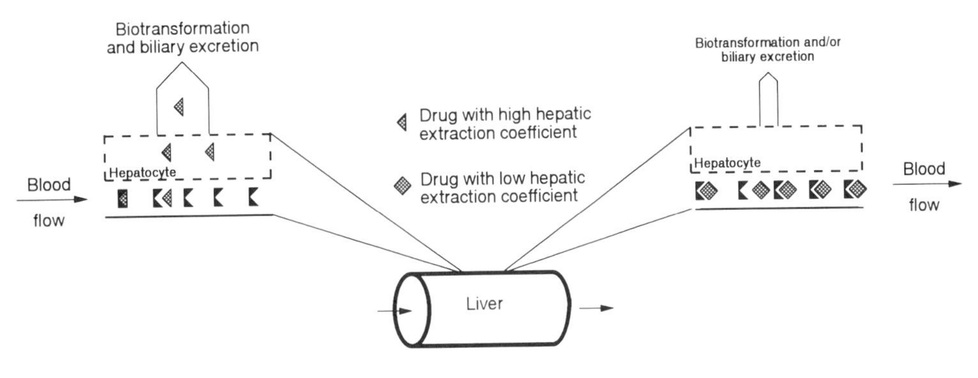

Fig. 9.14. Schematic representation of the steps involved in the hepatic elimination of a highly and a poorly extracted drug.

Under these conditions the larger portion of drug which reaches the liver through the hepatic artery and the portal vein is extracted (Fig. 9.13). This observation shows the analogy between the terms *hepatic extraction* and *hepatic clearance*. However, caution should be exercised when the drug follows the excretion route to the bile and afterwards is reabsorbed from the gastrointestinal tract. Obviously, in this case the drug will have a high hepatic extraction coefficient but the magnitude of its hepatic clearance will not be proportionally high since the drug reappears in the portal vein.

Equation (9.15) reveals that as E_h approaches unity (its maximum value) the value of the hepatic clearance is also increasing, approaching its maximum limiting value, i.e. the blood flow rate in the liver, Q_h. The magnitudes of the hepatic clearance for drugs with low E_h value can be determined from their low extraction coefficients. Following this reasoning, the drugs listed in Table 9.1 can be considered in terms of the relative contribution of blood flow rate and cellular events to the value of CL_h. For drugs with $E_h < 0.3$, the value of CL_h depends mostly on their uptake and biotransformation in the hepatocytes, in other words on the E_h value. For drugs with $E_h > 0.7$, hepatic clearance depends mostly on blood flow rate in the liver (accordingly, these drugs are characterized as *flow limited* or *perfusion limited*). For drugs with $0.3 < E_h < 0.7$, both the blood flow rate and the activity of hepatic enzymes contribute to the determination of the value of hepatic clearance.

By definition, the hepatic extraction coefficient can be expressed as the quotient $(C_1 - C_2)/C_1$ (equation (9.15)), where C_1 is the incoming concentration; in this particular case C_1 corresponds to the free concentration of drug in the blood which bathes the hepatocyte.† Drug bound to the plasma proteins is considered as a buffer which functions via the equilibrium between the free and bound drug.

† For drugs with extensive binding in plasma proteins and a high hepatic extraction coefficient ($E_h \approx 1$), total drug concentration is used as the incoming concentration.

Cytochrome P450

The liver possesses the ability to biotransform xenobiotic molecules in various ways; the system that handles the biotransformation reactions is called the *hepatic microsomal system*. This enzymatic system is associated with the smooth endoplasmic reticulum of the liver cells and is responsible for most biotransformation reactions. It can be isolated from the liver after homogenization of liver tissue, centrifugation at 12 000 × *g* for 30 min and further centrifugation of the supernatant for 1 h at 105 000 × *g*. The precipitate of the second centrifugation is the *microsomal fraction*, which contains the fragments of the endoplasmic reticulum formed during homogenization of the liver tissue. The main constituent of the microsomal fraction is a haemprotein (or, more accurately, a group of haemproteins) known as *cytochrome P450*.

Cytochrome P450 catalyses the insertion of an oxygen atom to an aliphatic or aromatic molecule. Its discovery goes back to 1958, when it was considered as an unusual pigment and not an enzyme. Its peculiar name derives from the observation that when carbon monoxide was flushed in an aqueous suspension of the microsomal fraction, a strong absorption peak was developed at 450 nm, resulting in the name pigment 450 (P450). Its recognition as haemprotein was made in 1964. P450 is the main constituent of the microsomal fraction, with a concentration almost 1 nmol/mg of microsomal protein.

All P450s isolated from various species consist of a polypeptide chain with molecular weight 45 000–55 000 and contain a non-covalently bound haem molecule. Most P450s show an absorption maximum in the region of 418 nm, which is shifted near to 390 nm when the substrate (drug) is bound.

The mechanism of the catalytic oxidation of drugs by cytochrome P450 has not been fully elucidated. Studies so far suggest a cycle of six steps, with some intermediates still in question since they have not been experimentally observed. The proposed cycle is depicted in Fig. 9.15.

Step 1: Based on the crystal structure analysis of P450s, the binding site resembles a small cavity, frequently called the *substrate pocket*. The key elements of the substrate

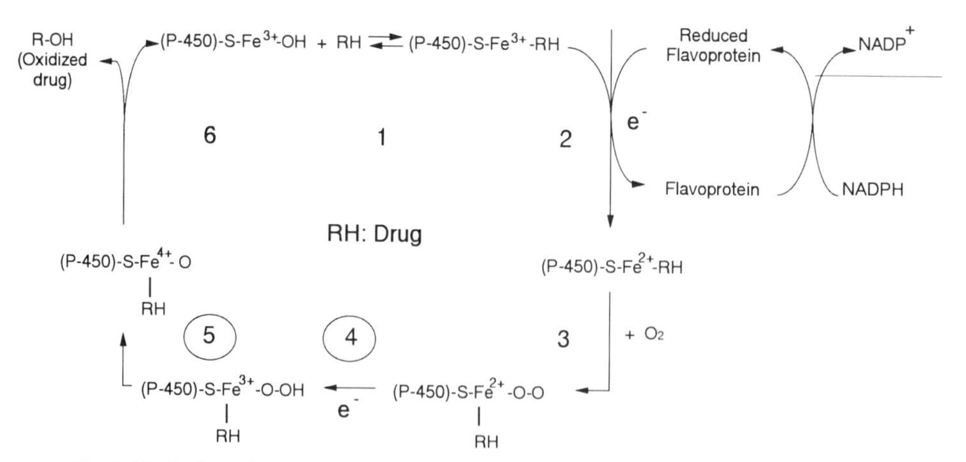

Fig. 9.15. Outline of the six-step electron transport chain involving cytochrome P450 in the oxidation of drugs by the microsomal system. The circled steps have not been directly observed.

pocket are the amino acid cysteine, and the iron atom of haem, which is coordinated with a water molecule. Upon binding of the substrate water molecules are liberated from the cavity.

Step 2: The bound form of the enzyme is reduced to Fe^{2+} by a flavoprotein, which is NADPH-cytochrome c reductase. The reductase is itself maintained in a reduced state by NADPH.

Steps 3 and 4: The reduction of Fe^{3+} in step 2 allows the coordination of the haem iron atom with O_2. After the oxygenation, a (hypothetical) ferric-peroxy intermediate is formed. The existence of this intermediate is based on the experimental observation that peroxides facilitate the hydroxylation reactions of P450 without the need for electron transfer steps.

Steps 5 and 6: Step 5 consists of cleavage of the peroxy O—O bond. The next step is the formation of the (hypothetical) enzyme ferryl-oxy Fe^{4+}—O intermediate. In this complex, the oxygen atom linked to the iron of haem has only six valence electrons. Its strong electrophilic character enables the abstraction of a hydrogen atom from a carbon atom in close proximity, thus creating a carbon radical; the latter is spontaneously transformed into the hydroxylated product.

The reactions catalysed by cytochrome P450, or generally by the hepatic microsomal enzymes, share the oxidative character illustrated in Fig. 9.15. These reactions can be classified in various categories, for each of which an example is given below.

1. Side-chain oxidation (aliphatic oxidation): Side-chain oxidations lead to alcohol formation. This can be shown with the oxidation of phenylbutazone:

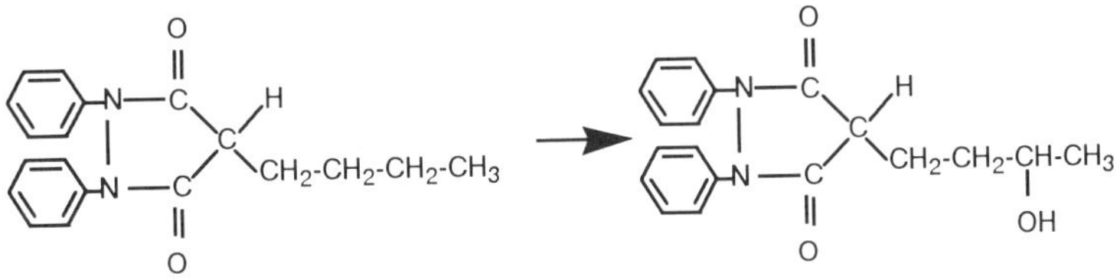

CH_2-CH_2-CH_2-CH_3 → CH_2-CH_2-CH(OH)-CH_3

2. Aromatic hydroxylation: The formation of *p*-hydroxy-phenytoin as the main metabolite of phenytoin is a typical example of aromatic ring hydroxylation:

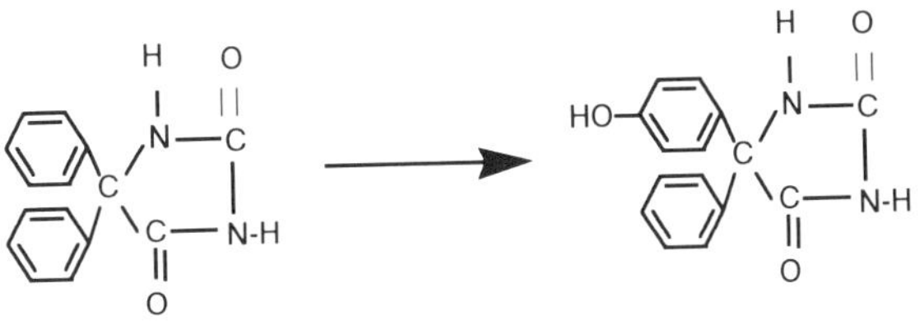

3. N-Dealkylation: Substituted amines can be subjected to *N*-dealkylation by conversion of the alkyl groups to aldehydes as, for example, in the demethylation of imipramine:

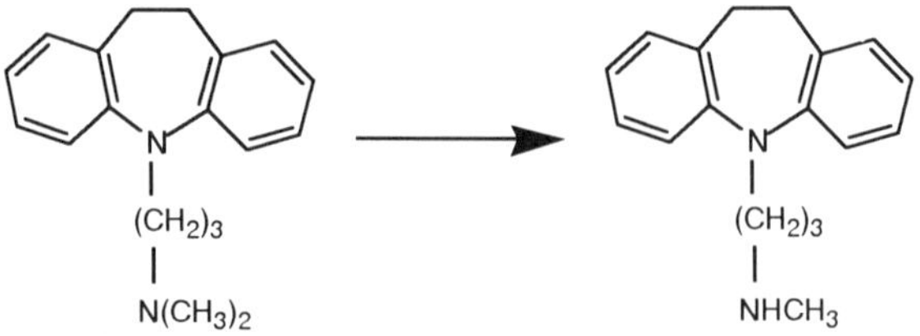

4. *O-Dealkylation*: The cleavage of the ether bond leads to the formation of phenols or alcohols. The biotransformation of phenacetin into paracetamol illustrates this type of reaction:

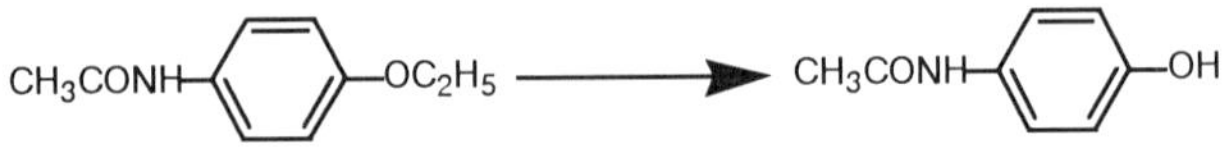

5. *S-Demethylation*: Methylmercaptans are usually demethylated to give the corresponding mercaptans. Thus, 6-mercaptopurine is the metabolite of 6-methylthiopurine:

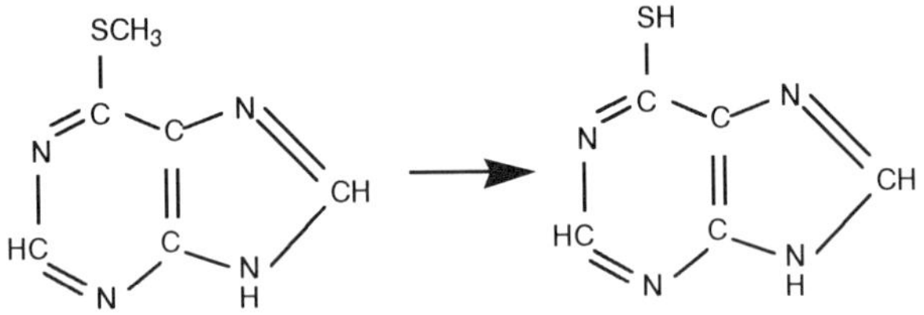

6. *Oxidative deamination*: The biotransformation of amphetamine to methylbenzylketone is a typical example of oxidative deamination:

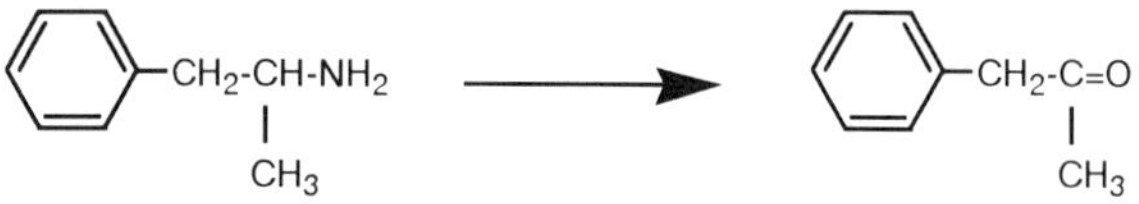

7. *Sulfoxide formation*: The oxidation of thioethers yields the corresponding sulfoxides, as shown for chlorpromazine:

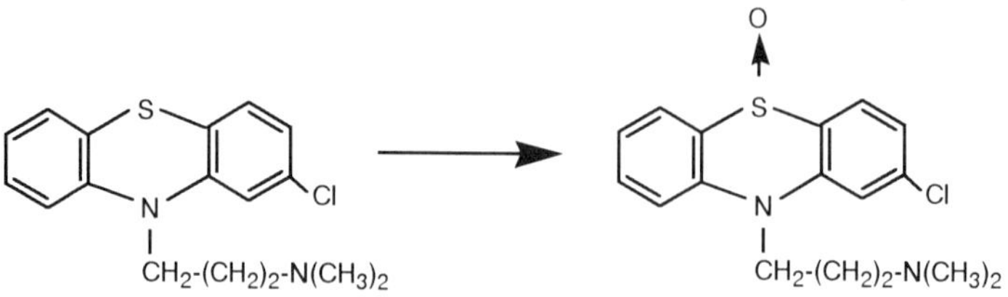

8. *Desulfuration*: The conversion of pentothal to pentobarbitone is a characteristic example of this reaction:

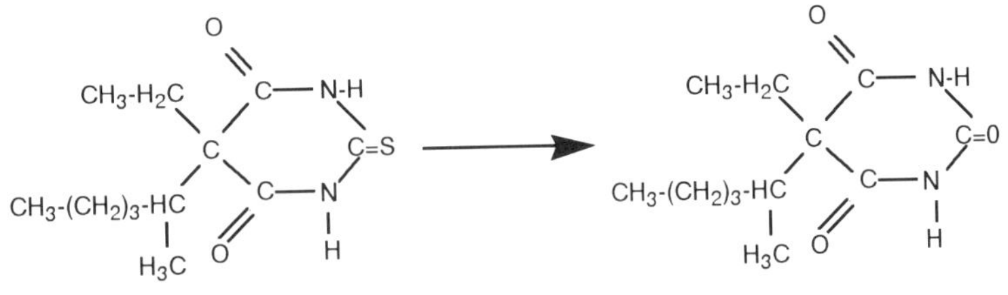

9. *N-Oxidation and N-hydroxylation*: Substrates for *N*-oxidation include secondary and tertiary amines; a classical example is the formation of the chlorpromazine *N*-oxide. Unsubstituted amides, amines and monosubstituted amines can be subjected to *N*-hydroxylation; an example of this type of reaction is the formation of phenylhydroxylamine from aniline:

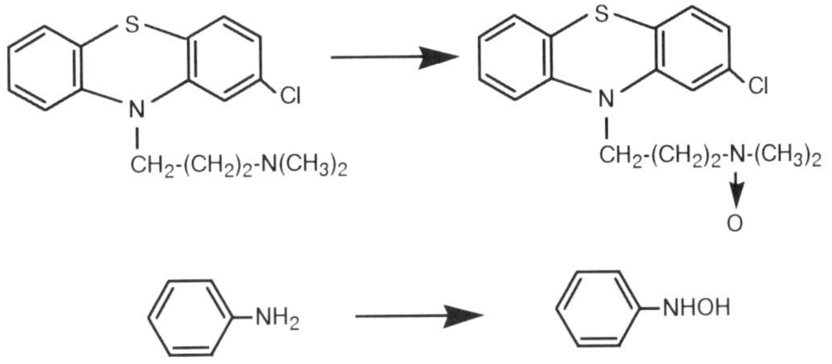

All the above oxidative reactions, as well as other biotransformations, such as reductions and hydrolyses, whether catalysed by microsomal enzymes or not, are characterized as *first-phase reactions*. The common characteristic for these reactions is that they either 'create' or 'unmask' a specific group in the drug's molecule, which is most commonly called a *handle*. In the majority of cases, biotransformation is completed with the *second-phase reaction*, where the metabolite's handle is conjugated with an endogenous compound. First- and second-phase reactions are shown in generalized form in Fig. 9.16. Of course in some cases the drug only undergoes a first-phase reaction. This can happen when the physicochemical properties (water solubility, lipophilicity, pK_a) of the metabolite (M_1 in Fig. 9.16) are sufficient to ensure rapid renal excretion. This type of behaviour is exemplified with the hydrolysis of pethidine to the corresponding water-soluble acid:

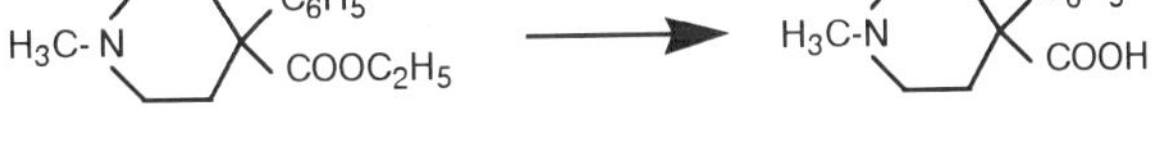

Similarly, sometimes only a second-phase reaction is observed (Fig. 9.16, $D_3 \rightarrow M_2$). For example, morphine is conjugated directly with glucuronic acid at the aromatic hydroxyl to yield an ethereal type glucuronide (see below).

The main conjugation reactions of the second phase are the formation of β-glucuronides and sulfate esters, methylations and acetylations (or, more generally, acylations).

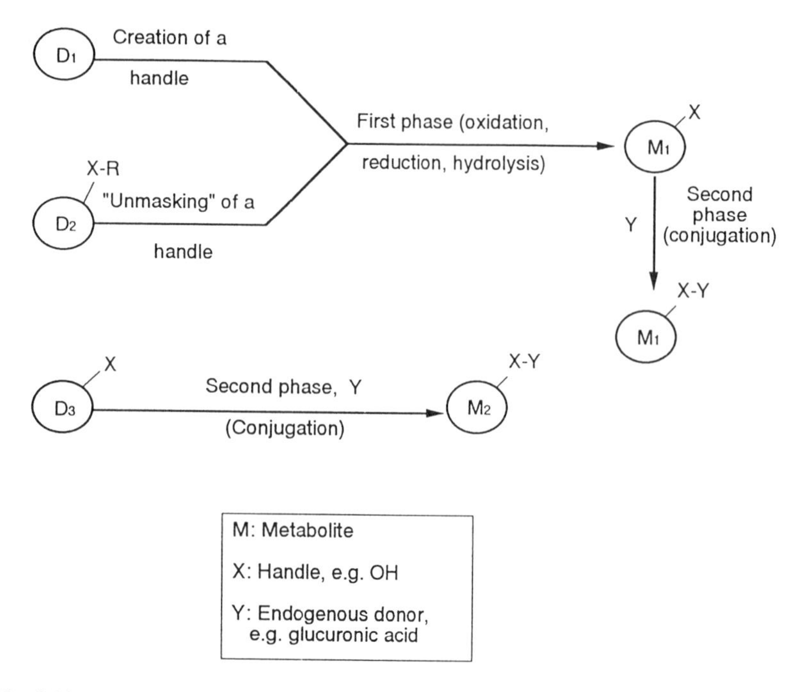

Fig. 9.16. Schematic representation of the two biotransformation phases for drugs D_1 and D_2. For drug D_3 the necessary 'handle' is pre-existing, allowing immediate conjugation.

1. β-Glucuronide formation: This large category of conjugations includes the formation of (i) etheric type *O*-glucuronides (e.g. paracetamol glucuronide), (ii) esteric type *O*-glucuronides (e.g. the glucuronide on the carboxyl group of salicylic acid), (iii) *N*-glucuronides and (iv) *S*-glucuronides. In all cases, the adduct of the conjugation is a derivative of β-D-glucuronic acid, which results from the reaction of the drug with uridine diphosphate-α-D-glucuronic acid. The reaction of glucuronidation is exemplified in Fig. 9.17 with the formation of an ethereal type glucuronide.

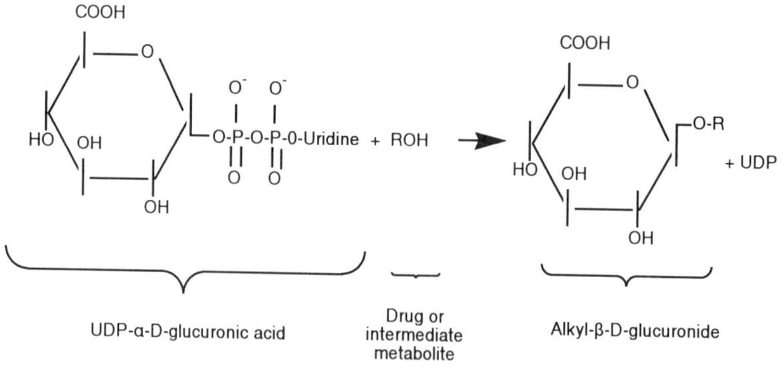

COOH — O — HO — OH — OH — O⁻ O⁻ — O-P-O-P-0-Uridine + ROH → COOH — O — O-R — HO — OH — OH + UDP

UDP-α-D-glucuronic acid — Drug or intermediate metabolite — Alkyl-β-D-glucuronide

Fig. 9.17. Formation of an etheric type β-glucuronide. UDP = uridine diphosphate.

Glucuronidation is an extremely common second-phase reaction in humans and other mammals for xenobiotic molecules. The reasons for the predominance of formation of β-glucuronides probably include the following:

— large amount of carbohydrates are available in the body, particularly glucose, which is a precursor for the synthesis of glucuronic acid;
— the polarity and hydrophilicity of the parent drug is dramatically enhanced after the formation of β-glucuronides. This is due to the presence of the hydroxyl groups as well as the acidic character of the carboxyl group ($pK_a = 3.5$). These features facilitate renal excretion of the glucuronides;
— the glucuronides are almost always less toxic than the parent drugs; and
— there is a vast number of compounds which are substrates for the uridine diphosphate-glucuronyltransferase.

2. *Methylations*: Compounds bearing the groups OH, NH, NH_2 or SH can be methylated by *S*-adenosylmethionine. This reaction is catalysed by methyltransferases.

3. *Acetylations or acylations*: Acetyl-CoA acts on amines to convert them to acetylated products. The formation of acylated derivatives involves the conjugation of drug with amino acids like glycine and glutamine. In this case, the conjugation takes place between the amine group of the amino acid and the carboxyl group of drug or the intermediate metabolite.

4. *Ethereal sulfate formation*: The endogenous donor of sulfate is the 3′-phosphoadenosine-5′phosphosulfate (PAPS), in accordance with the reaction:

OH — Sulfotransferase → OSO_3H

The main second-phase reactions are quoted in Table 9.2, along with the interactive groups and the endogenous donors.

Kinetics of drug biotransformation

As mentioned in section 2.3.2.1 the kinetics of drug biotransformation are described by the Michaelis–Menten equation:

$$u = \frac{V_{max} C_{sub}}{C_{sub} + K_M} \tag{9.16}$$

The graphic representation of equation (9.16) is shown in Fig. 9.18. The graph of Fig. 9.18 illustrates that the rate of biotransformation increases non-linearly with the concentration of the substrate, up to a maximum value, V_{max}. The Michaelis–Menten constant, K_M, can be estimated graphically; its value corresponds to the concentration of the drug

Table 9.2. Second-phase biotransformation reactions[a]

Conjugation reaction	Reacting groups	Endogenous donor
Glucuronidation	—OH, —NH_2, —COOH, —NH, —SH	UDP-glycuronic acid
Methylation	Ar—OH, —NH_2, —NH, —SH	*S*-Adenosylmethionine
Acetylation	Ar—NH_2, RNH_2, —SO_2NH_2	Acetyl-coenzyme A
Acylation (conjugation with glycine or glutamine)	Ar—COOH	Protein
Esterification	Ar—OH, $ArNH_2$, ROH	PAPS

[a] Ar = phenyl, R = alkyl.

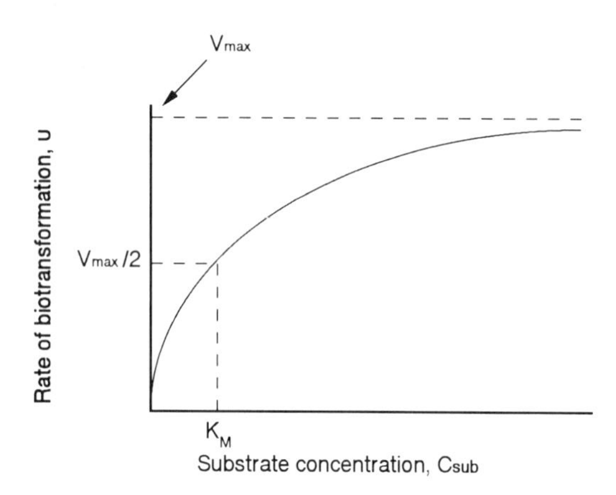

Fig. 9.18. Rate of biotransformation versus substrate concentration.

(substrate) which causes a biotransformation rate equal to $V_{max}/2$ (Fig. 9.18). The lower the K_M value, the greater the chemical affinity between the enzyme and the substrate.

Limits in the behaviour of equation (9.16) can be obtained by considering the relative magnitude of C_{sub} and K_M. When the concentration of drug is much smaller than K_M ($C_{sub} \ll K_M$), equation (9.16) becomes

$$u = \left(V_{max} / K_M\right) C_{sub} \tag{9.17}$$

This means that the rate of biotransformation is proportional to the concentration of the drug and therefore first-order kinetics apply. This behaviour is reflected in the initial part of Fig. 9.18, over which the rate of biotransformation increases linearly with drug concentration. For drug concentration values, on the same order with K_M, the rate u obeys the relationship in equation (9.16). In situations where C_{sub} is much larger than K_M ($C_{sub} \gg K_M$), equation (9.16) gives

$$u = V_{max} \tag{9.18}$$

In this case, the rate of biotransformation is not dependent on the drug concentration, and the kinetics are zero order. Equation (9.18) corresponds to the plateau of the curve in Fig. 9.18.

The changes in the kinetics can be related to interactions at the molecular level between the enzyme and drug. The rate of reaction increases initially in a linear relationship to drug concentration because at very low drug concentrations there are excess empty binding sites on the enzyme (first-order kinetics). At higher drug concentrations, the rate of biotransformation increases non-linearly until the binding sites on the enzyme are completely saturated. Thereafter, the rate of biotransformation remains constant and equal to V_{max}, regardless of increases in drug concentration (saturation kinetics). Michaelis–Menten kinetics, expressed in terms of drug mass, are also referred to as dose-dependent kinetics. In Table 9.3 a number of compounds which follow Michaelis–Menten kinetics are quoted.

Table 9.3. Some compounds which exhibit Michaelis–Menten biotransformation kinetics at therapeutic levels

Alcohol	Penicillamine
5-Bromo-2-deoxyuridine	Prednisolone
Bromouracil	Propoxyphene
5-Deoxy-5-fluorouridine	Propranolol
Diltiazem	Salicylates
5-Fluorouracil	Salicylamide
Hydralazine	Theophylline
Nicardipine	Phenytoin
Nitroglycerine	Verapamil

The Lineweaver–Burke equation

The plot of the Michaelis–Menten equation is not linear (Fig. 9.18). A number of linear transformations for equation (9.16) have been proposed, the most well-known of which is the Lineweaver–Burke equation:

$$1/u = \left(1/V_{max}\right) + \left(K_M/V_{max}\right)\left(1/C_{sub}\right) \tag{9.19}$$

A graphical representation of equation (9.19) is shown in Fig. 9.19.

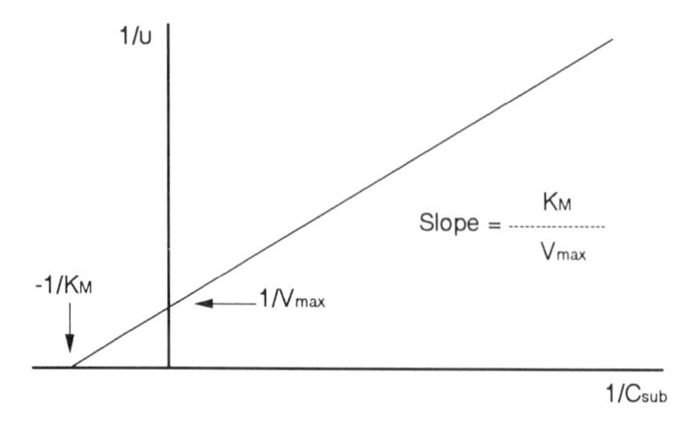

Fig. 9.19. Graphical representation of the Lineweaver–Burke equation. Estimates for K_M and V_{max} are obtained from the intercepts and the slope of the straight line.

Example 9.7: The following data were obtained in a biotransformation study using isolated microsomes:

Drug concentration C_{sub} (μg/ml)	*Biotransformation rate* u (μg/ml per minute)
0.10	0.270
0.20	0.400
0.40	0.530
0.60	0.600
0.80	0.640
1.0	0.670
1.5	0.710
2.0	0.730
4.0	0.760
8.0	0.780
16	0.790
20	0.790

Calculate the parameters V_{max} and K_M using the Lineweaver–Burke equation.

Answer: According to equation (9.19) the reciprocal values of the rates and concentrations should be calculated:

$1/C_{sub}$	$1/u$
10	3.70
5.0	2.50
2.5	1.89
1.7	1.67
1.2	1.56
1.0	1.49
0.67	1.41

0.50	1.37
0.25	1.33
0.12	1.28
0.06	1.26
0.05	1.26

The line of best fit, obtained by linear regression analysis, is

$$(1/u) = 1.25 + 0.25\,(1/C_{sub}) \qquad (R = 0.9998)$$

from which we calculate that

$$V_{max} = 0.80\ (\mu g/ml)/min \quad \text{and} \quad K_M = 0.20\ \mu g/ml$$

Example 9.8: During a pharmacokinetic study it was found that a drug is removed from the body exclusively by biotransformation and that the relationship expressing the decrease of the drug concentration in plasma is

$$\frac{dC_{sub}}{dt} = u = -\frac{V_{max}C_{sub}}{K_M + C_{sub}} = -\frac{0.60C_{sub}}{0.10 + C_{sub}}$$

where $V_{max} = 0.60\ (\mu g/ml)/h$ and $K_M = 0.10\ \mu g/ml$. Calculate the time required for the decline of drug concentration from 30 to 18 $\mu g/ml$.

Answer: Both concentration values are much larger than the value of K_M $(30 > 18 \gg K_M)$. Consequently, the decrease in drug concentration can be approximated using zero-order kinetcs:

$$u = V_{max} = 0.60\ \mu g/ml \text{ per hour}$$

The time required for the decrease of 12 $\mu g/ml$ $(30 - 18 = 12\ \mu g/ml)$ in the concentration is calculated from zero-order kinetics as

$$\frac{12}{0.60}\ \frac{\mu g/ml}{(\mu g/ml)/h} = 20\ h$$

Enzyme induction

A great number of compounds, among them many drugs, increase the enzymatic activity of the hepatic microsomal system. These compounds are called *enzyme inducers*. When the inducers are coadministered with a drug, an increase in the drug oxidation rate results. A number of changes are associated with enzyme induction and the most important of them are

(a) increase in both liver size and liver blood flow;
(b) increase in both total and microsomal protein per unit of liver weight;
(c) proliferation of smooth endoplasmic reticulum (as observed by electronic microscopy); and
(d) increased synthesis and decreased degradation of cytochrome P450 and most of the components involved in the oxidation cycle shown in Fig. 9.15.

These observations substantiate the view that enzyme induction is accompanied by increased protein synthesis. In accordance with this viewpoint, actinomycin D and ethionine, which reduce protein synthesis, have been found to block enzyme induction. Studies of enzyme induction have not yet revealed the structural requirements for efficient induction. As a rule of thumb, the inducing agent is lipophilic and is a substrate of the inducted enzyme system (see Table 9.4).

Table 9.4. Some inducers of the microsomal system

Barbiturates	Tranquillizers	Analgesics	Other
Phenobarbitone	Chloral hydrate	Antipyrine	Ethanol
Pentothal	Chlordiazepoxide	Phenylbutazone	Chlorinated pesticides
Barbitone	Glutethimide		Griseofulvin
Cyclobarbitone	Meprobamate		Phenytoin

The most thoroughly studied enzmye inducer is phenobarbitone, which can increase enzyme activity up to four times. Its powerful inducing effect, in comparison to other barbiturates and other inducers of similar structure, has not yet been explained.

An interesting source of enzyme induction is cigarette smoking. This enzyme induction is attributed to the tobacco constituents and their combustion products, i.e. 3-methylcholanthrene, 3,4-benzopyrene and nicotone. Thus, cigarette smokers have faster elimination rates for antipyrine and theophylline. It should be noted that smoking is a factor which is taken into account when theophylline dosage is calculated; in general, smokers require higher theophylline doses to maintain therapeutic drug levels.

Another example which shows that enzyme induction can have serious consequences in clinical practice is the inducing effect of phenobarbitone on dicoumarol levels (Fig. 9.20). The administration of phenobarbitone causes a fall in dicoumarol levels which is reflected by a proportional decrease in prothrombin time (a measure of anticoagulant effect). Accordingly, extreme caution must be exercised when dicoumarol and phenobarbitone are coadministered to avoid either failure of the anticoagulant therapy or haemorrhagic crises.

Enzyme inhibition

Due to the fact that a very large number of drugs share the cytochrome P450 enzyme system, it is not uncommon for a patient to receive two drugs which interact with the same enzyme site. Each of the two drugs acts as an inhibitor for the other's degradation, and the phenomenon is called enzyme inhibition. The various types of enzyme inhibition can broadly be divided into three categories:

(a) *Substrate competition*: This is the typical case when two substrates (drugs) compete with one another for the same enzyme.

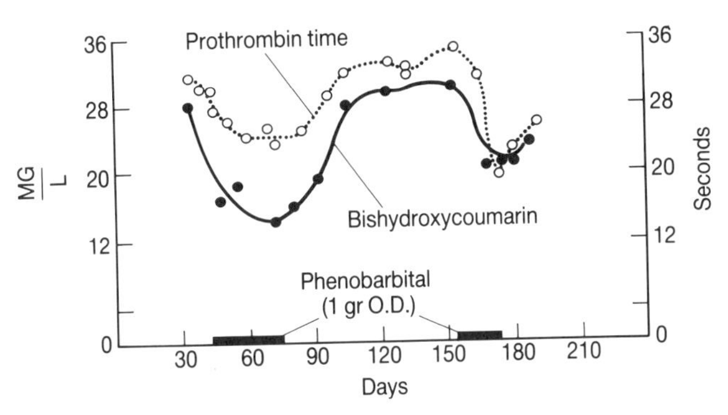

Fig. 9.20. The effect of phenobarbitone enzyme induction on (a) the biotransformation rate of dicoumarol (75 mg/d) and (b) prothrombin time. (Reproduced from *Clinical Pharmacology and Therapeutics* **6**: 420–429 (1965), with permission.)

(b) *Competitive or non-competitive inhibition*: The inhibitor decreases the affinity or the activity of the enzyme for the competitor.

(c) *Product inhibition*: This inhibition occurs when the metabolite interferes with enzymatic activity for the parent drug.

Inhibitory interactions are likely to be important clinically with drugs that have a narrow therapeutic range, e.g. anticoagulants, antiepileptics and hypoglycaemic agents. A typical example is the retardation of the rate of elimination of phenytoin by dicoumarol (Fig. 9.21).

Another interesting example of a clinically important interaction is the effect of phenylbutazone on warfarin plasma levels. Clinical observations have repeatedly shown that if during anticoagulant therapy with warfarin (10 mg/d) phenylbutazone is coadministered (100 mg/8 h), haemorrhagic crises occur. Since phenylbutazone does not have any anticoagulant activity, the interpretation of the interaction was initially associated with the ability of phenylbutazone to displace warfarin from the plasma proteins. This explanation was shown to be unlikely since many other compounds displace warfarin from its binding sites without enhancing its effect. The elucidation of the mechanisms involved was achieved during the mid-1980s when researchers studied the effect of phenylbutazone on the free plasma levels of *R*(+) and *S*(–) warfarin isomers using stereoselective methods. Warfarin is used as a racemic mixture, with the *S* isomer being five times more active than the *R* isomer. Also, warfarin is removed from the body almost exclusively by biotransformation and the *S* isomer is biotransformed more rapidly than the *R* isomer in humans. This means that soon after the administration of warfarin the ratio of the isomers is continuously changing with time in favour of the *R* isomer. Analysis of the data revealed that the effect of phenylbutazone on the *R* isomer is entirely due to its displacement from the plasma proteins, while the effect on the *S* isomer is mainly ascribed to the inhibition of biotransformation. Consequently, retardation of the elimination of the *S* isomer increased the free levels of this isomer which, when coupled with its intrinsic high anticoagulant activity, caused patients to haemorrhage (see Table 9.5).

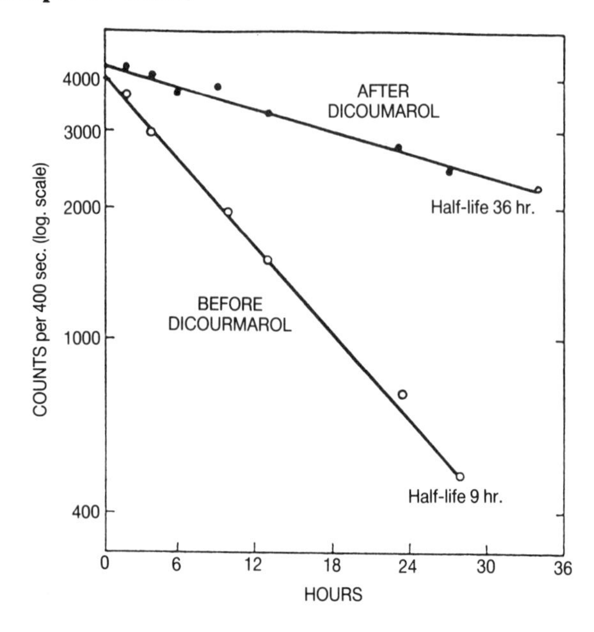

Fig. 9.21. The effect of dicoumarol enzyme inhibition (when administered in doses which reduced the activity of prothrombin by 30%) on the biotransformation rate of [^{14}C]phenytoin. (Reproduced from *Lancet* ii: 265–266 (1966), with permission.)

Table 9.5. Some inhibitors of the microsomal system

Allopurinol	Nortriptyline
Chloramphenicol	Perfenazine
Dicoumarol	Phenylbutazone
Disulfiram	Sulfaphenazole
Isoniazid	
Monoaminoxidase inhibitors (MAO)	

Effect of genetic factors on drug biotransformation

Studies of the effect of heredity on pharmacodynamic and pharmacokinetic characteristics of drugs constitute the subject of *pharmacogenetics*. A special branch of this field is concerned with the difference between individuals with respect to biotransformation rates of drugs. Although there is some inter-individual variability in biotransformation rates for most drugs, in certain cases the differences in drug biotransformation rate between groups of patients are extreme and genetically linked.† In such cases we refer to *polymorphism of biotransformation*. Under these circumstances, the frequency of two phenotypes‡ with very different metabolism depends on the incidence of the specific genes in the population.

† The formation of the protein part of the enzyme is regulated genetically.

‡ Phenotype is based on genotype, but in this case expression of the gene also relies on environmental factors.

Polymorphism of N-acetylation: This is the best-documented example of genetic polymorphism and has been studied in depth. The responsible enzyme is *N*-acetyltransferase, which catalyses the acetylation of amines and hydrazines. Isoniazid is the model compound for this type of polymorphism which exihibits two discrete groups of acetylators, termed slow and fast acetylators. The fast acetylators demonstrate a biotransformation rate of isoniazid almost three times higher than the slow ones. The half-life of isoniazid is 45–80 min for the fast and 140–200 min for the slow acetylators, respectively. The isoniazid polymorphism is clearly depicted in Fig. 9.22 as a frequency histogram of the 6 h post-dose plasma levels of 483 individuals who received the same dose. The histogram exhibits two maxima (bimodal distribution), with one group of the population having an average isoniazid plasma concentration of ~1 μg/ml, and the other group having a concentration of ~4.5 μg/ml. The individuals of the first group metabolize isoniazid faster than the individuals of the second group. The intermediate impact of this difference is that the fast acetylators require larger doses of isoniazid to maintain therapeutic drug levels. A greater frequency of peripheral neuropathy has been observed in the group of slow acetylators. This symptom is a side-effect of isoniazid therapy and is associated with the higher isoniazid levels. Polymorphism of *N*-acetylation is also displayed in the biotransformation of other drugs, such as sulfadimidine, procainamide

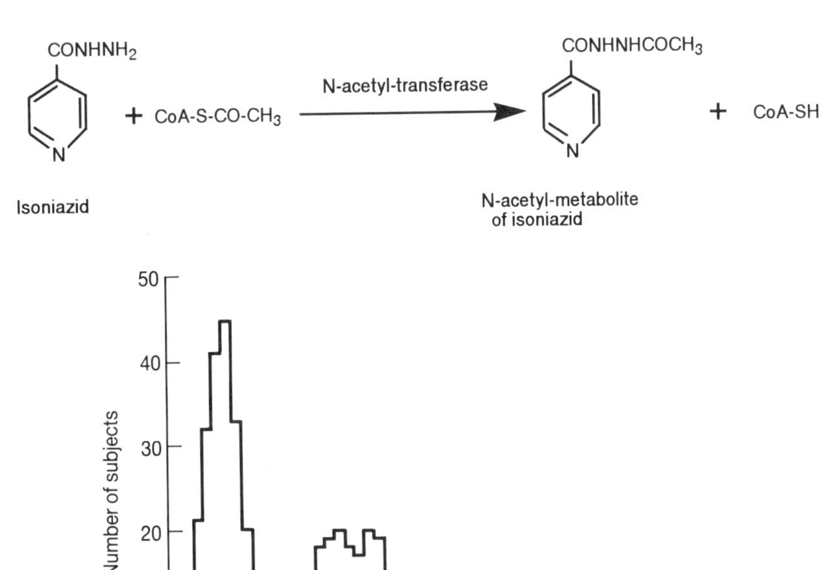

Fig. 9.22. Six hours post-dosing concentrations of isoniazid in plasma of 483 subjects, after per os administration of 9.8–10 mg/kg. (Reproduced from *British Medical Journal* 2: 485–491 (1960), with permission.)

and hydralazine. Population studies around the globe have shown that the slow acetylators constitute 55–60% of the population in Europe, 10% of the population in Japan and almost 100% of the Eskimo population.

Genetic factors and microsomal oxidation: The biotransformation of drugs, which is catalysed by microsomal enzymes, varies widely among individuals. The variables measured most frequently include plasma half-life, clearance and hepatic clearance. In the vast majority of cases only a single mode is observed in the frequency distribution of the studied variable for a given microsomal oxidation. This means that both environmental and genetic factors contribute to the variability and the influence of a gene cannot be discerned. Under these circumstances, the mode of the inheritance is 'polygenic', which means that an unknown number of genes at numerous loci control the transmission of the given microsomal oxidation. However, the impact of inheritance in phenomena under polygenic control can become evident with studies in selected families and in particular twins. For example, Fig. 9.23 shows that the rate of biotransformation of phenylbutazone is the same in identical twins, but differs in fraternal twins. Similar studies for the microsomal oxidation of antipyrine, dicoumarol and nortriptiline have shown that their biotransformation is also under a considerable measure of genetic control. The genetic effect on biotransformation has also been proved by the degree of enzyme induction caused by phenobarbitone on the antipyrine biotransformation rate. Again, in identical twins an almost identical increase in the antipyrine biotransformation rate is found, while significant differences are observed in fraternal twins.

Genetic polymorphism has been demonstrated for a small number of drugs with exceptionally high inter-individual variability in microsomal oxidation reactions. One of the best known is the debrisoquine polymorphism. Debrisoquine (D) is an antihypertensive agent which is biotransformed to the 4-hydroxy metabolite (4-HO-D) by one of the eight isoenzymes comprising cytochrome P450. A bimodal frequency distribution has been found for the metabolic quotient (D/4-HO-D), with efficient metabolizers (~90% of the population) having values of metabolic quotient in the range 0.1–10 and poor metabolizers (~10% of the population) having values between 12 and 100. Since other drugs are also biotransformed by the same isoenzyme, debrisoquine serves as a model compound, with more general significance. Numerous attempts have been made to find common patterns of microsomal oxidation, with two goals in mind. First, optimum dosage adjustment for a drug can be achieved by knowing the kinetics of another compound metabolized by the same enzymes. Second, insight into the mechanism(s) of the biotransformation of a large group of drugs can be gained. Several drugs, such as antipyrine, desipramine and phenylbutazone, have been tested for this purpose, and the use of a drug 'cocktail' has also been explored as a marker of enzymatic activity.

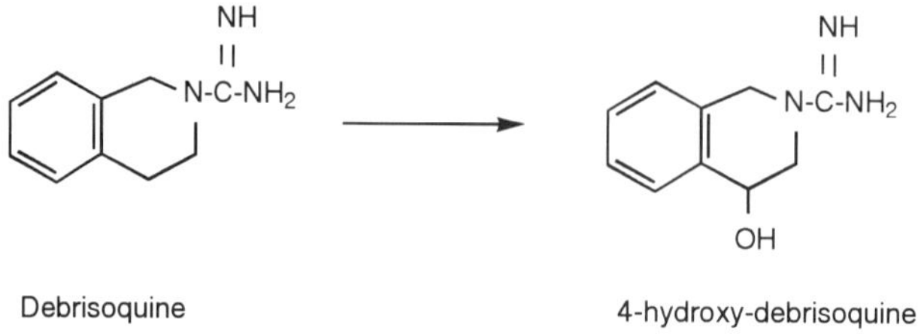

NH
||
N-C-NH_2 ⟶ NH
||
N-C-NH_2
OH

Debrisoquine 4-hydroxy-debrisoquine

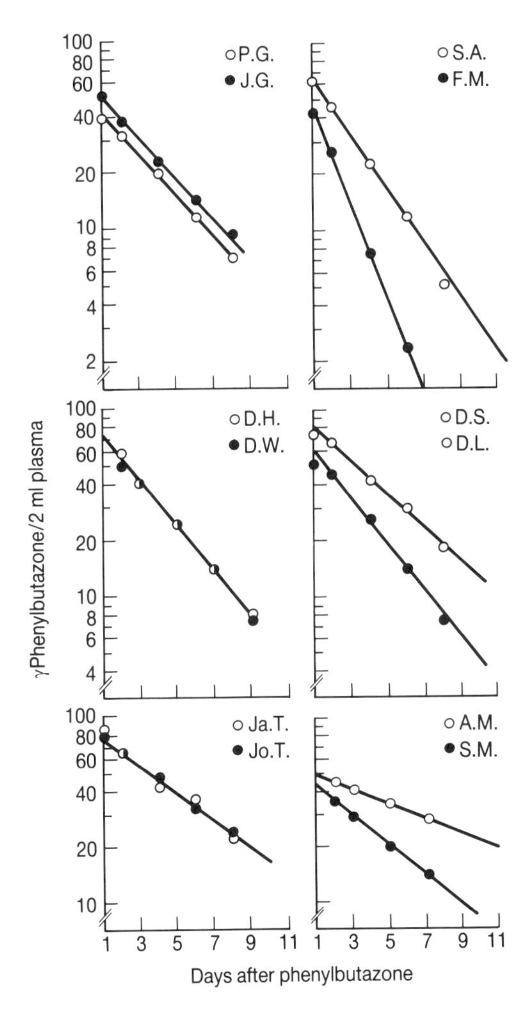

Fig. 9.23. Semi-logarithmic plots of phenylbutazone concentrations in plasma versus time, in three pairs of identical and fraternal twins. (Reproduced from *Science* **159**: 1479–1480 (1968), with permission.)

Finally, other genetic polymorphisms of microsomal oxidation different from the debrisoquine type have been found. This means that their genetic patterns are controlled by isoenzyme(s) different from the isoenzyme responsible for the oxidation of debrisoquine. Two such oxidation reactions exhibiting polymorphism are those for tolbutamide and mephenytoin.

9.3.3.2 Biliary secretion and enterohepatic circulation

In humans, the larger part of the bile secreted from the liver is stored temporarily in the gallbladder. About 250–1000 ml of bile passes through the gallbladder daily. When the bile resides in the gallbladder (the volume capacity of which is ~14–60 ml) it is continuously concentrated because of absorption of water and electrolytes through the gallbladder wall. Thus, the contents of the gallbladder bile become 5–20 times more concentrated during storage. Despite this concentration, the gall bladder bile continues to be isoosmotic with plasma, since its organic constituents (cholesterol, lecithin, bilirubin, bile salts) are relatively inactive osmotically.

During the interdigestive period (section 6.2) closure of the gall bladder sphincter prevents the gallbladder from emptying its contents into the duodenum. The longest storage period of bile in the gallbladder is observed during the night (Fig. 9.24). Even then, there is a continuous basal level of hepatic bile flow into the duodenum, due to the positive pressure gradient between the gall bladder and the bile duct. Discharge of gall bladder bile into the duodenum occurs in response to meal intake. The contractions of the gallbladder start within 20 min of a meal intake and the duration of emptying ranges from 20 to 105 min. Emptying is under humoral regulation by the polypeptide *cholecystokinin*. On the average 50–90% of the gall bladder content is emptied. The larger part of the bile is reabsorbed, mostly in the ileum. This phenomenon is termed *enterohepatic circulation* (Fig. 9.25)

Certain drugs and their metabolites are secreted from the liver into the bile, only to be reabsorbed from the intestine. Representative examples of drugs undergoing enterohepatic cycling are given in Table 9.6.

Drug secretion from the liver to the bile depends on the molecular weight, the charge and the lipophilicity of the drug. In all cases the molecular weight of the drug must be

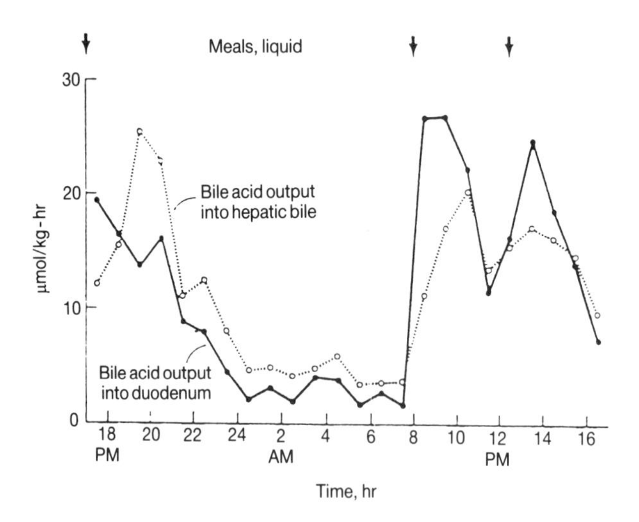

Fig. 9.24. Secretion rate of bile acids from liver to bile (······) and from both liver and the gallbladder to the duodenum (——), in five volunteers. When the secretion rate from the liver to the gallbladder is higher than the secretion rate of bile acids into the duodenum, bile acids accumulate in the gallbladder. In the second case bile acids are discharged from the gallbladder into the duodenum. (Reproduced from *Gastroenterology* 75: 879–885 (1978), with permission.)

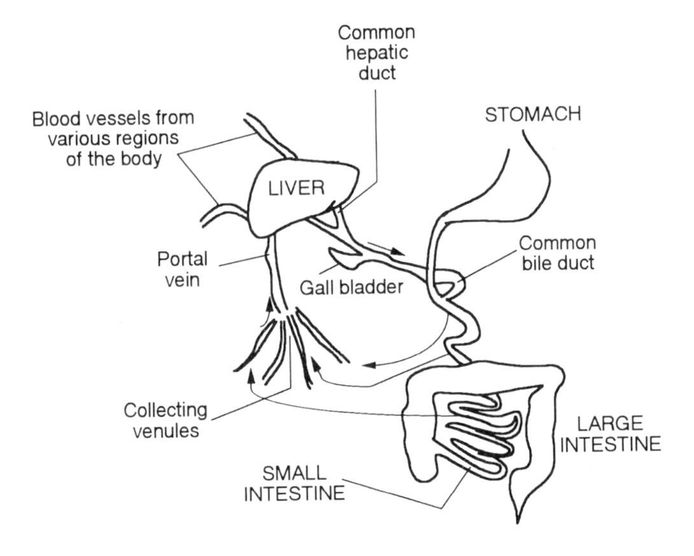

Fig. 9.25. Enterohepatic circulation.

Table 9.6. Some drugs which are excreted in the bile

Colchicine	Penicillin
Cardiac glucosides	Steroid hormones
Erythromycin	Streptomycin
Indomethacin	Tetracyclines
Quinine	Vinblastine

relatively high (>250). Nevertheless, general rules in regard to the drug physicochemical characteristics for the secretory mechanisms in the bile cannot be given with any degree of certainty. The transport of drugs which are weak bases or acids from liver to bile appears to be mainly accomplished by active mechanisms as illustrated by the competitive inhibition and the maximum transport rates often found in drug biliary excretion studies. However, the mechanism of secretion of large non-ionized molecules (cardiac glycosides and steroid hormones) has not been clarified as yet.

Reabsorption of drugs from the intestines depends on the factors discussed in chapter 6. Reabsorption of drug secreted in the bile results in an extension of its residence time in the body.

Evaluation of the extent of enterohepatic circulation of a drug in humans can be accomplished with *in vivo* pharmacokinetic studies. Animal studies (usually in rats) can also be performed. Experiments with animals offer the alternative of direct collection of bile for long time intervals which makes it possible to

(a) study in depth the effects of enterohepatic circulation on various physiological functions, e.g. fat absorption;
(b) directly calculate the fraction of drug that is not reabsorbed from the intestines.

9.4 FIRST-PASS EFFECT

In chapter 6 we mentioned that apart from the physical barriers the entry of drug in the general circulation can also be restricted by metabolic barriers. Pre-systemic biotransformation reactions comprise what we call today the *first-pass effect*. In the case of oral administration, this term can be applied to any biotransformation reaction that happens to a drug in the intestinal lumen, epithelia, portal blood or liver, *prior* to its arrival to the general circulation. We will focus our attention on the biotransformation reactions which take place in the gastrointestinal mucosa and the liver after per os administration. If a drug has a very significant first-pass effect in these two regions its oral administration will be inefficient. Under these circumstances, other routes of administration, e.g. transdermal or sublingual administration of nitroglycerin, are preferred.

9.4.1 Biotransformation in the gastrointestinal mucosa

The first-pass effect in the gastrointestinal (GI) mucosa becomes very significant when the rate of biotransformation is much faster than the rate of drug's permeation through the epithelial layer.

Typical classes of compounds with extensive biotransformation in the GI tract include most hormones and larger peptides. The extraction coefficients in the intestinal mucosa, E_i,† of representative drugs along with the corresponding hepatic extraction coefficients E_h are quoted in Table 9.7. The most important enzymes involved in the biotransformation of drugs in the mucosa of the intestines are quoted in Table 9.8. Note that in a limited number of cases, biotransformation in the GI mucosa can be utilized to advantage the design of prodrugs with more efficient delivery.

Table 9.7. Intestinal E_i and hepatic E_h extraction coefficients measured in *in vivo* studies

Drug	E_i (%)	E_h (%)	Species
Aspirin	47	33	Rat
	28	36	Dog
L-Dopa	46–62	0–8.5	Dog
Morphine	66	61	Rat
Propranolol	0	92	Dog
Salicylamide	42	36	Rat
Phenacetin	0	13	Rat

† When biotransformation in the GI mucosa is considered, the value of the extraction coefficient is always reflected in the corresponding value of clearance (section 9.3).

Table 9.8. Enzyme systems in the intestinal mucosa responsible for the biotransformation of drugs

Acetyltransferase	Ketosteroid reductase
Alkaline phosphatase	Monoaminoxidase
Glutathione *S*-transferase	Monooxygenases
Glucuronyltransferase	Dopa-decarboxylase
Disaccharidases	Xanthine oxidase
Esterases	Peptidases (amino and carboxypeptidases)
Sulfur transferases	P450

The mucosal enzymes are located on the luminal membrane, the cytoplasm and the lysosomes. The activity of the enzymes can be induced by the presence of food and other exogenous substances in the GI tract. The degree of activity of enzymes also changes longitudinally along the GI tract. For most enzymes, activity is higher in the duodenum and lower in the ileum; similarly, enzymatic activity is usually reduced on passing from the caecum to the colon. There is also a radial component to enzyme activity, with activity generally greater at the villous tip than in the crypt. In an analogous manner, the uptake of tetrapeptides and polypeptides is accompanied by an initial cleavage to dipeptides in the brush border, while a further cleavage takes place in the cytoplasm.

The conventional pattern of two-phase hepatic biotransformation reactions is also observed in the biotransformation reactions of the GI mucosa. The reactions of phase I are mainly oxidations and hydrolyses, e.g. aspirin and pivampicillin,[†] and are catalysed by cytochrome P450. The most common phase II reactions in this region are methylations, acetylations, formation of sulfate esters and glucuronides. Although there may be significant differences among species, most of the biotransformations in the GI mucosa have been observed in animals (Table 9.7). The study of biotransformations in the intestinal epithelial cells is carried out with homogenates of the GI mucosa of animals or cell cultures of human cancer cells, usually Caco-2 cells prepared from colonic epithelium (section 6.4).

9.4.2 Per os administration: first-pass effect in the liver

The liver is the most important site of the first-pass effect following oral administration of drugs, since the activity of cytochrome P450 enzymes in the GI mucosa is only 5–10% of the corresponding activity of the same enzymes in the liver. A prerequisite for a pronounced first-pass effect in the liver is a high value of hepatic extraction coefficient, i.e. $E_h \approx 1$. In this case, the whole quantity of drug is extracted from blood in the sinusoids and biotransformed in the hepatocytes. When the drug has a relatively high hepatic extraction coefficient, a number of factors related either to physiology or the characteristics of the formulation influence the magnitude of the first-pass effect. The most important of these are

† The hydrolysis of pivampicillin in the GI mucosa liberates the active drug, ampicillin (section 5.1).

(1) *Blood flow rate*: When the blood flow rate increases the mean free drug concentration in the sinusoids is also increased, resulting in a more efficient hepatic extraction. Blood flow rate in the liver is reduced when standing rather than sitting, while exercising, with age, with cardiovascular disease, and in hepatitis and cirrhosis, while it is increased during digestion and after administration of hydralazine.

(2) *Gastric emptying*: Rapid gastric emptying usually results in rapid uptake of drug from the intestinal mucosa, which in turn results in high drug concentrations in the portal vein. The net result of these changes will be an increase of the bioavailability of drug since the kinetics of the first-pass effect follow the principles of Michaelis–Menten kinetics, i.e. the enzymes become saturated. However, if the biotransformation has a wide concentration over which kinetics are essentially first order, rapid absorption will not affect the bioavailability.†

(3) *Rate of release of drug from the formulation*: Slow release of drug from the formulation results in low concentrations of drug in the blood reaching the portal vein. Consequently, biotransformation will be in the first-order region, implying maximum efficiency of metabolism and hence minimum bioavailability. Note that bioavailability after a controlled-release dosage form will be lower than that observed from the immediate-release dosage form only if levels achieved after the latter succeed in at least partially saturating the enzymes.

(4) *Protein binding of drug*: Extensive binding of drug to the plasma proteins reduces the portion of drug taken up from the hepatocytes. This general observation is not valid for all cases since drugs with a high percentage of binding may also have a high hepatic extraction ratio (see albumin receptor model, section 9.3.2). Other factors which affect the protein binding can also affect the enzymatic activity and/or the blood flow rate. For example, phenobarbitone increases the binding of propranolol and simultaneously causes enzyme induction and quite possibly increases the blood flow rate.

9.4.2.1 Assessment of first-pass effects in the liver

Studies for the evaluation of the first-pass effect in humans require measurements of the drug's concentration in blood prior to its entry and after its exit from the liver. Usually, the drug is coadministered with a compound whose hepatic uptake characteristics are known, e.g. indocyanine green.‡

Analysis of the experimental data is based on one of two models developed in the 1970s and shown in Fig. 9.26. These models are also used for the analysis of data in conventional hepatic biotransformation studies. Relevant equations for these two models can also be applied in experiments dealing with the first-pass effect in epithelial membranes. The prerequisite for the utilization of these relationships is that the biotransformation occurs only in the studied region.

† The type of kinetics and its effect on the bioavailability should be viewed in the light of the analysis presented for the Michaelis–Menten equation in section 9.3.

‡ Coadministered substances are usually used for determination of the hepatic function.

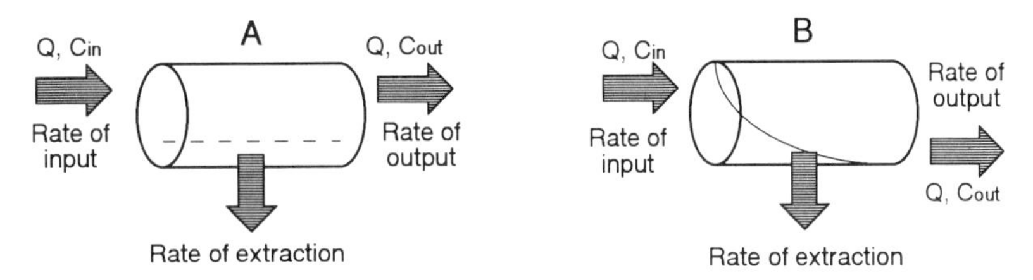

Fig. 9.26. The two models used for the study of first-pass effect and in general of the metabolic clearance. (A) The well-stirred model; (B) the parallel tube model. The term *metabolic clearance* is used here since the term *hepatic clearance* includes both the metabolic and biliary excretion. (Redrawn from *Acta Pharmaceutica Suecica* 23: 173–190 (1986).)

The well-stirred model

According to this model the liver is considered to be a well-stirred container (mixing tank), meaning that the free concentration of drug in all sinusoids corresponds to the concentration which is available for biotransformation (Fig. 9.26A). The concentration of drug in the vicinity of the enzymes is considered equal to the free concentration of drug in the venous blood. When this model was initially developed, first-order kinetics for the enzymatic activity were assumed. Today, this model is used for Michaelis–Menten kinetics as well. On the basis of this model, the fraction of drug which is *not* biotransformed in the liver, f_h, is given by the equation

$$f_h = Q_h/(Q_h + CL_h f_f) \tag{9.20}$$

where Q_h is the blood flow rate in the sinusoids, f_f is the fraction of the free drug in the hepatic channels and CL_h is the hepatic clearance, which is equal to V_{max}/K_M for the enzymatic system studied. The quotient V_{max}/K_M is frequently called intrinsic clearance. This quantity expresses the inherent ability of the biotransformation of the liver enzymes without the limitations from the blood flow rate which are imposed in the classical definition of clearance.

The parallel tube model

In this case the liver is modelled with a series of equal, parallel tubes with a constant enzymatic activity throughout their entire length (Fig. 9.26B). According to this model, the concentration of drug in the blood perfusing the tubes declines exponentially along the tubes. The fraction of drug which escapes biotransformation, f_h, is given by the equation

$$f_f = \exp[-(CL_h f_f)/Q_h] \tag{9.21}$$

The predictions based on these two models are similar when the bioavailability of drug is high; however, significant differences are observed with drugs of low bioavailability. In general, the parallel tube model underestimates the extent of bioavailability in comparison to the well-stirred model. An inherent problem associated with the use of these models is the proper expression of the 'real' concentration of drug in the hepatocytes. Normally, the free drug concentration is utilized; however, the role of the bound drug and the rate of dissociation of the protein–drug complex have not been clarified as yet. The data gathered so far have shown that both these models require modifications since they are not capable of predicting the extent of bioavailability when non-linear kinetics are encountered, when the blood flow rate has changed due to anastomoses of blood vessels, when the drug follows enterohepatic circulation or if the drug is biotransformed at more than one site, e.g. in the GI mucosa as well as the liver. In spite of these limitations, both models have been used successfully to predict the bioavailability of drugs with extensive first-pass effect in the liver, such as propranolol or lidocaine.

9.4.3 The influence of first-pass effect on bioavailability

Since the first-pass effect is mainly associated with the liver, drugs with medium or high hepatic extraction coefficients will exhibit medium and high first-pass effect, respectively. In other words, if drugs with $E_h > 0.3$ are administered per os, they will present reduced bioavailability due to their significant hepatic extraction. Fig. 9.27, constructed in accordance with Fig. 9.2, illustrates the effect of hepatic extraction on the bioavailability of drug. According to Fig. 9.27 the upper limit for the bioavailability of drug will be

$$\text{bioavailability} = F = 1 - E_h \tag{9.22}$$

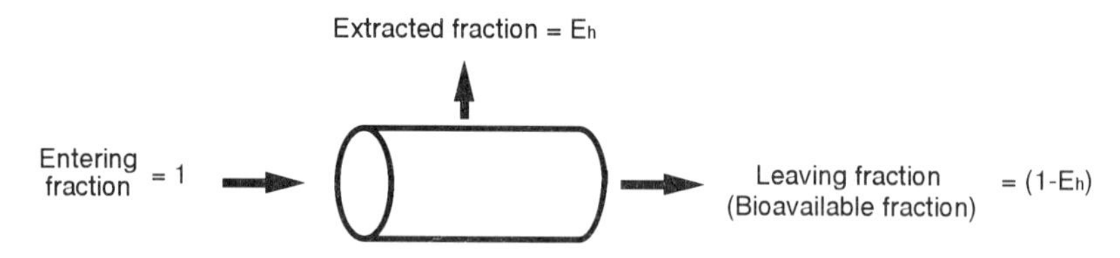

Fig. 9.27. Schematic representation of the impact of first-pass effect on bioavailability, assuming that all administered drug is absorbed across the GI mucosa.

For example, lidocaine with a value 0.7 for E_h will present a maximum of 30% bioavailability; however, it could be even less if one takes into account formulation and/or solubility factors (chapter 4). Because of the large number of factors influencing the enzymatic activity as well as the first-pass effect, the bioavailability of drugs with a significant first-pass effect may present great variability. Larger doses will be required for orally administered drugs with very significant first-pass effect in order to achieve plasma concentrations similar to those obtained after intravenous administration. This is true even when there is complete uptake of drug from the GI epithelium; in such a case there is an explicit discrepancy between the fraction absorbed (= 1) and the systemic bioavailability ($\ll 1$) (section 3.1).

The dose-dependent influence of first-pass effect on bioavailability can be interpreted on the basis of Michaelis–Menten kinetics and the concept of metabolic clearance. According to the fundamental definition of clearance in section 9.1, the metabolic clearance can be expressed by the equation

$$\text{metabolic clearance} = (\text{rate of biotransformation/incoming concentration})$$
$$= (V_{max} C_{sub})/(K_M + C_{sub})/C_{sub}$$

Therefore

$$\text{metabolic clearance} = V_{max}/(K_M + C_{sub}) \tag{9.23}$$

The conventional units, [volume/time], accompany the metabolic clearance, since V_{max} corresponds to the maximum rate of biotransformation of the administered dose, e.g. [mass/time], while K_M and C_{sub} are expressed in concentration units. Equation (9.23) shows that the metabolic clearance decreases with an increase in the incoming concentration, C_{sub}, in the liver. The maximum value of metabolic clearance is observed when $C_{sub} \ll K_M$ and corresponds to the intrinsic metabolic clearance, V_{max}/K_M.

The experimental results for alprenolol are in complete agreement with the theoretical analysis. Higher bioavailability of alprenolol has been found when dosage is increased. This experimental finding is the result of saturation of the enzymatic activity ($K_M \ll C_{sub}$) at higher doses, which reduces the first-pass effect. Accordingly, the value of the hepatic extraction ratio, E_h, in equation (9.15) is lower at higher doses. In some cases a reduction of the first-pass effect on bioavailability can be achieved. For instance, the administration of the semisuccinate ester of propranolol caused a dramatic increase of propranolol plasma levels due to reduction of the first-pass effect. However, attempts to reduce the first-pass effect may induce other problems. In the case of orally administered peptides biotransformed by proteases in the GI epithelium, the administration of protease inhibitors to suppress the biotransformation of peptides may allow the uptake of non-desirable substances of peptide structure like enterotoxins.

FURTHER READING

Breimer DD. Interindividual Variations in Drug Disposition: Clinical Implications and Methods of Investigation. *Clin. Pharmacokinet.* **8**: 371–377 (1983).

Cafruny EJ. Renal Tubular Handling of Drugs. *Am. J. Med.* **62**: 490–496 (1977).

Campbell DB. Stereoselectivity in Clinical Pharmacokinetics and Drug Development. *Eur. J. Drug Metab. Pharmacokinet.* **15**: 109–125 (1990).

Colburn WA. Pharmacokinetic Analysis of Concentration Time Data Following Administration of Drugs that are Recycled in the Bile. *J. Pharm. Sci.* **73**: 313–317 (1984).

Fabre G, Combalbert J, Berger Y and Cano JP. Human Hepatocytes as a Key In Vitro Model to Improve Preclinical Drug Development. *Eur. J. Drug Metab. Pharmacokinet.* **15**: 165–171 (1990).

Garceau Y, Davis I and Hasegawa J. Plasma Propranolol Levels in Beagle Dogs after Administration of Propranolol Hemisuccinate Ester. *J. Pharm. Sci.* **67**: 1360–1363 (1978).

George CF. Drug Metabolism by the Gastrointestinal Mucosa. *Clin. Pharmacokinet.* **6**: 259–274 (1981).

Goresky CA and Schwab AJ. Flow Cell Entry and Metabolic Disposal: Their Interactions in Hepatic Uptake. In: *The Liver: Biology and Pathobiology*, Arias IM, Jacoby WB, Popper H, Schachter D and Shafritz DA (eds), 2nd edn, pp. 807–831, Raven Press, New York (1988).

Klaassen CD and Watkins JB. Mechanisms of Bile Formation, Hepatic Uptake, and Biliary Excretion. *Pharmacol. Rev.* **36**: 1–67 (1984).

Kuipers F, Havinga R, Bosschieter H, Toorop GP, Hindriks FR and Vond RJ. Enterohepatic Circulation in the Rat. *Gastroenterology* **88**: 403–411 (1985).

Levy RH, Boddy AV. Stereoselectivity in Pharmacokinetics: A General Theory. *Pharm. Res.* **8**: 551–556 (1991).

McLean AJ and Morgan DJ. Clinical Pharmacokinetics in Patients with Liver Disease. *Clin. Pharmacokinet.* **21**: 42–69 (1991).

Pacifici GM and Viani A. Methods of Determining Plasma and Tissue Binding of Drugs: Pharmacokinetic Consequences. *Clin. Pharmacokinet.* **23**: 449–468 (1992).

Pond SM and Tozer TN. First Pass Elimination: Concepts and Clinical Consequences. *Clin. Pharmacokinet.* **9**: 1–25 (1984).

Poulos TL. Cytochrome P450: Molecular Architecture, Mechanism and Prospects for Rational Inhibitor Design. *Pharm. Res.* **5**: 67–75 (1988).

Rowland M, Benet LZ and Graham GG. Clearance Concepts in Pharmacokinetics. *J. Pharmacokinet. Biopharm.* **1**: 123–136 (1973).

Sernka T and Jacobson E. *Gastrointestinal Physiology: The Essentials*, Ch. 11, Williams and Wilkins, Baltimore (1979).

Vessel ES. The Antipyrine Test in Clinical Pharmacology: Conceptions and Misconceptions. *Clin. Pharmacol. Ther.* **26**: 275–286 (1979).

Wilkinson GR and Shand DG. A Physiological Approach to Hepatic Drug Clearance. *Clin. Pharmacol. Ther.* **18**: 377–390 (1975).

PART IV

10

Statistical treatment of experimental data

Objectives

After completing this chapter the reader will be able to perform the following statistical treatments:

— *Testing for the equivalence of means*
— *Simple linear regression analysis*
— *Correlation*

An important component of any scientific study is the statistical analysis of the results. Even in physical and chemical experiments, minor variations in technique result in some variation in the data obtained. In the life and health sciences, variation in response to experimental protocols is increased because of the inherent variability in biological parameters. Here, especially, appropriate statistical analysis is crucial to extraction of meaningful conclusions. This last chapter of the book describes the basic statistical procedures used in biopharmaceutics for analysing experimental data. The information provided is introductory and the references in the bibliography at the end of the chapter are provided for those who wish to read further about these and other methods.

10.1 TESTING FOR THE EQUIVALENCE OF MEANS

10.1.1 Definitions

10.1.1.1 Normally distributed data

The *sample mean*, denoted by $\overline{X}$, is a measure of the location of the data and it is defined by

$$\overline{X} = \frac{\sum_{i=1}^{n} X_i}{n} \tag{10.1}$$

where

$$\sum_{i=1}^{n} = x_1 + x_2 + x_3 + \ldots + x_n,$$

the sum of the n sample data points. The sample mean can be used as an unbiased estimator of the population mean, μ, when this is not known.

The *sample standard deviation*, denoted by SD, is a measure of the scatter of the data and it is defined by

$$\mathrm{SD} = \left[\frac{\sum_{i=1}^{n} (X_i - \overline{X})^2}{n-1} \right]^{1/2} \tag{10.2}$$

Another measure of the dispersion is the *variance* and it is defined by the square of the standard deviation, SD^2. If the population is normally distributed, the standard deviation of the sample represents a confidence interval in which 16% of the observations have values higher than $\overline{X} + \mathrm{SD}$ and 16% lower than $\overline{X} - \mathrm{SD}$ (16th percentile).† Thus, 68% of values lie in the range $(\overline{X} - \mathrm{SD})$ to $(\overline{X} + \mathrm{SD})$.

The *standard error of the mean*, a measure of the uncertainty in the estimate of the mean, can be computed from the standard deviation of means of random samples of the same size drawn from the original population:

$$\mathrm{SEM} = \frac{\mathrm{SD}}{n^{1/2}} \tag{10.3}$$

If the variance of a normally distributed population is known, then the distribution of $\overline{X}$ is known, and probabilistic statements can be made. However, usually the variance of the population is unknown and therefore it is estimated by the sample variance. In this case, the sampling distribution is not normal and a *t-distribution* on $n - 1$ degrees of freedom‡ is used. The percentiles of the t-distribution depend on the sample size as well as on the level of significance chosen; they can be easily obtained from tables. The plot of the t-distribution tends to become identical to the normal distribution plot as the sample size increases.

10.1.1.2 Testing for normality of the distribution

Various ways for testing normality are available. Practically, if the frequency distribution is multimodal, i.e. there are more than one peak, or the standard deviation is approximately as high as the mean (and the variable can take either positive or negative values

† Often the $\overline{X} \pm 2\mathrm{SD}$ confidence interval is used. This interval includes the 95% of the members of the sample (2.5% of values are lower than $\overline{X} - 2\mathrm{SD}$, while 2.5% of values are higher than $\overline{X} + 2\mathrm{SD}$).

‡ The degrees of freedom are equivalent to the number of independent observations, n, minus the number of parameters of the distribution which are calculated from the observations (i.e. in this case the degrees of freedom are $n - 1$, since the population mean is not known).

but not both), then the distribution deviates from normal. A more objective way is to plot the cumulative frequency distribution on normal probability paper (normal probability plot). Such a plot yields a straight line only in cases where the distribution is normal. Alternatively, in cases where the sample size is big ($n > 20$) certain statistical tests may be used such as χ^2 *goodness of fit* or the *Kolmogorov–Smirnoff test*. Details on these tests can be found in textbooks of statistics cited in the bibliography at the end of the chapter.

Unfortunately most of the time sample sizes are small and the evaluation of the normality is based on the judgement of the researcher rather than on concrete evidence.

10.1.1.3 Non-normally distributed data

In cases where the population values are not symmetrically distributed about the mean, the *median* describes the data better than the mean. The median is defined as the location at which half the members of the population fall below the value and half fall above the value. In cases where data are normally distributed, the mean and median are the same. The median is calculated after the values are ranked. If the number of observations is even the median is the average of the two central values. Measures that are used for describing dispersion of non-normally distributed data include the *data range* which is defined by the difference between the maximum and the minimum observed values and the *interquartile range* (25th percentile value to 75th percentile value).

Example 10.1: Dissolution $t_{50\%}$ (min) values of nine tablets from the same batch are the following:

45.8, 46.3, 47.3, 44.8, 43.9, 44.9, 43.1, 44.1 and 46.4

What is your estimate for the $t_{50\%}$ of this batch?

Answer: Since this sample has a small standard deviation compared to the individual values (SD = 1.4 min), the sample mean would give a satisfactory estimate of the $t_{50\%}$. More reliable evidence for the normality of the distribution of the population can be given by the plot of the cumulative frequency distribution† of the values (%) as a function of $t_{50\%}$, on normal probability paper (Fig. 10.1) (the linearity of which can be tested using linear regression analysis, as shown later in this chapter). Thus

$$\bar{X} = (45.8 + 46.3 + 47.3 + 44.8 + 43.9 + 44.9 + 43.1 + 44.1 + 46.4)/9$$
$$= 45.2 \text{ min},$$

and

$$t_{50\%} = 45.2 \ (\pm 1.4) \text{ min}.$$

The fact that the median is very similar to the mean value (44.9 min and 45.2 min, respectively) provides further evidence that the distribution of the population is normal.

† Initially values are ranked in ascending order. The percentage cumulative frequency, $p(x_i)$, is then calculated:

$$p(x_i) = \frac{\text{number of observations} \leq x_i}{n+1} \times 100 = \frac{i}{n+1} \times 100$$

x_i is the value of the ith observation and n is the total number of observations.

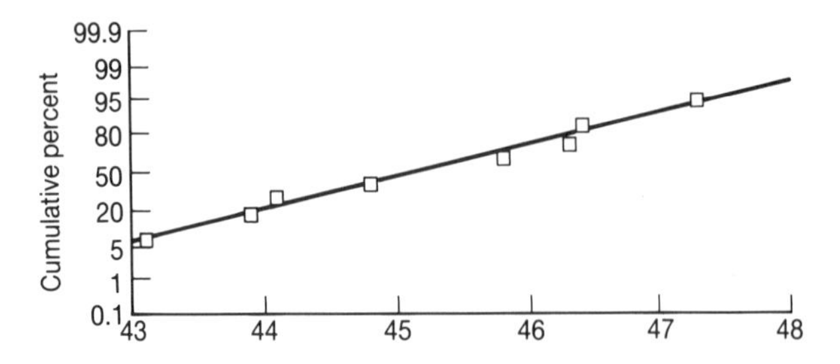

Fig. 10.1. Plot of the data of Example 10.1 expressed as cumulative frequency of values (%) as a function of $t_{50\%}$ on normal distribution paper, which converts the shape of the cumulative normal distribution plot to a straight line.

Example 10.2: Gastric pH values of 11 healthy young Americans in the fasted state were measured radiotelemetrically and found to be

5.8, 3.4, 1.5, 1.4, 1.6, 1.7, 7.1, 1.9, 1.5, 1.6 and 1.9.

What is your estimate for the pH of healthy young Americans in the fasted state according to this sample?

Answer: The standard deviation of the sample is 2.0, i.e. high compared to the mean value (2.7). In addition, the difference between mean (2.7) and median (1.7) is wide, suggesting that the frequency distribution is not normal. Thus it would be more accurate if the estimate was based on the median than on the mean. Therefore, the best estimate for the pH of healthy young Americans in the fasted state according to this sample is 1.7.

10.1.2 Evaluating the significance of differences

The type of test for the identification of difference between two or more samples depends on the distribution of the values in the population and the relationship between the samples. Table 10.1 provides a summary of the most frequently used statistical hypothesis-testing procedures in biopharmaceutics. As seen in this table, two experimental aspects are important for deciding which is the most appropriate test: the type of the experiment and the scale of measurement.

Examples used in this book usually involve comparison of two samples. Therefore the following discussion refers to procedures that are followed for testing statistically significant differences between two samples by taking into account the mode of distribution.

10.1.2.1 Comparing two samples from normally distributed populations (parametric tests)

In this case the *t-test* is used. There are three types of comparisons with *t*-test:

(a) comparison of a sample mean with the true population value;
(b) comparison of two sample means from paired observations (dependent samples), i.e. of a response which is measured before and after a change in the conditions of the experiment using the same sample (e.g. comparing two drug formulations by studying the same subjects on two occasions);

Table 10.1. Summary of some statistical methods to test hypotheses in biopharmaceutics

Type of experiment	Scale of measurement		
	Interval[a]	Ordinal	Nominal[b]
Two treatments/ different individuals	Unpaired t-test	Mann–Whitney rank-sum test	Chi-square/ contingency table
More than two treatments/different individuals	ANOVA	Kruskal–Wallis statistic	Chi-square/ contingency table
Two treatments/ same individuals	Paired t-test	Wilcoxon signed-rank test	McNemar's test
More than two treatments/same individuals	Repeated-measures ANOVA	Friedman statistic	Cochrane Q
Association between two variables	Regression analysis/ Pearson product–moment correlation	Spearman rank correlation	Contingency coefficient

[a] Data are considered that belong to normally distributed populations.
[b] Not frequently applied biopharmaceutical problems.

(c) comparison of the means of two unpaired samples (independent samples). In this case the sample sizes may not be equal (e.g. comparing absorption of a drug in a group of men versus a group of women).

In all cases t values are calculated and then the possibility that the difference between the means is significant is determined from statistical tables based on the *t-statistic*. The t-statistic represents the minimum value of the ratio

$$t = \frac{\text{difference of the means}}{\text{standard error of the difference of the means}} \tag{10.4}$$

at which two means can be statistically equivalent. If the analysis is performed using a personal computer software package the level of significance is usually provided. The equations which are used in all three cases of t-test are given below:

(a) When only one sample exists and the mean of a sample is compared with the known population mean, μ, equation (10.5) is used:

$$t = \frac{(\bar{X} - \mu)}{SD/(n)^{1/2}} \tag{10.5}$$

The value of t is compared with the t-statistic for $n - 1$ degrees of freedom.

(b) When the observations (measurements) are paired then the comparison of the means is based on the following equation:

$$t = \frac{\bar{X}_1 - \bar{X}_2}{SD_{(X1i - X2i)}/(n)^{1/2}} \tag{10.6}$$

$SD_{(X1i - X2i)}$ is the standard deviation of the n differences, $(X_{1i} - X_{2i})$, with $i = 1, 2, \ldots, n$. The value of t is compared with the t-statistic for $n - 1$ degrees of freedom.

(c) When two unpaired samples are compared t value is calculated as follows:

$$t = \frac{\bar{X}_1 - \bar{X}_2}{\left\{\left[\frac{SD_1^2(n_1 - 1) + SD_2^2(n_2 - 1)}{(n_1 + n_2) - 2}\right]\left[\frac{1}{n_1} + \frac{1}{n_2}\right]\right\}^{1/2}} \tag{10.7}$$

with $(n_1 + n_2) - 2$ degrees of freedom. SD_1 and SD_2 are the standard deviations of samples 1 and 2, respectively.

Example 10.3: In six subjects a reference solution formulation was administered orally. The areas under the plasma concentration versus time plots from time zero to infinity following the administration were:

$$AUC_{ref}, \mu g\ h\ ml^{-1}: E_1 = 60.0, E_2 = 71.0, E_3 = 75.0, E_4 = 64.0, E_5 = 77.0,$$
$$E_6 = 81.0.$$

After a washout time sufficient to ensure total elimination of drug from the subjects, a test tablet formulation which contained the same dose of the drug was administered orally to the same group of subjects. Blood samples were withdrawn at the same time intervals and the new AUCs from time zero to infinity were

$$AUC_{test}, \mu g\ h\ ml^{-1}: E_1 = 70.0, E_2 = 70.0, E_3 = 83.0, E_4 = 65.0, E_5 = 80.0,$$
$$E_6 = 82.0.$$

Is the extent of absorption (based on the AUC data) different between formulations?

Answer: The mean ±SD values of AUCs were $71.3 \pm 8.0\ \mu g\ h\ ml^{-1}$ for the first and $75.0 \pm 7.6\ \mu g\ h\ ml^{-1}$ for the second formulation, respectively. According to equation (10.6), it is found that $t = 2.057$. Statistical tables show that in order a difference to be significant at the 0.05 level† the minimum t value for $6 - 1 = 5$ degrees of freedom is 2.571. Thus the difference between the AUC values after administration of the two formulations is not statistically significant. The reader should bear in mind that in real

† The 0.05 level is considered as the cut-off level of significance and corresponds to a 95% confidence interval.

practice comparison of parameters derived from *in vivo* experiments are usually performed with statistical tests, other than the *t*-test, which takes into account the internal subject variability. More information can be obtained from the references at the end of chapter 3.

Example 10.4: $t_{50\%}$ (min) values for the dissolution of 12 tablets of an antihypertensive drug are the following:

43.4, 41.1, 40.8, 41.2, 44.7, 43.5, 40.8, 41.9, 40.4, 47.2, 42.0 and 45.8.

What would your estimate for $t_{50\%}$ be? Is $t_{50\%}$ of these tablets different from the $t_{50\%}$ of the tablets of the Example 10.1?

Answer: The $t_{50\%}$ is calculated to be 42.7 ± 2.2 min. Using equation (10.7), it is found that $t = 2.922$ with $(12 + 9) - 2 = 19$ degrees of freedom. Since for 19 degrees of freedom $t_{0.05} = 2.093$ it can be concluded that the difference is significant at the 0.05 level.

10.1.2.2 *Comparing two samples from non-normally distributed populations (non-parametric tests)*

The *t*-test is usually referred to as a parametric test because it is based on estimates of two population parameters (mean and standard deviation). In order for a parametric method to be applied the population values must be normally distributed around the mean. If not, parametric methods are not reliable because mean and standard deviation do not provide representative information for the population.† In such cases the appropriate tests are non-parametric so-called because they are not based on the values of calculated parameters, but on the ranks of the individual data.

The non-parametric equivalent of the paired *t*-test is the *Wilcoxon signed rank test*. When two samples are not paired the non-parametric equivalent of the unpaired *t*-test is the *Mann–Whitney rank-sum test* (Table 10.1). The procedure for each case is presented below by example.

Wilcoxon signed rank test

If in Example 10.2 the same subjects had their gastric pH measured in the fed state as well as in the fasted state, the significance of the difference of pHs between the two states could be tested with the Wilcoxon signed rank test. Briefly (Table 10.2), in the Wilcoxon test the magnitude of each observed change is ranked beginning with 1 for the smallest change and without taking into account the sign of the differences. Equal differences are assigned the same rank number equivalent to the average of the numbers that they would have been assigned if these differences had not had the same value. Zero differences are not taken into account. The signs of the changes are attached to each rank and the sum of the signed ranks constitutes the *W* criterion. The minimum value of the *W* criterion for the difference to be significant with a specific probability can be found in relevant statistical tables. Decision on the significance of the difference can be also made with the z_w statistic (especially when the sample is big and the minimum *W* criterion cannot be found in tables). The z_w is calculated according to the following equation:

† In drug absorption and disposition studies the sample size is usually small (less than 20), making it difficult to determine whether the population distribution is normal.

Table 10.2. Application of Wilcoxon's signed rank test on the effect of food on gastric pH of 11 young healthy Americans

Subject	pH in fasted state	pH in fed state	Difference	Rank of difference	Signed rank of difference
1	5.8	6.8	–1.0	1	–1
2	3.4	6.9	–3.5	5	–5
3	1.5	4.5	–3.0	4	–4
4	1.4	6.7	–5.3	10.5	–10.5
5	1.6	5.2	–3.6	6	–6
6	1.7	7.0	–5.3	10.5	–10.5
7	7.1	5.0	+2.1	3	+3
8	1.9	7.1	–5.2	9	–9
9	1.5	3.4	–1.9	2	–2
10	1.6	5.9	–4.3	7	–7
11	1.9	6.8	–4.9	8	–8
					$W = 60$

1 = smallest magnitude, 10.5 = largest magnitude.

$$z_w = \frac{|W| - 0.5}{\left[\frac{n(n+1)\,(2n+1)}{6} - \sum \frac{(\tau_i - 1)\,\tau_i(\tau_i + 1)}{12}\right]^{1/2}} \tag{10.8}$$

where n is the number of subjects, τ_i is the number of tied ranks in the ith set of ties, and Σ indicates the summation over all the sets of tied ranks. In cases where there are no ranks with the same value, the second term of the denominator of equation (10.8) is eliminated. The value of z_w is compared with the t-statistic for infinite degrees of freedom.† Thus for the example of Table 10.2 z_w is calculated as follows:

$$z_w = (60 - 0.5)\big/\left[(11 \times 12 \times 23/6) - (1 \times 2 \times 3/12\right]^{1/2} = 2.646$$

Since the t-statistic with infinite degrees of freedom at the 0.05 level is 1.960, it is concluded that the gastric pH changes when subjects are fed a meal are significantly different.

Mann–Whitney test

The steps that are followed when the Mann–Whitney test is applied are similar to the Wilcoxon signed rank test. Table 10.3 shows gastric pH values from the sample of Example 10.2 as well as the values from 12 other subjects of at least 65 years of age. The intent of the analysis is to assess differences in gastric pH with ageing. Observations from

† This procedure is followed since the distribution of the z_w values is approximately normal with zero mean.

Table 10.3. Application of the Mann–Whitney test to the assessment of the effect of age on fasted gastric pH

Young adults		Elderly	
pH values	Rank	pH values	Rank
5.8	22.0	3.4	19.5
3.4	19.5	1.4	7.5
1.5	10.0	2.1	18.0
1.4	7.5	1.2	4.5
1.6	12.5	1.2	4.5
1.7	14.5	1.1	1.5
7.1	23.0	1.5	10.0
1.9	16.5	1.2	4.5
1.5	10.0	1.7	14.5
1.6	12.5	1.1	1.5
1.9	16.5	1.2	4.5
		4.0	21.0
	$T = 164.5$		

1 = smallest magnitude, 23 = largest magnitude.

both samples are ranked according to their magnitudes. If two or more members of the sample have the same values they are assigned the same rank number. The assigned rank number is, as in the Wilcoxon test, the average of the ranks they would have been assigned if there had been no tie. The sum of the ranks in the smaller sample constitutes the T criterion (if both samples are the same then the sum of either one is computed). It should be noted that apart from the T criterion tables sometimes provide the value of the U criterion. The U criterion is related to the T criterion by the following equation:

$$U = T - n_s(n_s + 1)/2$$

where n_s is the size of the smaller sample or the common size of both samples. As with the Wilcoxon test, tables do not give the corresponding T or U values for large samples (usually when $n_s > 8$), and z_T may be calculated from the following equation:

$$z_T = \frac{\left|T - n_s(N+1)/2\right| - 0.5}{\left[\dfrac{n_s n_b (N+1)}{12} - \dfrac{n_s n_b}{12N(N-1)} \sum (\tau_i - 1)\, \tau_i(\tau_i + 1)\right]^{1/2}} \qquad (10.9)$$

$N = n_s + n_b$ and τ_i, have been defined in equation (10.8). The z_T value is compared with the t-statistic for infinite degrees of freedom. For the example of Table 10.3, z_T is calculated as follows:

$$z_T = [(164.5 - 132) - 0.5]/[264 - 0.02174 \times 120]^{1/2} = 1.979$$

Since z_T at the 0.05 level is 1.960 it is concluded that gastric pH is significantly different in elderly people.

10.1.2.3 Comparing more than two samples

The most appropriate tests to analyse data when there are more than two samples are summarized in Table 10.1.

The parametric test used when data are normally distributed is the analysis of variance (ANOVA).† ANOVA may be either factorial or on a repeated-measures basis. When only one factor is tested ANOVA is called one-way or single factor. An example for such type of analysis would be the effect of four viscosity (the factor under investigation) levels on the rate of gastric emptying of a fluid, using a parallel design. However, ANOVA could also be two-way, three-way, etc. If in the cited example the level of glucose in the fluid (second factor) was taken into consideration, as well as the viscosity, the analysis would become two-way. The bioequivalence testing of three drug formulations using a cross-over design (i.e. each subject receives each of the three formulations) represents a typical repeated-measures ANOVA.

When the distribution is not normal, non-parametric tests must be applied. The equivalent of the factorial ANOVA is the *Kruskal–Wallis test* (factors are assumed independent from each other) and the non-parametric equivalent of repeated-measures ANOVA is the *Friedman test.*

10.2 SIMPLE LINEAR REGRESSION ANALYSIS

10.2.1 The regression line

In the previous examples, statistical evaluation involved only one variable. What if two variables are simultaneously considered? For example in biopharmaceutics it is very common for one variable (amount of drug dissolved, plasma drug level, etc.) to be studied versus time. In this case fitting of an equation to the data is the most usual approach. The specific objectives are:

(a) to estimate the value of the parameters of the function $y = f(x)$; or
(b) to assess if a specific type of function describes satisfactorily the relation between variables y and x.

The first objective can be accomplished using *regression analysis*, while the second is assessed by *correlation* (discussed separately later in this chapter). Even though many biopharmaceutics equations are not linear, they can usually be transformed to a linear relationship. Thus, the discussion which follows considers linear fitting only.

Simple linear regression analysis is a statistical technique which is used to determine the relationship between the two variables x and y based on the best fitting of a straight

† ANOVA can be also applied to two samples in cases where several sources of variability affect the data. A typical example is a two treatment crossover or bioequivalence study where period, sequence, and/or carryover effects may affect the significance of the formulation differences.

line to the data X_i and Y_i (where $i = 1, 2, \ldots, n$ and n is the number of data pairs). A straight line is described by the following equation:

$$y = A + Bx \tag{10.10}$$

where y is the dependent variable (on the ordinate axis), x is the independent variable (on the abscissa axis), A is the intercept on the abscissa and B is the slope of the line. As shown in Fig. 10.2, the values of the intercept and slope define the line. Since data almost never compose an ideal line (due to experimental error) a line is drawn through the data in such a way that the total variability between the data and the line is minimized.

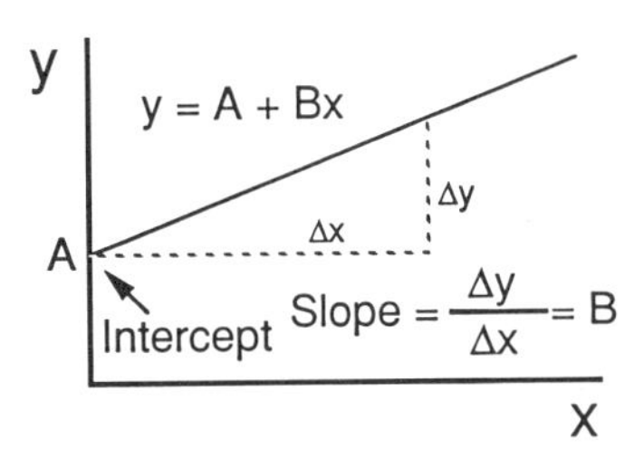

Fig. 10.2. Characteristics of a straight line.

In earlier examples in this chapter the variability in a population about the mean was estimated with the standard deviation, or the variance, by computing the sum of the squared deviations from the mean and then dividing it by the sample size minus 1. The same concept is used for measuring the variability of the data points around the line of best fit. The line is drawn in such a way that the sum of squared differences between the observed values of the dependent variable and the value calculated from the line for the equivalent value of the independent variable is minimized (Fig. 10.3). For this reason, the procedure is often called *the method of least-squares regression.* The resulting line is called the *regression line* of the dependent variable on the independent variable. Its equation is equation (10.10). The intercept A is given by

$$A = \frac{(\Sigma Y_i)(\Sigma X_i^2) - (\Sigma X_i)(\Sigma X_i Y_i)}{n\Sigma X_i^2 - (\Sigma X_i)^2} \tag{10.11}$$

and the slope is given by

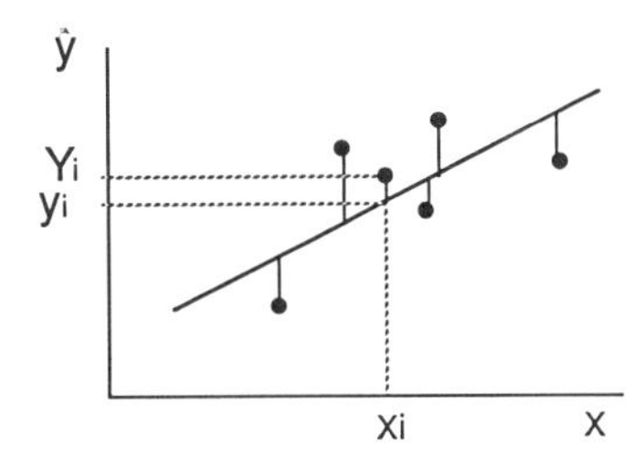

Fig. 10.3. The regression line. Dots correspond to experimental data, Y_i, and the intercepts of the perpendicular extensions to the regression line correspond to values which are predicted from the regression line for the corresponding value X_i.

$$B = \frac{n(\Sigma X_i Y_i) - (\Sigma X_i)(\Sigma Y_i)}{n\Sigma X_i^2 - (\Sigma X_i)^2} \tag{10.12}$$

in which X_i and Y_i are the coordinates of the ith pair of the sample ($i = 1, 2, \ldots, n$).

10.2.2 Statistical characteristics of the regression line

Assuming there is no error involved in the measurement of X_i, that the distribution of Y_i is normal, and that the variance, $(SE_{y,x})^2$, of the experimental data around the regression line is independent of the value of Y_i, $(SE_{y,x})^2$ can be calculated using

$$(SE_{y,x})^2 = \frac{\Sigma(y - Y_i)^2}{n-2} \tag{10.13}$$

The square root of the variance, $SE_{y,x}$, is called the standard error of the estimate. Based on the standard error of the estimate the variances of the intercept and the slope can then be calculated:

$$(SE_a)^2 = (SE_{y,x})^2 \left[\frac{1}{n} + \frac{\overline{X}^2}{\Sigma(X_i - \overline{X})^2} \right] \tag{10.14}$$

$$(SE_b)^2 = \frac{(SE_{y,x})^2}{\Sigma(X_i - \overline{X})^2} \tag{10.15}$$

SE_a and SE_b are called the standard error of the estimators of the slope and intercept, respectively. The significance of the difference of A and B from the true theoretical value for the intercept or the slope, respectively, may also be calculated.

If the theoretically expected value, a, is known, the estimator of the intercept may be compared with a using the t-test:

$$t = \frac{a - A}{SE_a} \tag{10.16}$$

for $n - 2$ degrees of freedom. Most of the time it is of more interest to compare the estimator of the slope, B, with the theoretical value of the slope, b. In this case the t-statistic is calculated by the following equation:

$$t = \frac{b - B}{SE_b} \tag{10.17}$$

at $n - 2$ degrees of freedom. In many cases it is also of interest to compare the slopes of two regression lines. This test can be performed using the t-statistic according to the following equation:

$$t = \frac{\text{difference of regression slopes}}{\text{standard error of difference of regression slopes}}$$

for $n = n_1 + n_2 - 4$ degrees of freedom. The standard error of difference of two regression slopes is calculated from

$$\left[(\mathrm{SE}_{b1})^2 + (\mathrm{SE}_{b2})^2\right]^{1/2}$$

where SE_{b1} and SE_{b2} are the standard errors of the estimators of each slope.

It should be mentioned that the tests described by equations (10.16) and (10.17) are not very robust. For this reason, such comparisons are frequently made using the confidence intervals for the estimated values of intercept and slope using the following equations:

$$b \pm (\mathrm{SE}_b)\, t_{n-2(p=0.025)} \tag{10.18}$$

$$a \pm (\mathrm{SE}_a)\, t_{n-2(p=0.025)} \tag{10.19}$$

where $t_{n-2(p=0.025)}$ is the minimum value of the t-statistic for $n-2$ degrees of freedom for which the difference is significant at the 0.05 (or 0.025 two-tailed) level. In addition, the confidence interval for a value y, which is calculated from the regression equation for a set $X_i = X_0$, is given by the following equation:

$$y \pm t_{n-2(p=0.025)} \left\{ (\mathrm{SE}_{y,x})^2 \left(\frac{1}{n} + \frac{(X_0 - \overline{X})^2}{\Sigma X_i^2 - (\Sigma X_i)^2/n} \right) \right\}^{1/2} \tag{10.20}$$

The following example illustrates estimation of the slope and the intercept, and calculation of the variance of the estimators.

Example 10.5: A drug is non-reversibly transported from compartment I (initial concentration $C_{\mathrm{I}0} = 46.0\ \mu\mathrm{g/ml}$) to compartment II. The concentration of the drug in compartment I at various time intervals is given below:

C_{I} (μg/ml):	39.8	20.9	11.5	5.00	2.50	1.10
t (h):	1	4	8	12	16	20

What are the statistical characteristics of the transport rate constant?

Answer: The equation which describes the change of concentration in compartment I as a function of time is similar to equation (2.6):

$$\ln C_{\mathrm{I}} = \ln C_{\mathrm{I}0} - k_1 t \tag{10.21}$$

Based on equation (10.21), $\ln C_{\mathrm{I}}$ and t are logarithmically related and, therefore, the experimental data are transformed as follows:

$\ln C_{\mathrm{I}}$:	3.83	3.68	3.04	2.44	1.61	0.92	0.10
t:	0	1	4	8	12	16	20

Fig. 10.4 graphically depicts $\ln C_I$ as a function of time.† Based on equations (10.11) and (10.12) (and after replacing Y with $\ln C_I$ and X with t) the following values are obtained:

Intercept: $a = \ln C_{I0} = 3.845$

Slope: $b = -0.185$

and $k_1 = 0.185h^{-1}$

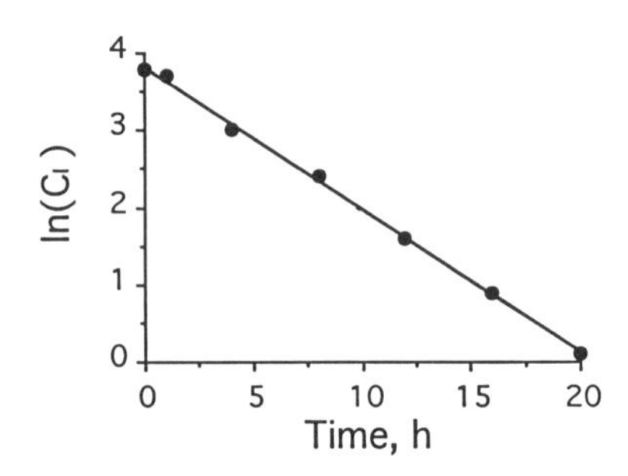

Fig. 10.4. $\ln C_I$ versus time for the data of Example 10.5. The line passing through the data is the regression line.

According to equation (10.15) the standard error of the estimate of the slope is $SE_b = (0.00279/349.43)^{1/2} = 0.00282$. From tables it can be found that the t-statistic for $7-2=5$ degrees of freedom at the 0.05 level is 2.571. Therefore, a 95% interval estimate of the slope is (according to equation (10.18)) given by

$$0.185 \pm 2.571 \times 0.00282 = 0.185 \pm 0.007$$

The t-statistics for the significance of both the intercept (compared to the true value $\ln(46.0) = 3.829$) and the slope (compared to zero) are calculated by equations (10.16) and (10.17):

$$t = |3.829 - 3.845|/SE_a = 0.016/[0.00279(0.143 + 75.94/349.43)]^{1/2} = 0.505$$

$$t = |0.185 - 0|/0.00282 = 65.6$$

These values indicate that the estimator of slope for 5 degrees of freedom is statistically different from zero, whereas for the intercept the value is not statistically different from the true value.

† The regression analysis is preferably applied to the equation in its original form (equation (2.7)). However, since non-linear fitting requires the use of a personal computer, equation (2.7) is often logarithmically transformed for convenience, even though a source of error (due to the rounding of the resulting numbers) may be introduced.

10.2.3 Measuring the adequacy of the linear model

The confidence with which a response can be predicted based on regression analysis depends on how the regression analysis was conducted and whether or not the basic assumptions required for the technique have been met.

Some of these assumptions have already been mentioned in the discussion of equation (10.13). The most important is the choice of an accurate form for the relationship which is to describe the experimental data. Second, the variance of the *residual or error values* must be constant. *Residuals* are calculated from the difference between the experimental value and the estimated value by the equation of the regression line. This assumption may be tested by plotting the residuals as a function of the independent variable. The residuals must be normally distributed. Third, the dependent variable must be an exclusive function of the independent variable. Finally, the independent variable must not be associated with any type of experimental error. In biopharmaceutics, the most common variables which are used as independent variables (time, weight, temperature, dose, etc.) are considered errorless. However, sometimes this criterion is not met. A typical example is the Scatchard plot (section 7.2.3.1), where error is associated with both variables.

To test whether the assumptions inherent in a regression analysis are valid, one relies mostly on residual (or error) patterns. Ideally, the *plot of residuals or errors* as a function of the independent variable should resemble Fig. 10.5A. Values should be randomly distributed on both sides of the line which passes through the zero residual point. If the residual plot resembles Fig. 10.5B, i.e. a curvature is apparent, the equation which has been selected to describe the phenomenon has a systematic error and needs to be modified. Fig. 10.5C shows how this plot will look if the variance of the residuals is reduced with increasing the independent variable. This situation is often observed in standard curves where very low concentrations approach the detection limit and the variance of the

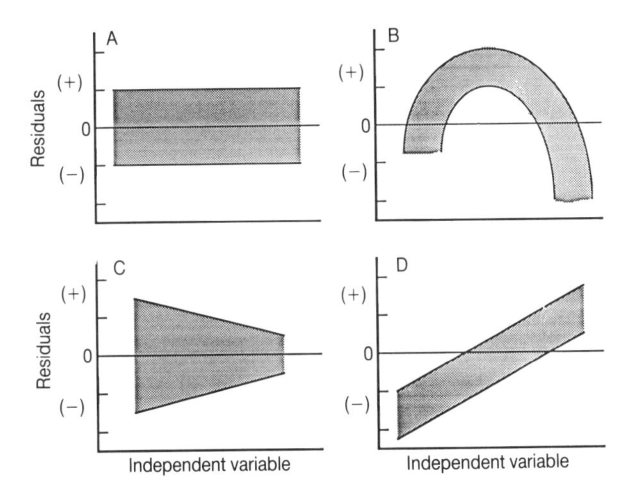

Fig. 10.5. Plots of residuals of various hypothetical linear regression analyses: (A) the basic assumptions for the application of the linear regression analysis apply; (B) the equation fitted to the data is not adequate and it should be of higher order; (C) observations do not have constant variance and depend on the independent variable; and (D) the residuals are not independent and most likely depend on one more variable which has not been taken into account.

measurement (absorbance, peak height, peak area, etc.) is higher than the variance at higher concentrations. In such situations fitting can be improved with the addition of a weighting factor, typically the inverse of the variance. Finally, Fig. 10.5D shows how the plot of residuals looks when the dependent variable is not only a function of the independent variable. Such a situation may be observed when the absorbance of standard solutions varies with time due to instability of the drug in the solutions. In these cases the regression equation is usually modified so that the inclusion of an additional parameter (in our example this is the period for which each sample is kept before measurement) is taken into account. Fig. 10.6 illustrates the plot of residuals for the data of Example 10.5.

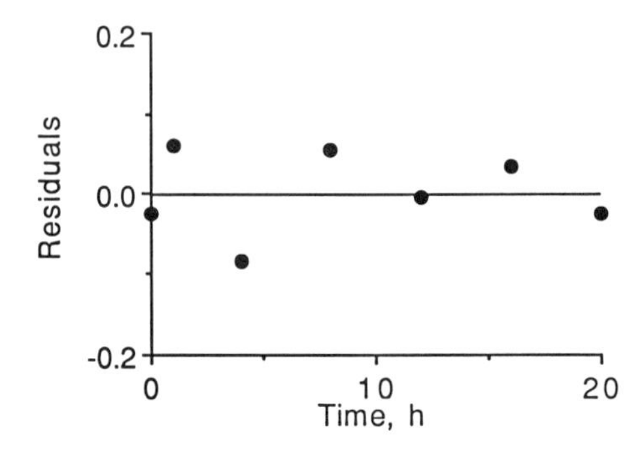

Fig. 10.6. Plot of the residuals for the data of Example 10.5.

It should be noted that apart from the plot of residuals the reliability of the results of a regression analysis can be tested with ANOVA, where the number of samples is the number of the estimated parameters (in case of linear analysis these are two: slope and intercept) and the sample size is the number of pairs of experimental data.

10.3 CORRELATION

10.3.1 Definition

Regression analysis specifies the relationship between the dependent and the independent variable. However, it does not give any information about the strength of the relationship. This information can be gained from the correlation of the data. In some cases the strength of the relationship may be the most important aspect of the statistical analysis.

The strength of the relationship between the dependent and the independent variable is assessed with the *correlation coefficient*. The correlation coefficient, R, may vary from −1 to +1 and, as shown in Fig. 10.7, the closer to +1 or −1 the stronger is the correlation (Fig. 10.7). The sign indicates whether the two variables change in a direct ($R > 0$) or inversely proportional manner ($R < 0$).

There are two types of correlation coefficients. The first is called the *Pearson product–moment correlation coefficient* and it is a measure of correlation of two variables whose values are assumed that have been drawn from normally distributed populations.

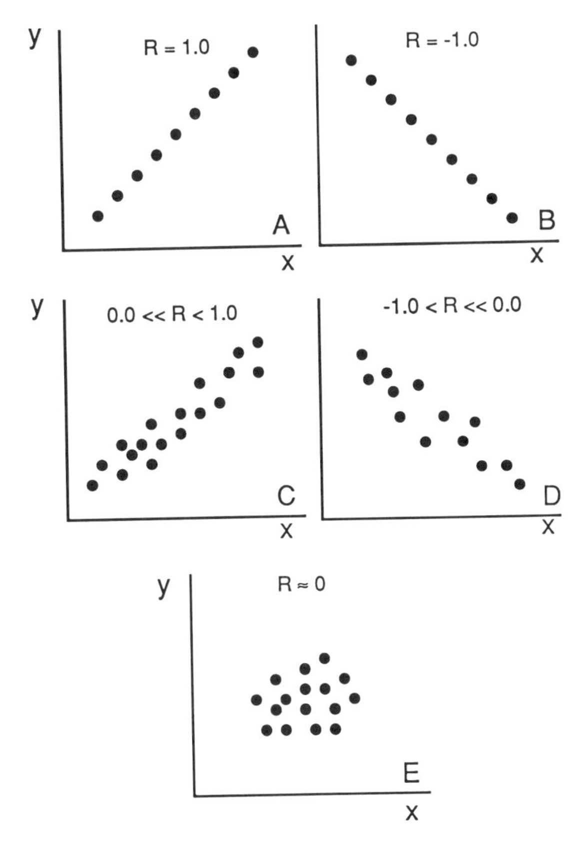

Fig. 10.7. The higher the absolute value of the correlation coefficient, the less scattered are the data and the stronger is the correlation between the two variables.

In contrast, when the data for both variables are in the ordinal scale, the correlation coefficient is called *Spearman rank correlation coefficient*. In biopharmaceutics the Pearson product moment correlation coefficient is most often used and can be calculated from the following equation:

$$R = \frac{\Sigma(X_i - \bar{X})(Y_i - \bar{Y})}{\left[\Sigma(X_i - \bar{X})^2 \Sigma(Y_i - \bar{Y})^2\right]^{1/2}} \tag{10.22}$$

The correlation coefficient calculated from equation (10.22)† shows the strength of the linear relationship of two variables, x and y, whose values are normally distributed. The

† A more facile computational form of this equations is the following:

$$R = \frac{n\Sigma X_i Y_i - \Sigma X_i \Sigma Y_i}{\left\{\left[n\Sigma X_i^2 - (\Sigma X_i)^2\right]\left[n\Sigma Y_i^2 - (\Sigma Y_i)^2\right]\right\}^{1/2}}$$

n is the number of the experimental pairs.

value of the correlation coefficient remains the same if the dependent variable is interchanged with the independent variable.

As mentioned earlier, the significance of differences in either the slope or the intercept from a theoretical value can be tested using the t-test. Similarly, the significance of the correlation coefficient can be tested with a t-test:

$$t = \frac{R}{\left\{(1-R^2)/(n-2)\right\}^{1/2}} \tag{10.23}$$

with $n-2$ degrees of freedom.

10.3.2 Comparison of linear regression analysis and correlation

The correlation coefficient is related to the slope of the regression line, b, as follows:

$$R = b\frac{\mathrm{SD}_X}{\mathrm{SD}_Y} \tag{10.24}$$

where SD_X and SD_Y are the standard deviations of the experimental data X and Y, respectively. Based on equation (10.23), if the slope is zero, then there is no correlation between the two variables. Similarly, if there is no correlation the slope of the regression line is zero.

It is important to note that a knowledge of the value of correlation coefficient does not give any further information on the adequacy of the fitting, because the correlation coefficient is not a measure of the linearity. It simply provides an indication of the strength of the relationship.† This means that values close to ±1 do not necessarily mean the equation which best fits the data is linear. Conversely, values close to zero do not always imply lack of correlation but may indicate that the relationship of the two variables is not linear. Since the correlation coefficient is often misused in the literature by interpreting it as a measure of the linearity rather than the strength of the relationship, a few examples are given below.

Table 10.4 contains three sets of hypothetical data. Based on the value of the correlation coefficient (as calculated from equation (10.22)) no correlation exists for set A ($R_A = 0.063$) whereas for set B correlation is very good ($R_B = 0.977$). However, if we take a look at the plots (Fig. 10.8A and B) it becomes clear that neither set A nor set B profiles are linear. Any attempt to compare the correlations using a linear correlation coefficient is not valid. It should be noted that although in this example the non-linearity is visually apparent this may not be so apparent in many data sets. In cases where data are not linearly related, relevant conclusions can be drawn from the plot of residuals. For the data of set C (Table 10.4) the correlation coefficient is relatively high ($R_C = -0.970$) and statistically significant at the 0.05 level. However, since data for a wide range of values are missing, the hypothesis that the relationship is linear for values $3 < X < 10$ may be wrong.

† Obviously if one knows the exact relationship of two variables and the adequacy of fitting, more information is already available than would be required for the assessment of the correlation of the two variables.

Table 10.4. Three hypothetical set of data for which the assessment of the correlation with the linear correlation coefficient is misleading

Set A		Set B		Set C	
X	Y	X	Y	X	Y
2	0.3	4	15	1	23
3	3.2	8	66	2	25
4	4.1	12	138	3	20
5	2.9	16	260	10	10
6	0.1	20	412	11	9

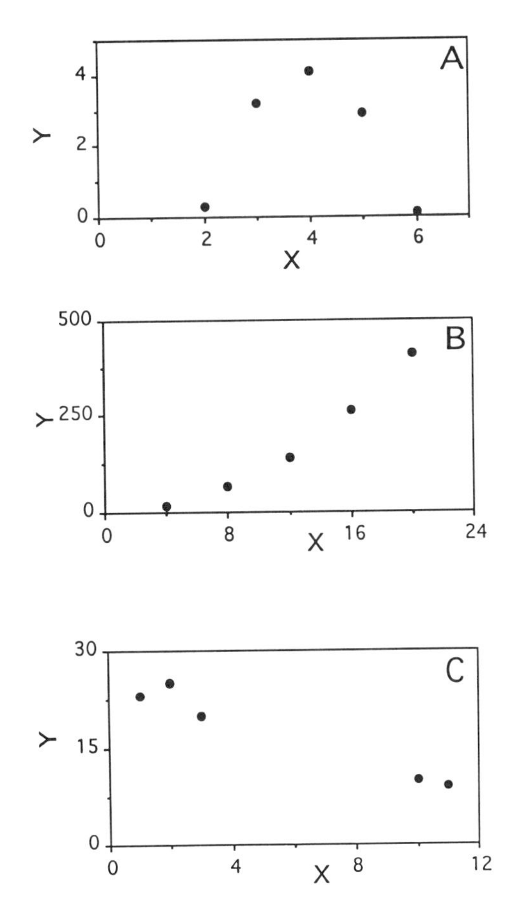

Fig. 10.8. Plots of data of Table 10.4, indicating the problems which may result from the incorrect interpretation of correlation coefficient. (A) Set A, (B) set B, and (C) set C.

In conclusion, the interpretation of a calculated correlation coefficient requires the use of residual plots to verify that the relationship being tested adequately describes the data.

FURTHER READING

Beloto RJ Jr and Sokoloski TD. Residual Analysis in Regression. *Am. J. Pharm. Educ.* **49**: 295–303 (1985).

Bolton S. *Pharmaceutical Statistics: Practical and Clinical Applications*. Marcel Dekker, New York (1984).

Box GEP, Hunter WG and Hunter JS. *Statistics for Experimenters: An Introduction to Design, Data Analysis, and Model Building*. Wiley, New York (1978).

Chatfield G. *Statistics for Technology* (2nd edn), Wiley, New York (1978).

Dixon WJ and Massey FJ Jr. *Introduction to Statistical Analysis* (3rd edn), McGraw-Hill, New York (1969).

Glantz SA. *Primer of Biostatistics*. McGraw Hill, New York (1981).

Sokal RR and Rohlf FJ. Biometry: *The Principles and Practice of Statistics in Biological Research* (2nd edn), Freeman, New York (1981).

Thakur AK. In: *Pharmacokinetics: Mathematical and Statistical Approaches to Metabolism and Distribution of Chemicals and Drugs*, Pecile A and Resigno A (eds), NATO ASI Series, Vol. 145, Plenum Press, New York (1988).

Wentworth WE. Rigorous Least Squares Adjustment: Application to Some Non-Linear Equations, I and II. *J. Chem. Educ.* **42**: 96–103, 162–167 (1965).

Index